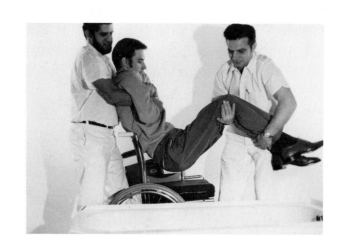

PHYSICAL

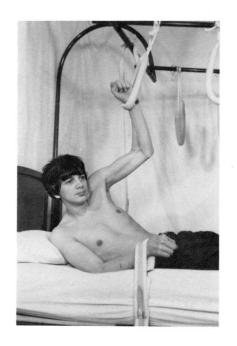

MANAGEMENT

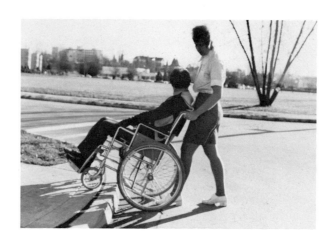

Cover photograph by Carol Hussey, B.F.A.

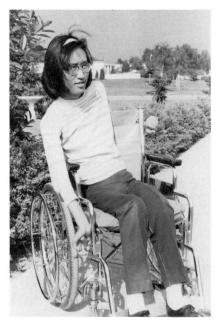

FOR THE
QUADRIPLEGIC PATIENT

JACK R. FORD, R.G.

Head Remedial Gymnast, G. F. Strong Rehabilitation Centre,
Vancouver, British Columbia

BRIDGET DUCKWORTH, M.A.O.T., O.T.R.

Occupational Therapist, G. F. Strong Rehabilitation Centre,
Vancouver, British Columbia

 F. A. DAVIS COMPANY, Philadelphia, Pa.

Library of Congress Cataloging in Publication Data
Ford, Jack R
Physical management for the quadriplegic patient.
Bibliography: p.
1. Tetraplegia. 2. Paralytics—Rehabilitation.
I. Duckworth, Bridget, jt. author. II. Title.
[DNLM: 1. Quadriplegia—Rehabilitation. WL400 F699p
1974]
RC406.T4F67   617'.375   74-3422
ISBN 0-8036-3675-X

Preface

This manual is written primarily for the use of paramedic students, nurses, and therapists who work with traumatic quadriplegic patients. Technical terminology has been avoided as much as possible in anticipation of the manual's being used also by the quadriplegic patient and his family. A glossary has been added for further clarity.

The style is in note form with steps well illustrated for quick and easy reference. It is designed this way so that it may be used as a working manual. There is no mention of level of injury; the level often is meaningless in regard to physical ability. The patient with a lower level lesion and many complications may not perform as well as the patient with a higher lesion. For this reason, methods have been put in sequence, outlining the method used by the most able patient and progressing to that used by the less able patient. The methods outlined are interchangeable and may be varied considerably. Clarity and space demand that all variations are not described under each method.

There is a growing population of quadriplegic people. This is due to both an increased accident rate and an increased survival rate. These factors demand that a book of this type be available to aid the quadriplegic individual in realizing his maximum capability and bring him back to living a useful and satisfying life.

The manual is written for the person who should be capable of becoming independent but does not forget the one who will not be able to reach this goal. It is hoped that the chapter on the care of the dependent patient will help the latter patient and his family solve the problems that will arise.

We have given minimal reference to social and psychological factors concerning the patient and his family; this does not mean they are regarded lightly. They may well be the most important factors in successful rehabilitation. It is our feeling, however, that there is already extensive literature on emotional adjustment to disability. More specialized information on marital adjustment can be found in literature on cord injury.

We have covered in detail the physical methods of self-care which have been successfully used by many patients at the G. F. Strong Rehabilitation Centre, Vancouver, British Columbia, Canada.

Acknowledgements

We would like to express our deep gratitude

to the management and staff of the G. F. Strong Rehabilitation Centre, Vancouver, Canada, for their active cooperation and encouragement,

to the Vancouver Foundation for their financial support,

to the many interested individuals and agencies for their support,

to Sidney Licht, M.D., for his encouragement,

to our publishers for the advice received.

We would especially like to thank the 56 quadriplegic patients who so kindly demonstrated the methods for this book. Their willing assistance made this publication possible.

Contents

1 *Introduction and Biomechanical Principles*

CORRELATION WITH THE HOME

Early contact with the patient's family may clarify issues and enable self-care methods to be correlated with the layout of the home. If the methods envisaged and the physical layout of the home are incompatible, the home may be modified or the self-care methods changed.

The patient's family should be shown what the patient will be able to do when he has reached a reasonable degree of efficiency. As soon as the required equipment has been determined, it should be set up in the home so that it can be used during preliminary weekend and holiday visits by the patient.

Follow-ups after the patient has returned home permanently will disclose any previously unforeseen difficulties and should encourage the patient to maintain his skills.

PROGRESSION

An adequate exercise program prescribed by the physician to condition remaining muscles is a prerequisite to the learning of transfer techniques. Lighter self-care techniques (eating, washing, etc.) should be started as soon as the medical status permits. Encouragement is given at first by establishing easy self-care goals that are sure to be accomplished. A patient should not be asked to attempt an activity unless it is known that he can accomplish at least part of it.

When a patient begins self-care training, a considerable amount of equipment may be necessary. As he approaches peak performance, the equipment should be reduced to a minimum.

All equipment must be safe, stable, and reliable. The helper must be in a position to prevent falls. If the helper has to change position while the patient is transferring, he should first make sure the patient is in a safe position. The patient must have confidence in the helper's ability to prevent him from falling before he can put full effort into self-care training.

Suggestions and questions by the patient should be encouraged. Thus he is involved in his own self-care program, his interest is aroused, and he learns to solve problems and adapt to situations that may arise later.

1

As the condition of the patient improves, both his exercise program and his self-care program should become more vigorous.

When a task has been accomplished, the patient must be encouraged to continue it as a practical daily activity. This builds up his tolerance so that he can progress to other demanding skills. As the patient's ability to look after himself increases, his exercise program may be cut back to allow more time for practical application of his self-care skills. Once a person has accomplished all his self-care, he will find little need for extra exercise.

Self-care, in itself, is physically demanding for a quadriplegic patient and, at first, very time consuming. When he has become proficient in his self-care, he should have reduced the time required to a practical level, allowing time for work and social activities.

MECHANICS

The body, with all its bones and joints, may be regarded as a series of levers and hinges. Therefore it would be reasonable to apply mechanical principles to create mechanical advantages.

LEVERS

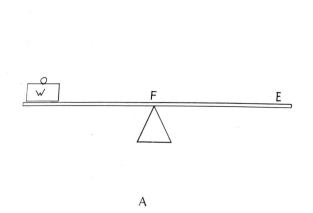

A

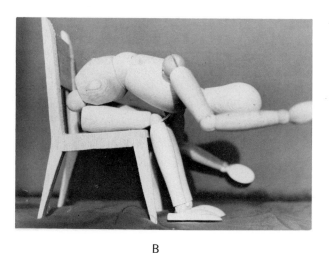

B

FIGURE 1-1

1st Class Lever (Fig. 1-1A)

When a seated person leans forward, his knees form a fulcrum and his head and shoulders help to counterbalance the weight of his lower trunk and thighs (Fig. 1-1B). This reduces the weight of the lower trunk and thighs on the chair by the weight of his chest, head, and shoulders.

2nd Class Levers (Fig. 1-2A)

To reduce the effort required to lift a weight, a fulcrum may be utilized. The manikin has placed an arm under one leg with the wrist resting on the other knee

FIGURE 1-2

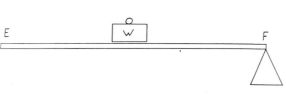

A

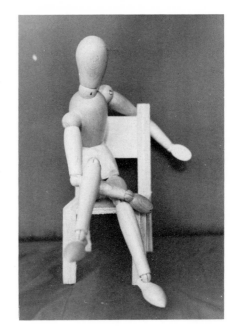

B

FIGURE 1-3

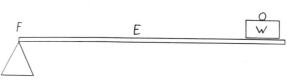

A

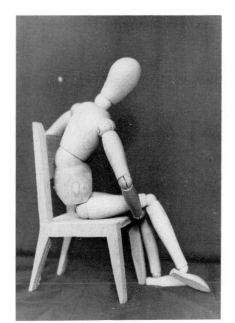

B

as a fulcrum (Fig. 1-2B). "Effort" or straightening the arm will lift the leg. A patient may use this leverage to cross his legs.

3rd Class Levers (Fig. 1-3A)

The hip joint forms the fulcrum, the leg forms the lever, and the effort is applied by the arm to lift the weight of the lower leg (Fig. 1-3B).

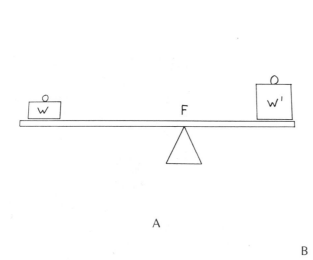

A

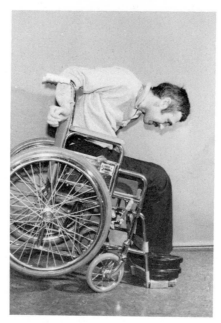

B

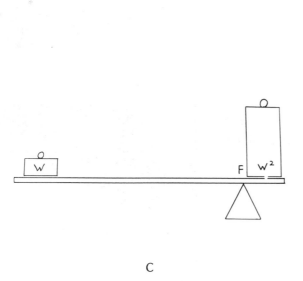

C

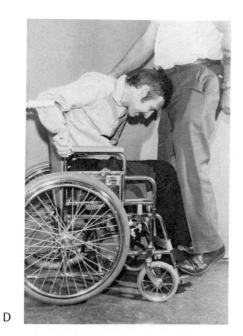

D

FIGURE 1-4. *A*, First class lever; *B*, With castors turned back, 40 pounds on the footrest will tip the wheelchair; *C*, With castors turned forward the fulcrum is moved forward; *D*, Thus, 210 pounds on the footrest will not tip the chair.

In Figure 1-4 the wheelchair can be regarded as a first class lever, or balance scale, with the castors forming the fulcrum (Fig. 1-4A). With a 150 pound man in the chair, if the castors are turned back, 40 pounds of weight placed on the footrest will tip the chair (Fig. 1-4B). With the castors turned forward, the fulcrum is about four inches further forward, thus increasing the wheelbase (Fig. 1-4C), and a 210 pound man can stand upright on the footrests without tipping the chair forward (Fig. 1-4D). For this reason castors must be turned forward for stability in transfers or for leaning forward in the chair while the feet remain on the footrests.

A platform was made with a cutout to accommodate a scale of the same height (Fig. 1-5). The wheelchair was placed on the platform. The helper stood on the scale to obtain and compare the effort used for the two following methods of moving a patient back in the chair.

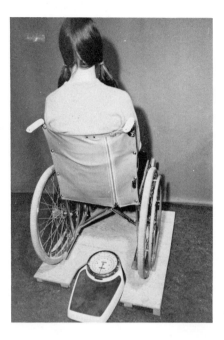
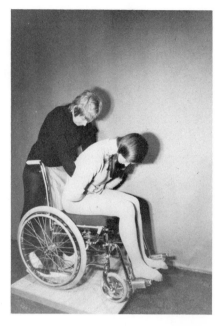

FIGURE 1-5

METHODS

Lever Method with Poor Mechanical Advantage

A, Lever method with poor mechanical advantage;

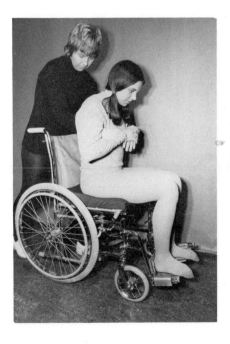
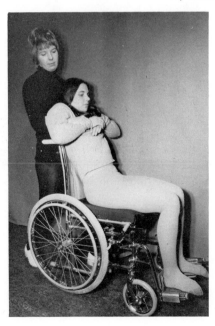
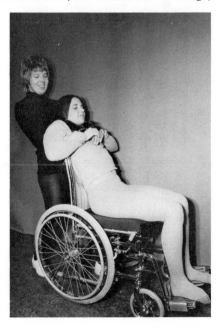

FIGURE 1-6.

5

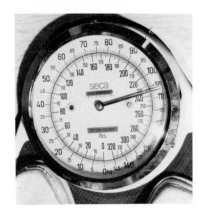

In Figure 1-6A the helper slides his hands under the patient's axillae, and holds the patient's wrists with a flat hand hold. He now lifts the patient to slide him back in the chair. The weight registered on the scales is 230 pounds (Fig. 1-6B).

In this move the helper's back is hyperextended because a good deal of lift is lost in elongating the patient's back and elevating his shoulder girdle. The patient cannot be moved properly in the chair because the top of the chair back acts as a fulcrum and tends to hold him forward. This lift is not only difficult for the helper; it may be quite uncomfortable for the patient, particularly if he has a weak shoulder girdle.

B, Weight registered during experiment.

Lever Method Utilizing Maximum Mechanical Advantage

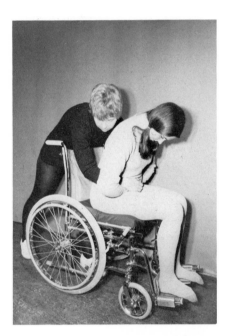
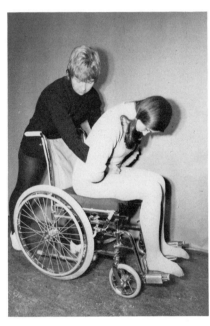
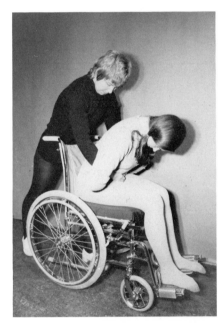

A

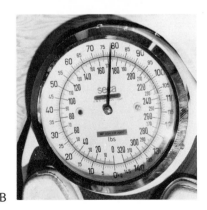

In Figure 1-7A the helper places the patient's hands over his lower abdomen. The helper's hands are placed over the patient's hands with his forearms under the patient's rib cage. The patient is flexed forward. The fulcrum of the lever is the point where the forearms hug under the rib cage. The effort is exerted at the helper's upper arm by a shrug of his shoulders and the pressure is applied at the symphysis pubis as the helper's arms straighten and force the patient back. This is a most effective first class lever as shown by the pressure on the scale of 170 pounds (Fig. 1-7B).

FIGURE 1-7. *A*, Lever method utilizing maximum mechanical advantage; *B*, Weight registered during experiment.

B

6

PENDULUM (Fig. 1-8A)

Pendular movements may be used to advantage, the result being dependent on the placement of the fulcrum. In Figure 1-8B the patient swings beyond the point beneath the fulcrum by taking advantage of the placement of the fulcrum. The lift must be high enough to clear at the low point of the arc if the pendulum is used on a flat surface. In this instance the feet are moved across first so that they assist rather than retard the swing.

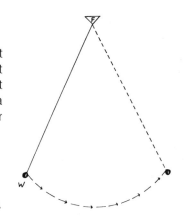

FIGURE 1-8   A

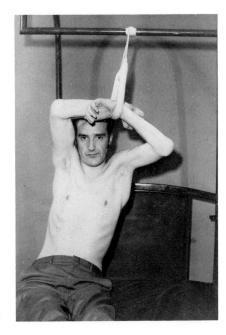
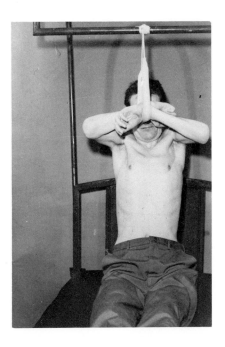
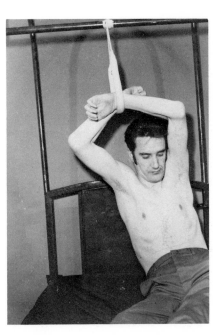

B

MOMENTUM

Momentum is a property of a moving body that can be used to advantage. An example is the attempt to throw a forearm into a sling when the triceps muscle is not working. In Figure 1-9A the arm is flung into the sling so that the elbow has no time to bend. If a patient reaches for the sling slowly his forearm drops before his hand is in position (Fig. 1-9B). Because of his momentum, a patient moving fast with vigor will move easily.

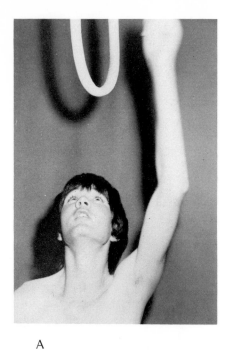

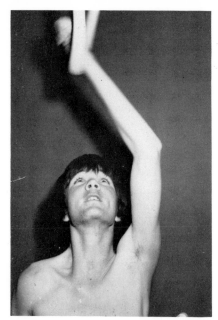

A

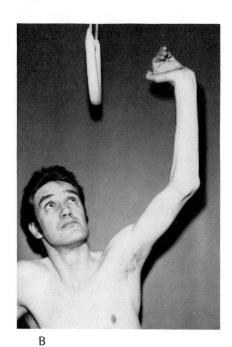

B

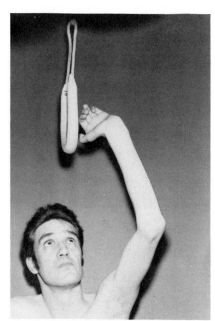

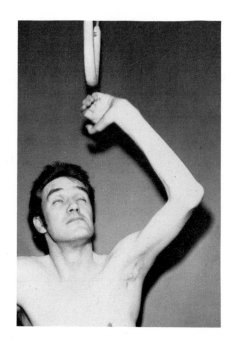

FIGURE 1-9. *A*, Fast movement; *B*, Slow movement.

FRICTION

As shown in Figure 1-10 a great deal less weight or "effort" is required to move an object sliding on a smooth surface such as nylon than is required on a rough surface such as cotton. Therefore, nylon draw sheets and cushion covers are frequently used and patients are advised to wear nylon-cotton pants rather than

8

corduroy or jeans when learning transfer techniques. If hands should slip when pushing on a slippery surface, moistening the heel of the hand with the tongue is often the solution.

If these basic mechanical principles are understood, the reasons underlying the methods explained in the manual will be clear, and variations, combinations, and new methods will evolve more easily.

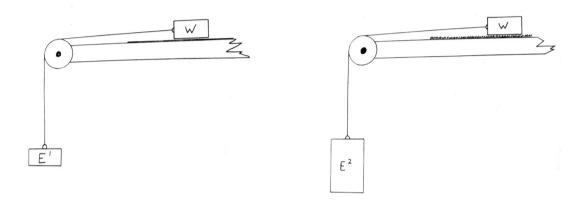

FIGURE 1-10

MAJOR PROBLEMS THAT MAY BE ENCOUNTERED DURING TRAINING

Nearly every quadriplegic patient has a period of depression before he accepts his disability. This manifests itself in many ways such as apathy, aggression, overcheerfulness, and unrealism. The patient may not be able to apply himself fully to learning his self-care until he has at least partially accepted his disability.

Previously existing medical complications, such as cardiac problems, poor vision, psychiatric illness, psychological problems, or old age, may preclude complete independence.

Medical complications such as skin breakdown or urinary infections may delay training and cause frustration to the patient.

Although some spasm can be useful, excessive spasm may require treatment by a physician. Sometimes positioning may be worked out to prevent triggering unwanted spasm.

Excessive flaccidity of muscles and ligaments or lack of joint range can greatly interfere with the application of mechanics to movement. Body build, such as emaciation, obesity, or disproportionate build, can also interfere with the application of mechanics.

Loss of position sense in upper extremities can make self-care difficult because the patient does not know where an arm is when it is not in sight, for example when he attempts to pull up the back of his pants.

A person with no athletic inclination may have difficulty in learning transfer techniques which require good coordination.

Head injury is often masked by the severity of the primary injury. This may be suspected if a patient has undue difficulty in learning or retaining self-care techniques.

Social and psychological aspects are inseparable from the physical. Reasonable long term goals must be set to give the patient an incentive. Prospects of living with his family, working, or driving a car are goals which easily make the difference between a patient with ambition and a patient without.

2 *Wheelchair*

Mobility and Propelling

THE WHEELCHAIR

The most suitable wheelchair for the quadriplegic patient is the standard adult chair of the foldable tubular X-frame type. This chair's flexibility allows good contact of the wheels with the floor. A flat metal double X-frame has the disadvantage of rigidity, which on uneven surfaces could leave one wheel not touching the ground, thus making it impossible for the patient to propel the chair.

EQUIPMENT

Arm rests should be removable, executive, upholstered. Foot rests are swing away and adjustable with brakes of the push-away lever type (permitting the patient to apply the brakes with the same movement used in propelling the chair). Front castors have 8 inch solid grey rubber tires. (Most suitable for uneven surfaces.) Rear tires are grey pneumatic with 1⅜ inch diameter or solid grey rubber. (Black tires will mark floors.)

Cushions may be foam rubber 3 inch thick No. 3 density with cloth covers. (Do not use plastic covers as they do not absorb moisture and may cause excessive perspiration.) Other cushions (air cushions, gel cushions, water cushions, etc.) may be selected later since each individual's skin seems to react differently to a variety of cushions. (The cushion which suits everyone has yet to be invented.) The foam rubber cushion is tolerated well by a majority of patients and is certainly the easiest to use while learning to transfer. When the patient becomes proficient at transferring he may be able to use a cushion of his choice. Nylon cover over a cloth cover will facilitate movement in the chair. A 3/8 inch tempered hardboard, cut to fit within the frame of the seat is inside the cushion cover under the cushion. Velcro strips, 2 inches wide, are sewn from front to back on both sides of the bottom of the nylon cushion cover with opposing strips sewn to the seat of the chair. It is easier to launder the cushion covers if the hook velcro is sewn to the chair.

One or two detachable leg straps are fastened with velcro or a post and loop, one behind the ankle (Fig. 2-1) and another optional at about midcalf. These prevent the feet from becoming caught behind the foot rests. Individual heel straps are not

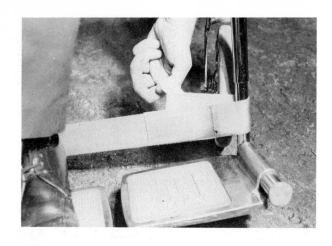

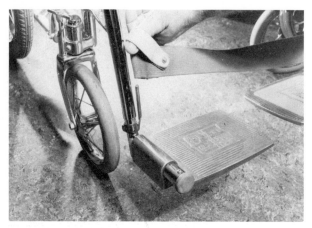

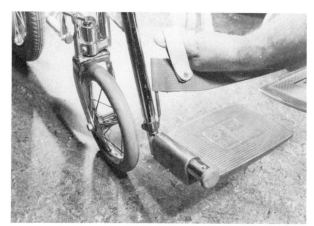

FIGURE 2-1

recommended for the quadriplegic patient because the metal uprights which retain the heel straps are hazardous. A patient, learning to lower his legs, may drop a foot onto them and cause trauma. In addition, the straps must be pushed forward before the foot rests can be folded up.

SPECIAL EQUIPMENT

Brake extension which is removable for additional leverage if required.

A safety belt of 2 inch webbing may be attached to the second retainer screw on both sides of the back. It may be fastened in front with a regular buckle, a car safety-strap buckle (Fig. 2-2), a hook, or a velcro D-ring fastening. Thumb loops may be sewn to the straps to make fastening possible.

A tibial strap for the patient with gross extensor spasms of the back, who sometimes slides out of a waist safety strap. A strap across the tibial tuberosities is attached to the front upright of the wheelchair arm (Fig 2-3A). If extensor spasms are of the knees only, the strap can be attached to the frame of the leg rests (Fig. 2-3B).

12

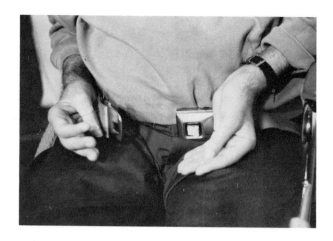

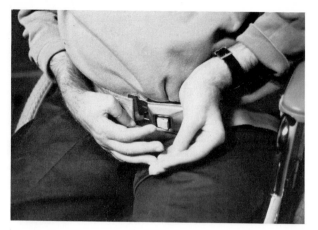

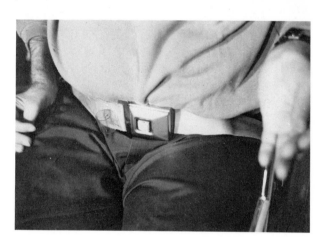

A

FIGURE 2-2

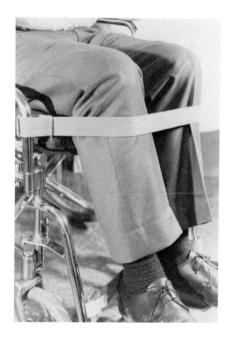

B

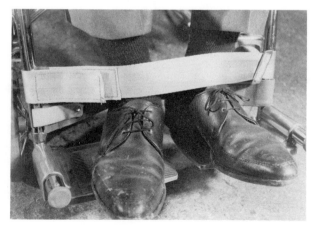

FIGURE 2-3

13

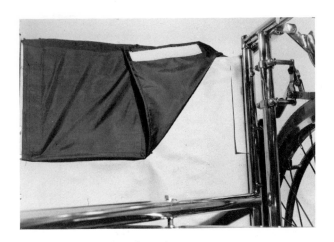

FIGURE 2-4

If the patient must slide out of the back or front of the chair, a nylon flap may be sewn to the top edge of the cushion with a soft velcro strip sewn to the free end (Fig. 2-4). An opposing strip of velcro is sewn to the underside of the wheelchair seat; this prevents the cushion from rolling up during transfer.

Detachable backs. Although zipper backs are commercially available, they are very difficult for a quadriplegic to fasten. Therefore, it is necessary to have a back that is removable on one side and fastened by a full length contoured metal clip, which fits onto the front of the upright and is secured by a small pin (Fig. 2-5).

Swivel backs will sometimes enable the patient to change position more easily in the chair (Fig. 2-6). The position of the swivel on the uprights must be carefully adjusted.

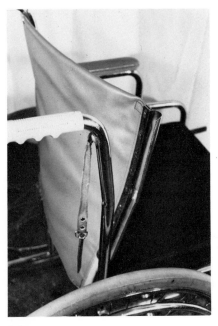
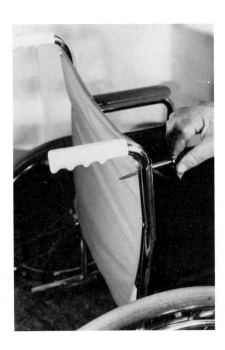
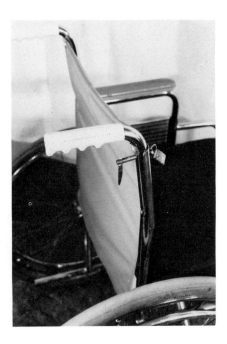

FIGURE 2-5

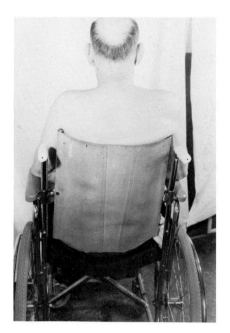
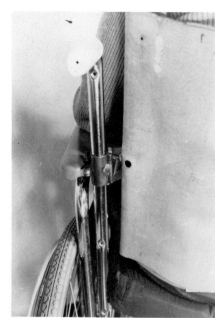

FIGURE 2-6

A wheelchair tray is of use to the majority of quadriplegics. The advantages of the tray shown in Figure 2-7 are simple attachment, stability, and appearance. Two ⅜ inch holes are drilled in executive arm rests just in front of the pad and on the curve to accommodate the rods. The rods consist of ⅜ inch cold rolled steel 16 inches long, flattened at one end and bent at 90°, 5 inches from the other end. The flattened end is drilled and bolted to the tray to line up with the chair arms. The rods are then placed in the holes in the chair arms to ensure a good fit before bolting them permanently into position under the tray using electrical cable straps. The tray is made of ½ inch plywood covered with Arborite or Formica, finished with aluminum edging to form a small lip around the tray. The tray may be made to fold (Fig. 2-8).

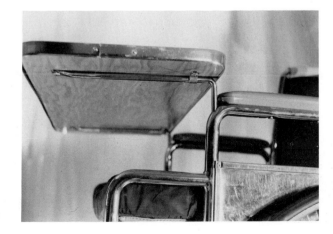
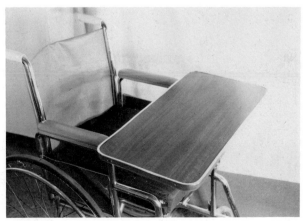

FIGURE 2-7

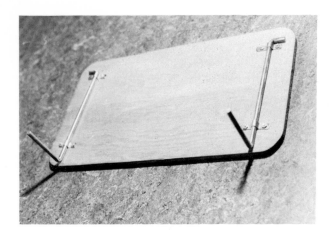 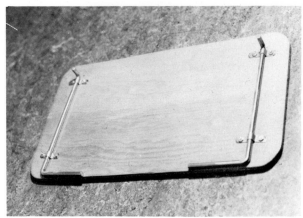

FIGURE 2-8

POSTURING THE PATIENT

Correct posturing of the patient in the chair is essential for efficient operation of the wheelchair.

The chair must be adapted to his leg length before the patient can position himself. The weight of the patient's thighs should be distributed evenly along the length of the cushion when the patient is sitting with his back, including his sacrum, in contact with the back of the chair. This weight is distributed by adjustment of the height of the foot rest.

Only occasionally will it be necessary to order a custom-built chair, i.e. for the unusually tall patient. Measurement charts are available from the dealers.

At first a patient may need a high back. This must be removable (Fig. 2-9) because it will interfere with his scapular action, making both propulsion of the chair and self-care activities difficult. A simple method of extending the chair back, providing comfort and stability, is easily constructed. Aluminum tubing of a diameter to fit over the wheelchair tubing is split down its length for 4 inches. The top of the cut is contoured to fit the curve of the pushing handle, thereby forming a continuation of the chair back upright. An envelope of leather or other material is sewn to fit over the uprights and overlap the chair back; this envelope is placed over the uprights before attaching them to the chair.

A reclining back may be required; however, this will interfere grossly with independence, making the application of most mechanical principles ineffective.

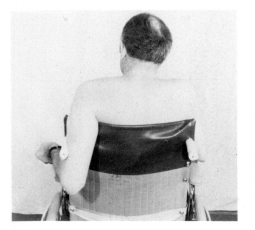

FIGURE 2-9

16

Although a wheelchair seat slopes down towards the back, the patient who sits slumped on his sacrum may require a greater slope to help his posture. This can be accomplished by making the cushion into a wedge shape, higher at the front than the rear. This also helps prevent such a patient sliding forward out of the chair.

In order to create a flat surface to aid transfer, balance, and posturing, 1/4 inch tempered hardboard may be placed under the cushion inside the cover. This must be 1-1/2 inches inside the seat rails on either side to obviate interfering with the mechanism of the chair.

The natural sag of the wheelchair seat sometimes causes the knees to slide together (Fig. 2-10). This is not desirable because it disturbs balance. If the previously mentioned tempered hardboard under the cushion does not correct this tendency, a saddle formed by placing a roll of foam rubber under the centre front of the cushion will correct it.

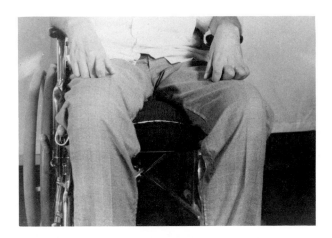
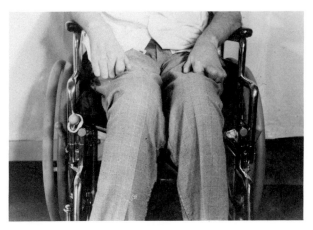

FIGURE 2-10

The emaciated patient may have a tendency to pressure areas caused by the back of the chair rubbing on his spinous processes. If this occurs, pads, 3 inches wide of 1 inch foam rubber are leather covered and sewn from the top to the bottom of the chair back with a 2 inch space between them (Fig. 2-11).

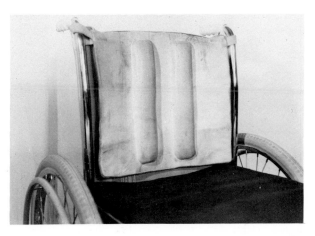

FIGURE 2-11

SELF-POSITIONING

MOVING BACKWARD

The patient, when moving back in the chair, leans forward and transfers part of his weight from his buttocks to his feet. Some of the body weight is placed forward of the knees, which act as a fulcrum. The mechanical advantage gained by this position will enable the buttocks to be levered up and pushed back with the help of shoulder flexion.

Method 1. (Fig. 2-12) In this method the patient places the palms of his hands on his wheels and leans forward so that, by depressing his shoulder girdle and flexing his shoulders, he will take the weight off his buttocks and move them back.

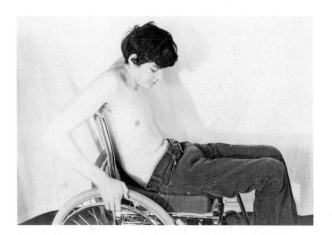
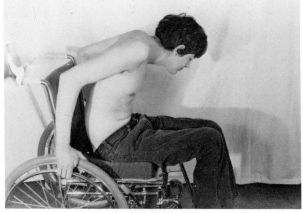
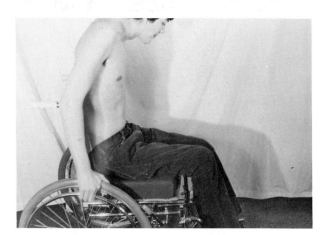
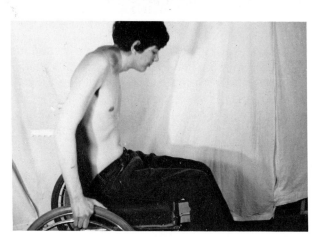

FIGURE 2-12

Method 2. (Fig. 2-13) With this technique, the patient places his arms outside the armrests, positioning his thumbs against the inside of the front of the armrests. By flexing his elbows, he pulls his trunk forward; then, flexing his shoulders, he pushes his buttocks back into the chair. A continuation of shoulder flexion will push him to the upright position.

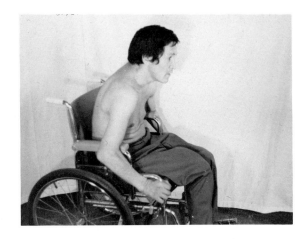
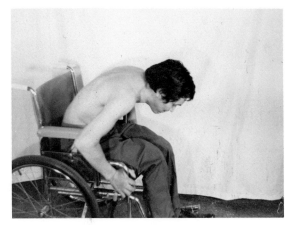
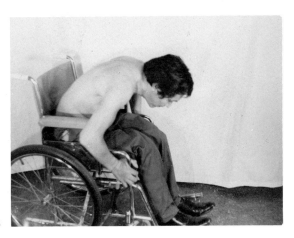
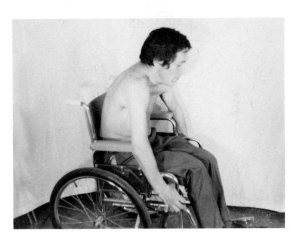

FIGURE 2-13

Method 3.   (Fig. 2-14) In this case the patient puts his arms inside the chair arms and places his thumbs against the inside of the front of the armrests. He moves back in the wheelchair, using the same technique as in Method 2. To sit up, he places his elbows on the armrests and works his elbows towards himself as far as possible, using adduction of the shoulders initially and protraction of the shoulders as he progresses to the upright position. He extends his neck quickly to gain momentum as he nears the upright, throwing him past his point of balance against the back of the chair.

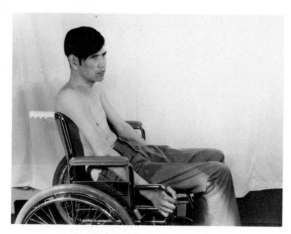

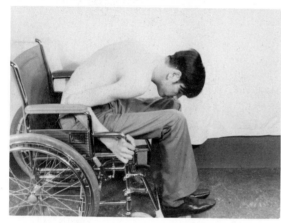
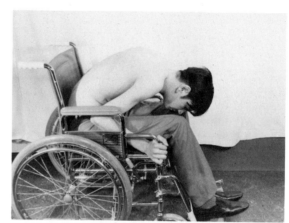

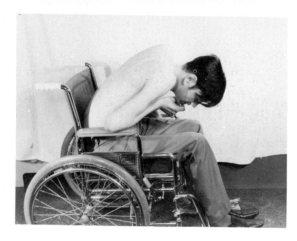
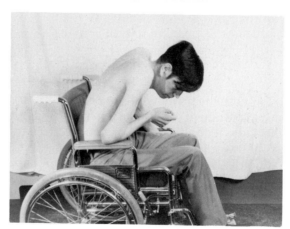

FIGURE 2-14

Method 4. (Fig. 2-15) Placing both extended wrists over the back of the chair, the patient flexes his trunk forward as far as possible. Flexion of the elbows will both pull the patient back into the chair and sit him up. Purchase is increased by the patient's sliding his hands down the back of the chair as he comes to a sitting position.

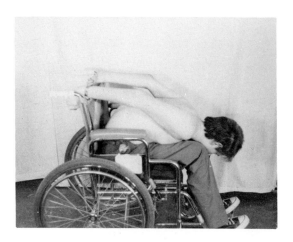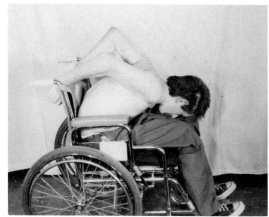
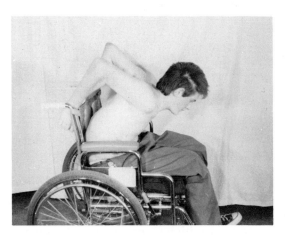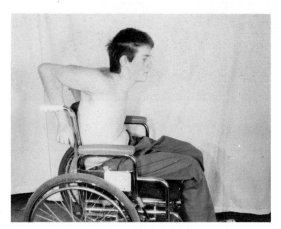

FIGURE 2-15

Method 5. (Fig. 2-16) The patient, who is unable to sit up using any of the previous methods, places one arm over the back of the chair and positions his wrist under his knee or chair arm to flex his trunk forward. The arm over the chair back is flexed at the elbow to move himself back in the chair. The other arm is used simultaneously to push against the armrest. Since there is some tendency to twist to one side using this method, the patient may have to repeat the action using the opposite arm over the chair back.

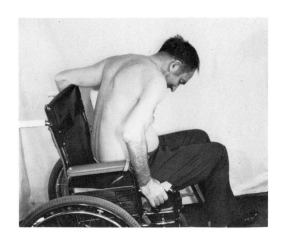

FIGURE 2-16

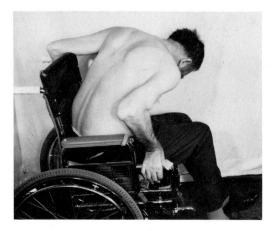

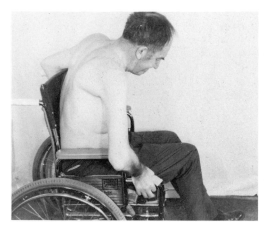

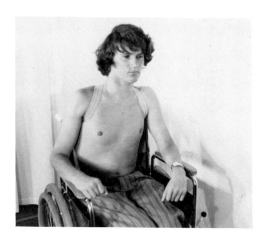

An aid, which is very useful in training the quadriplegic in trunk mobility and the development of confidence, is made in the following manner. Two loops of light elastic are fixed to the first screw from the top of the wheelchair back on each side. The loops are placed around the shoulders of the patient, the left loop around the right shoulder and vice versa (Fig. 2-17A). These act as spring assists in lateral and forward trunk movements and eliminate the danger of falling (Fig. 2-17B). The tension can be decreased by elongating the loops as the patient becomes more adept.

FIGURE 2-17

A

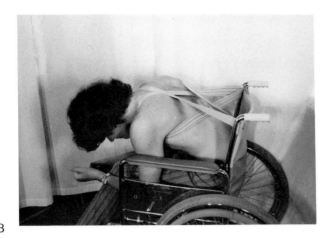

B

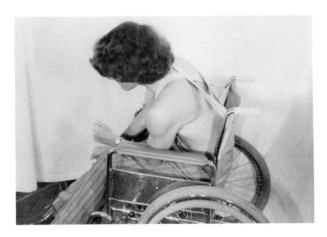

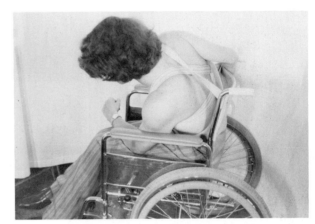

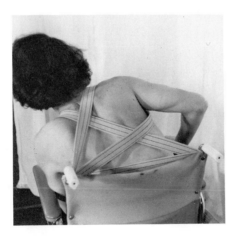

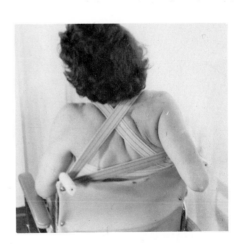

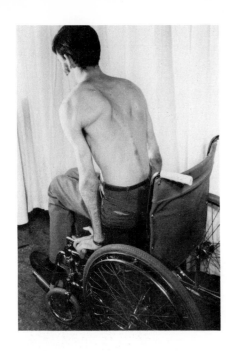 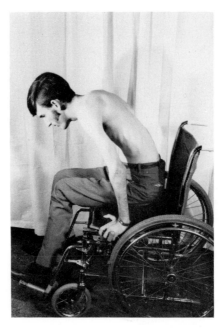

FIGURE 2-18

MOVING FORWARD

Method 1.   (Fig. 2-18) In this method the patient places both palms on the wheels and locks his elbows. By depressing his shoulder girdle and extending his neck and shoulders sharply he throws his buttocks forward in the chair.

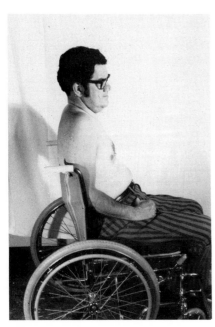 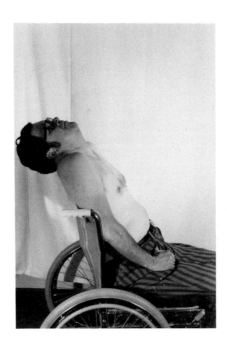

FIGURE 2-19

24

Method 2. (Fig. 2-19) A simple method, the patient puts his thumbs in his pants pockets or belt tabs and places his elbows against the chair back as close to his body as possible. He pushes his buttocks forward in the chair by extending his wrists, upper trunk, and neck.

Method 3. (Fig. 2-20) Simultaneously the patient extends his neck and throws both arms up and over his head. This gives sufficient momentum to slide his buttocks forward on the chair.

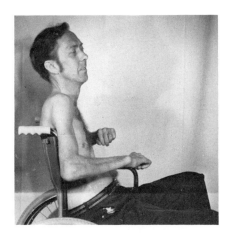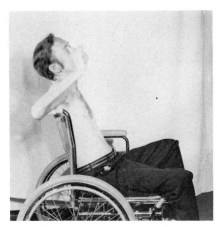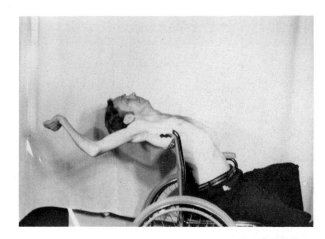

FIGURE 2-20

Method 4. (Fig. 2-21) One arm is hooked around the pushing handle of the chair; the patient flexes this shoulder to pull the trunk over and into rotation and extension. This action relieves the weight from the opposite buttock and tends to move it forward. This forward movement may be enhanced by either swinging the free arm forward vigorously or by pushing against the arm or wheel of the chair. The action is repeated using opposite arms and alternated until the desired position is reached.

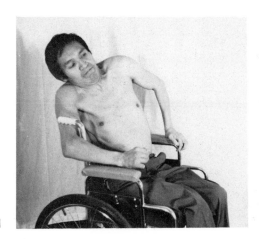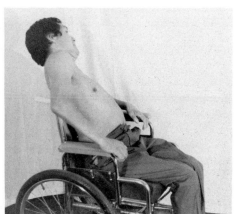

FIGURE 2-21

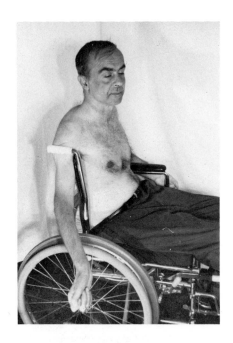
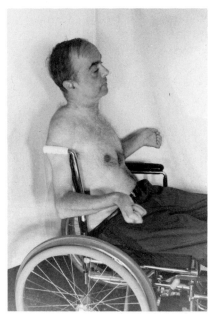
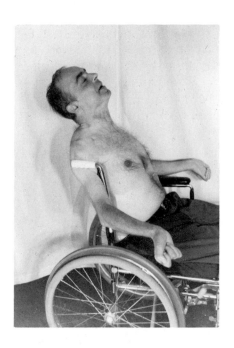

FIGURE 2-22

Method 5. (Fig. 2-22) Using this technique, the patient swings both arms behind the pushing handles of the chair. When he flexes his shoulders vigorously he will extend his trunk over the back of the wheelchair, making it into a fulcrum and levering his buttocks forward.

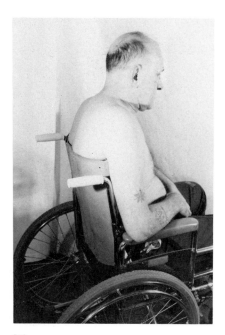
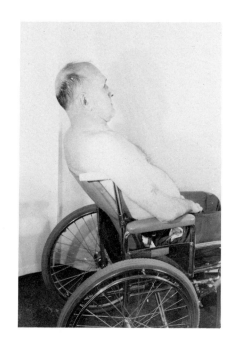

FIGURE 2-23

26

Method 6.   (Fig. 2-23) Extension of neck and shoulders will rock the patient back, causing the bottom of the swivel back to swing forwards. This relieves some weight from his buttocks and slides him forwards. A stop should be placed so that the patient who cannot adequately control the movement will not slide forward too far. This stop may be a length of leather running between the two back uprights and behind the swivel back uprights, near the top.

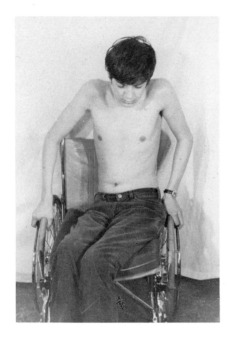
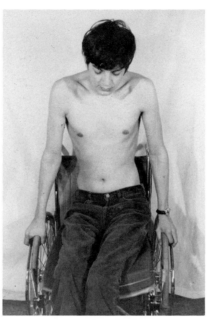
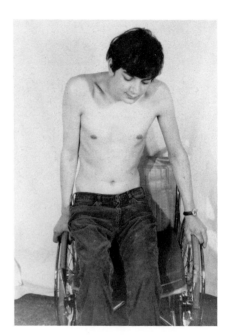

MOVING ACROSS THE CHAIR SEAT

Method 1.   (Fig. 2-24) Some patients can do a straight arm pushup on the wheels of the chair. In this situation the patient leans forward until he reaches his point of balance. He does his pushup using his shoulder depressors, thus enabling him to swing his buttocks laterally. When he is learning this movement he starts by swinging his trunk from side to side in pendulum fashion. This enables him to move further because of the developed momentum.

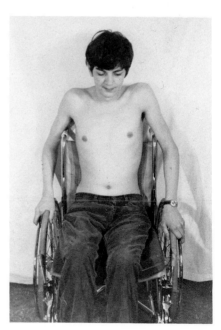

FIGURE 2-24

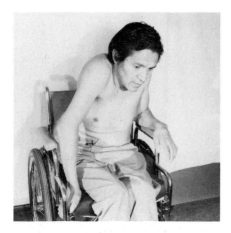
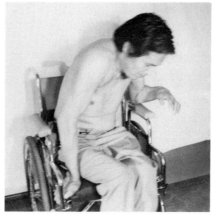
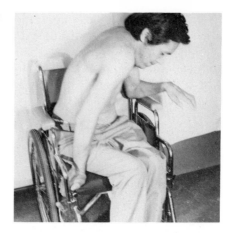

FIGURE 2-25

Method 2. (Fig. 2-25) The patient places a forearm on the inner side of the armrest and leans over this arm. He puts the other hand on the wheelchair cushion at midthigh level and locks the elbow. By depressing both shoulders and flexing his trunk forward and over the armrest, some of the pressure is relieved from the buttocks and they are levered sideways and back.

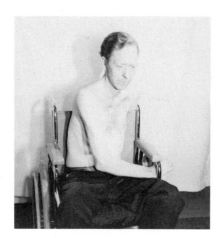

Method 3. (Fig. 2-26) Placing one arm over the chair back, the patient hooks his elbow under the pushing handle. The other arm is positioned across his body with the thumb web hooked into the chair front upright. This causes him to twist and lean over the armrest with his forearm resting on his thighs. By throwing his trunk forward and flexing both shoulders, his buttocks will move back and towards the opposite side of the chair.

FIGURE 2-26

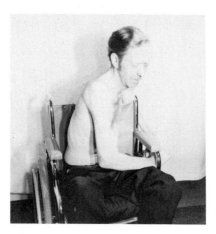
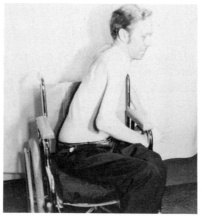
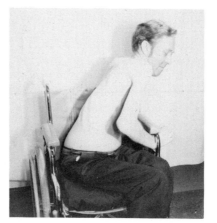

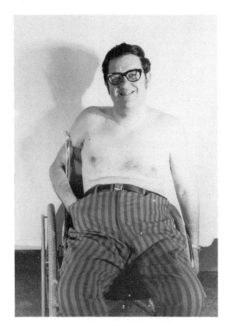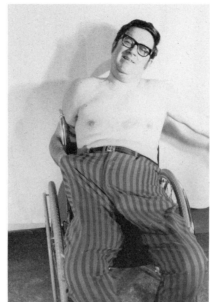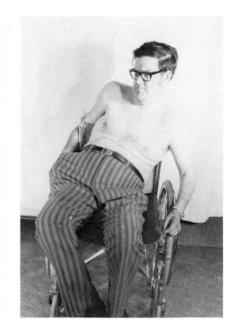

FIGURE 2-27

Method 4. (Fig. 2-27) This is a particularly useful method for a patient who is wearing a splint on one hand. The patient places one arm over the chair back, hooks his elbow around the pushing handle, and puts his hand into his pants pocket. By throwing his weight over the chair back and simultaneously rotating his shoulder externally he will lever his buttocks over. This also ensures that the pants are wrinkle-free beneath the buttocks.

PROPELLING THE CHAIR

The patient must be correctly positioned in the wheelchair before he is ready to learn the techniques of propelling the chair.

WHEELING FORWARD

The patient places the heels of both hands on the drive rims as far back as possible. His shoulders are internally rotated and his elbows slightly flexed initially. A pushing action is developed by adduction and external rotation of the shoulders (Fig. 2-28). The upper trunk is extended to maintain balance as the hands move forward. Patients are inclined to move their hands only a short distance until they have learned to synchronize these movements. Greater speed and balance will be developed with practice.

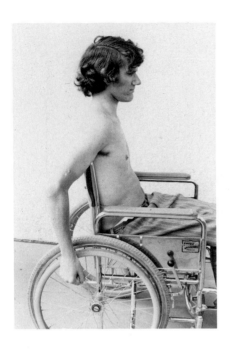
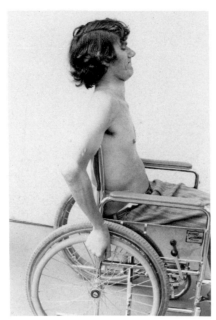
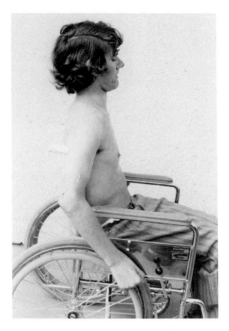

FIGURE 2-28

In some cases a patient is unable to maintain balance in the chair while wheeling and cannot tolerate a safety belt across the chest. In such instances he may wheel while placing one or both arms behind the pushing handles (Fig. 2-29). However, this restricts his shoulder flexion and causes him to lose a considerable amount of driving power.

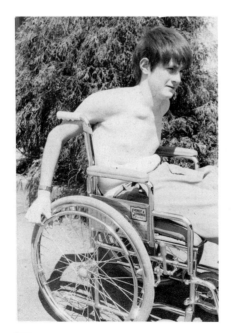
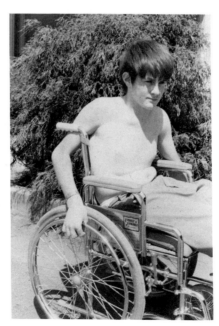

FIGURE 2-29

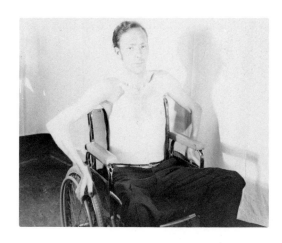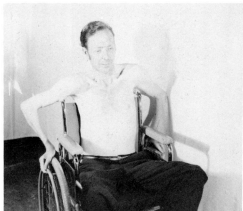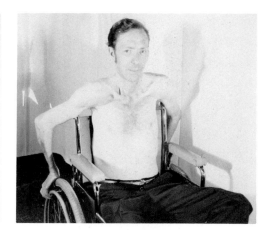

FIGURE 2-30

WHEELING BACKWARD

The patient who uses drive rims will back up by placing his hands as far forward as he can reach, with elbows slightly flexed. With his back resting against the back of the wheelchair, he adducts and internally rotates his shoulders while he elevates and retracts his shoulder girdle (Fig. 2-30). This develops a pulling action that will not cause him to fall forward.

Some patients who use this technique also extend the upper trunk to gain additional pull and maintain balance (Fig. 2-31).

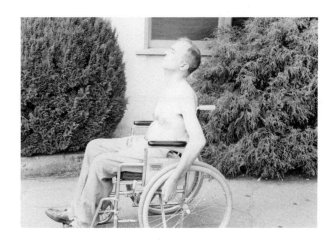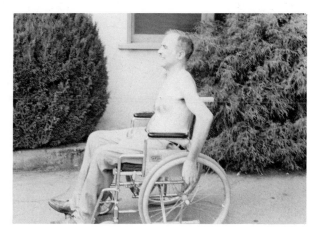

FIGURE 2-31

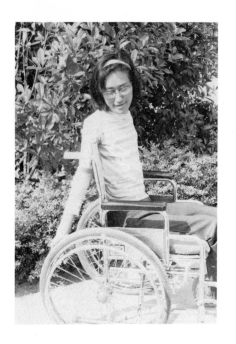

The patient who is unable to maintain balance while wheeling backward must additionally place one or both arms over the back of the wheelchair. He places the heel of this hand against the inside of the tire; his shoulder must be externally rotated and elevated (Fig. 2-32). To develop a push, he abducts and depresses his shoulder.

HAND POSITIONS

If the patient's hands slip on the drive rims, the drive rims may be taped temporarily. This may indicate the need for commercially available plastic-covered rims or rubber-covered rims. Note the hand position change as the shoulders rotate externally (Fig. 2-33). To cover the rims with rubber, the drive rims are removed from the hangars and cut through. One inch surgical tubing is slipped on to the rim, and pulled back from the cut, which is then silver soldered. Sufficient tubing is used to ensure a tight butt fit when it is released. The rims are now remounted.

FIGURE 2-32

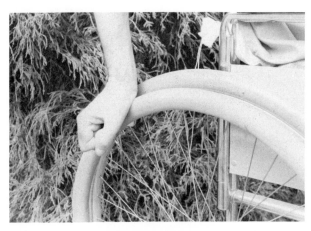

FIGURE 2-33.

A, Forward

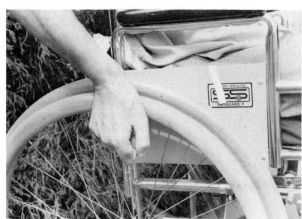

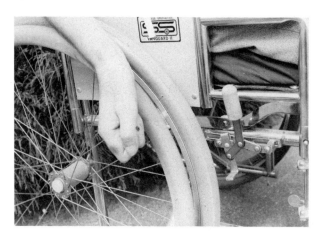

32

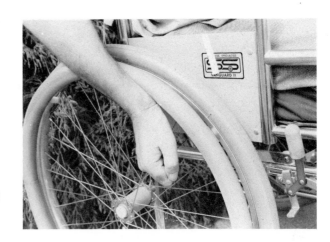

B, Backward

The patient who is unable to obtain sufficient purchase on the drive rims may push directly on pneumatic tires (Fig. 2-34). He may wear pusher mitts to protect his hands and gain friction. The spacers between the drive rims and the wheels are removed, and the drive rims bolted directly to the hangars. The drive rims are retained to prevent the fingers from becoming caught in the spokes.

FIGURE 2-34

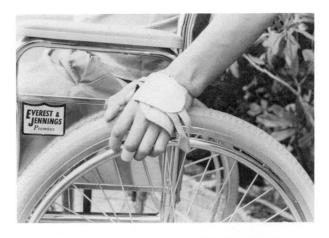
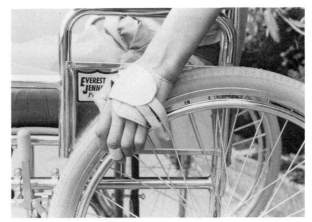

A, Forward

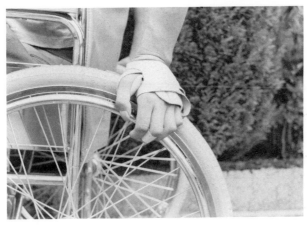
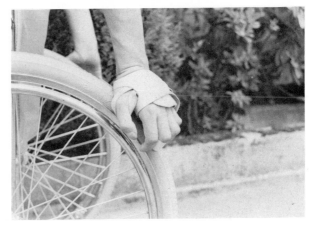

B, Backward

Pusher mitts (Fig. 2-35) are made of cowhide with a velcro fastening and a hook velcro or rubber pushing surface (see Appendix). There is a thumb loop at either end with a hole to fit over the thumb at about a third of the distance from the end. The first loop is slipped over the thumb so that the pusher mitt lies over the back of the hand. It is then brought up over the palm of the hand, the thumb is inserted into the hole, and the mitt is fastened.

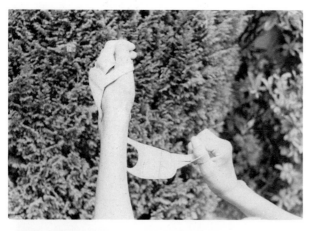

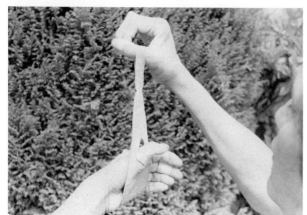

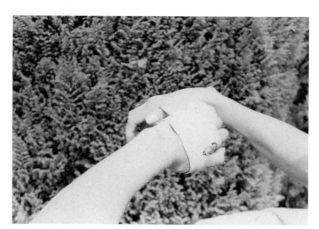

FIGURE 2-35

The patient who is unable to gain friction on the tire or rim may push on wide spacers. The patient places his thumb webs on the drive rims with his thumbs against the spacers (Fig. 2-36). It is possible to propel the chair using this method even though the shoulder adductors may be weak. To adapt the wheelchair, replace the four 3/4 inch spacers with eight 1-1/2 inch spacers.

Vertical lugs may be added if the patient is unable to position his hand to utilize spacers (Fig. 2-37). Eight to twelve lugs will be necessary. They should be

34

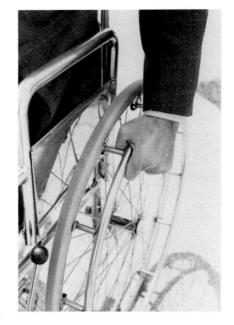

FIGURE 2-36

A, Forward   *B*, Backward

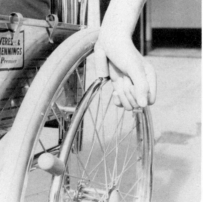
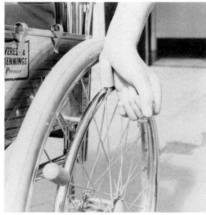
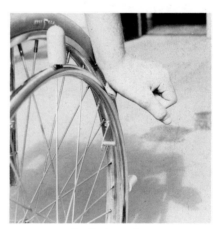

FIGURE 2-37

A, Forward   *B*, Backward

covered with rubber brake handle tips. Horizontal lugs are not recommended as they are hazardous and widen the chair.

A moulded splint, extending from behind the metacarpophalangeal (MP) joints to half way up the forearm, will stabilize a flail wrist. Pushing hooks, appropriately positioned and bent for the individual patient, are attached to the moulded splint (Fig. 2-38). The patient can push against spacers, wide spacers, or against vertical lugs inside or outside the drive rim.

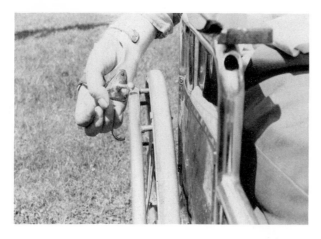
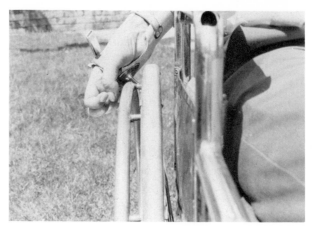

FIGURE 2-38.
A, Forward;

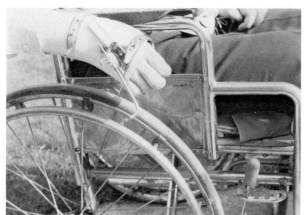
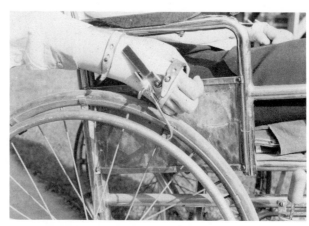

B, Backward.

The patient who is unable to propel a chair by any of the aforementioned methods will require an electrically driven wheelchair. This may be driven using a removable joystick (Fig. 2-39). Special adaptations may be required, i.e. a head-stick (Fig. 2-40) a mouthstick, or a ballbearing rocker splint (Fig. 2-41). Prescription of this chair should be avoided where possible since the weight of the chair makes transport difficult up stairs or in a car.

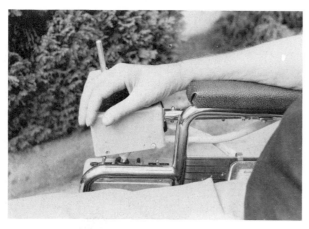
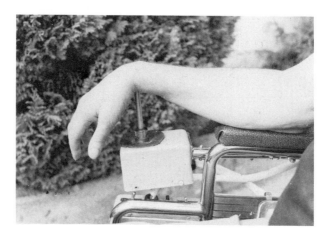

FIGURE 2-39

36

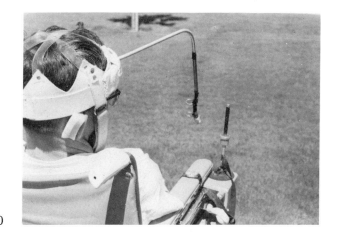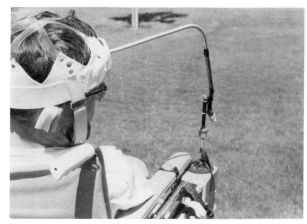

FIGURE 2-40

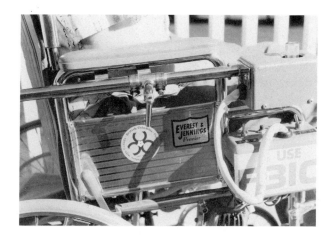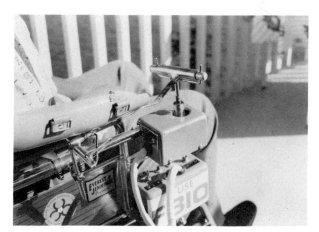

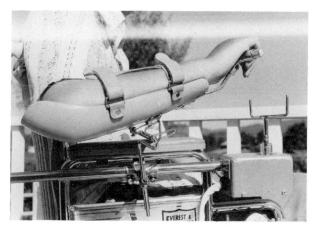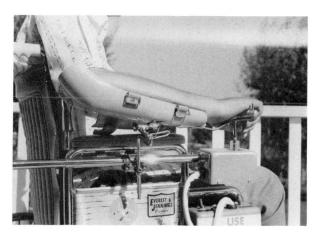

FIGURE 2-41

37

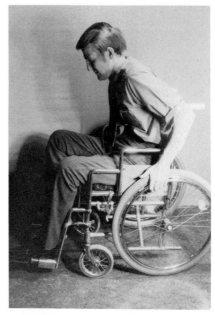
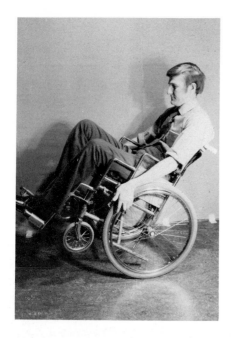

FIGURE 2-42

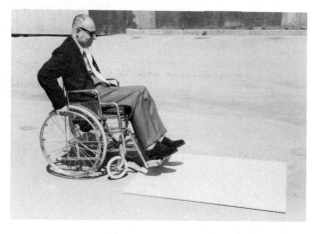

FIGURE 2-43

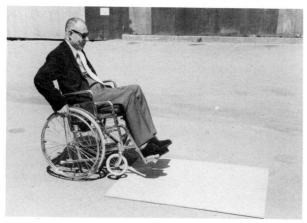
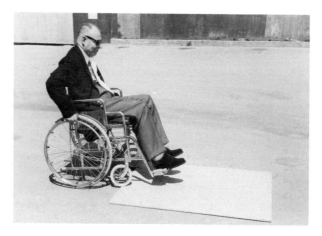

JUMPING OR BALANCING THE CHAIR

Some quadriplegics are able to jump the front castors over small obstacles such as carpet edges or weather strips. The chair must be rolled back slightly before pushing sharply forward to lift the front wheels (Fig. 2-42), but the castors must remain in the trailing position. The patient with a low lesion and with good strength and balance may learn to balance his chair, a great advantage in clearing obstacles and managing rough ground (Fig. 2-43). To balance the chair the patient must sit well back. He maintains the chair in the balanced position by slight counteracting wheel movements, pushing forward if the wheels drop and back if they should lift too high.

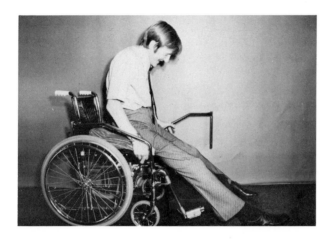
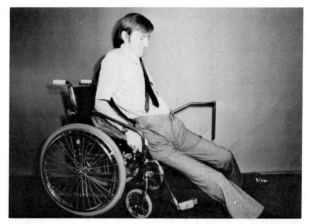
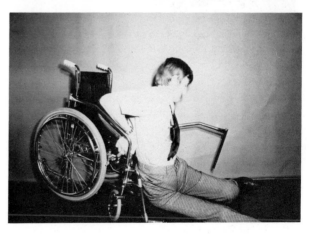

FIGURE 2-44

GETTING IN AND OUT OF THE CHAIR TO THE FLOOR

When moving from the chair to the floor (Fig. 2-44), the patient wheels forward to turn the castors back and applies the brakes. He turns one armrest so that

39

it projects forward of the chair. He puts his feet ahead of the footrests and drops a cushion on the footrests. He slides to the edge of his chair until the chair tips forwards and lowers himself the remaining short distance.

In getting back into the chair (Fig. 2-45), the patient lifts himself onto the cushion on the footrests. He grasps the projecting wheelchair arm and places the other hand against the inside of the other wheelchair arm. Strength, skill, and balance are required for the lift back into the wheelchair.

To replace the cushion (Fig. 2-46), the patient puts his foot on a high leg retainer strap and pushes the cushion well under his raised knee. When he does a pushup the cushion springs partially under him; he can square the cushion by doing a pushup and actually place the cushion with his buttocks.

To replace a foam cushion, the cushion is folded in half and wedged between the arm of the chair and the hip. A pushup on the folded cushion and the opposite armrest will flip the cushion under him. It is squared into position again by using the buttocks.

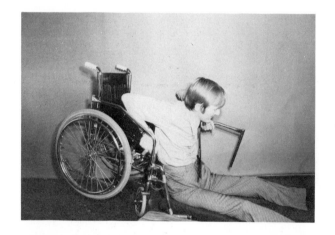
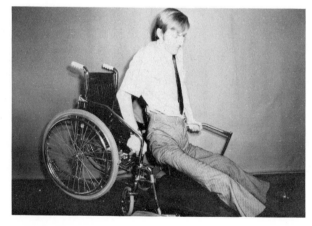
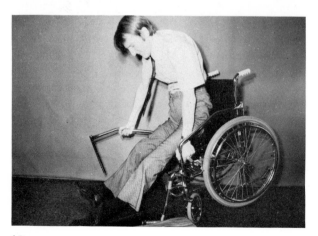
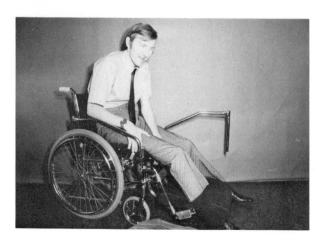

FIGURE 2-45

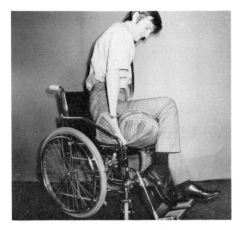

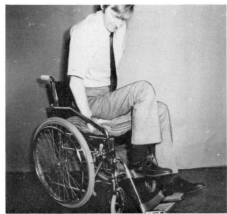

FIGURE 2-46

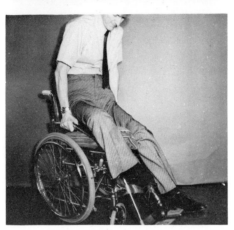

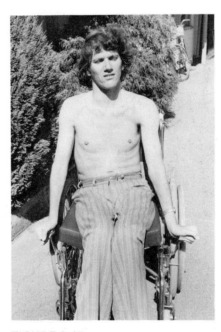

FIGURE 2-47

BRAKES

Applying

Pushing forward on the brakes is the preferred movement for locking. Many patients apply their brakes simultaneously, using the same movement as in wheeling—flexion of the shoulder with adduction and external rotation (Fig. 2-47). To maintain balance some patients apply a brake with one hand using the other arm as a counterbalance (Fig. 2-48). A patient may hook one elbow over the pushing handle and use it as an anchor point to develop more momentum to push against the brake (Fig. 2-49).

The hand position is determined by the degree of external rotation required and the presence or absence of wrist extensors. Wrist extension and/or external rotation can be used to flick the brakes on (Fig. 2-50). The heel of the hand or the fingers push against the brake when elbow flexion and external rotation of the shoulder are used to apply the brakes (Fig. 2-51).

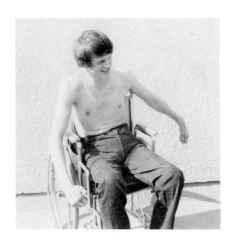

FIGURE 2-48

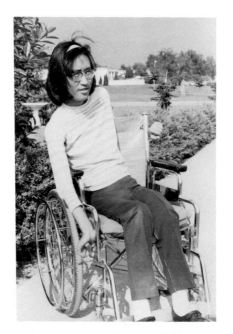

FIGURE 2-49

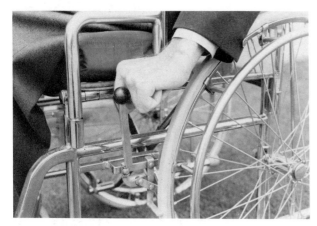

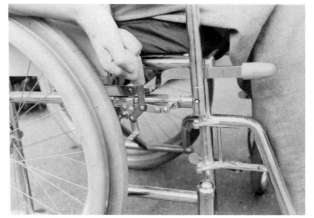

FIGURE 2-50

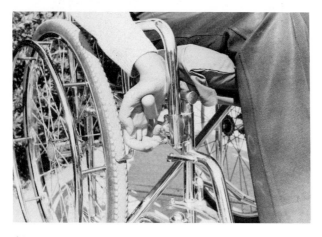

FIGURE 2-51

Releasing

The same methods of maintaining balance while applying the brakes are used for release, except that the maintenance of balance is made more difficult by the pulling action. The brakes may be released simultaneously usually using adduction and internal rotation of the shoulders (Fig. 2-52). The brakes may be released using a chopping action, hitting the side of the hand against the brake handle (Fig. 2-53).

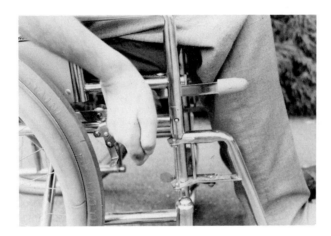

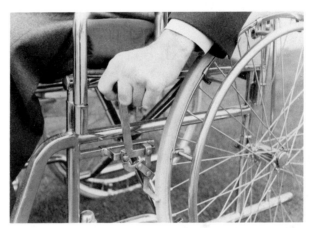

FIGURE 2-52

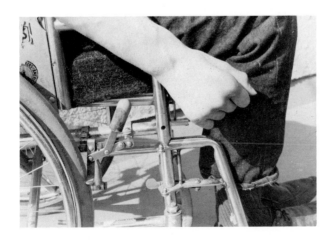

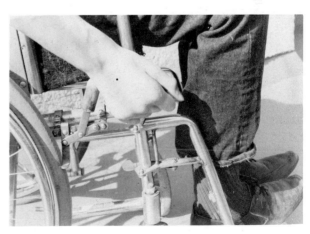

FIGURE 2-53

MAINTENANCE

The necessity of weekly maintenance should not be overlooked since the wheelchair is the equivalent of legs to a quadriplegic. The following must be done once weekly:

The chrome should be cleaned with a type of cleaner that leaves a waxy finish and which, when polished, provides a protective coating.

Lint should be removed from around the axles with a bottle brush.

The upholstery should be washed with mild soap and water.

The wheels should be checked for loose spokes and worn bearings. Pneumatic tires should be tested for correct pressure.

A few drops of light oil should be applied to the bearings at the hubs. Care must be taken not to apply too much oil because it will cause dripping and gathering of lint.

The patient himself should do as many of these tasks as he can depending on the severity of his disability. He will be more efficient if he works from a firm padded surface on the floor. Regular maintenance will reduce the number of costly repairs and the inconvenience of being without a wheelchair.

3

Bed Mobility and Transfers

BED AND EQUIPMENT

The bed should be a sturdy metal to facilitate the attachment of necessary equipment. It should have an open panel head and foot to allow the patient to insert a hand to pull himself up the bed. The bed must have rubber-tipped legs to prevent the bed from sliding. The mattress must be the same height as the wheelchair cushion when both are compressed equally. (Some patients must have a deliberate slope to assist them in one direction provided they are efficient when travelling in the opposite direction.)

Plywood may be bolted directly to the bed frame.

The mattress should be firm and spring-filled, facilitating movement on the bed.

Toe space must be allowed at the foot of the bed for prone lying; this may necessitate an extra long bed.

A footboard will take the weight of the covers from the feet when the patient is supine. The elimination of weight on the feet will facilitate movement in bed.

A nylon contour sheet will be an advantage to patients who must move by sliding. The sheet should be a tight fit to prevent wrinkling and should have a conventional sheet beneath it to absorb moisture.

Bed hooks are required to attach the front of the chair to the bed and, occasionally, to prevent the rear wheels from sliding (Fig. 3-1). (A rope with a hook made out of a coat hanger can be used for assessment purposes.) More complicated hooks can be used with automatic spring locks. It is desirable to use foldaway hooks, so that the bed can be made without any hazardous projections. (See Appendix.)

A leg retainer board (Fig. 3-2) will provide leverage and prevent the legs from falling off the bed during transfer. The top must be padded with 1 inch foam rubber and covered.

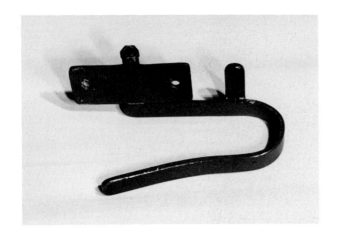

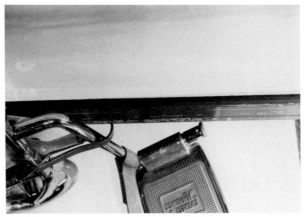

FIGURE 3-1

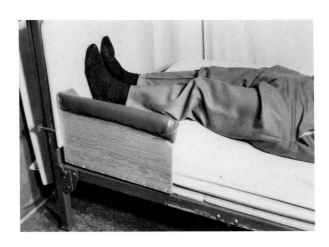

FIGURE 3-2

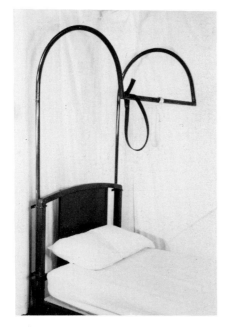

OVERHEAD EQUIPMENT

If an overhead bar is required it must be strongly constructed and may be attached to either the bed frame or the wall behind the bed (Fig. 3-3). The bar should run the full width of the bed and be approximately above the elbows of the patient when his arms are by his side. The minimum height of the bar should be just beyond arms reach when the patient is sitting. Final adjustments must be made to suit the individual patient.

FIGURE 3-3

A projection from the centre of the bar runs horizontally toward the foot of the bed for no more than half the length of the bed (Fig. 3-4). A longer projection requires attachment at the foot of the bed (Fig. 3-5).

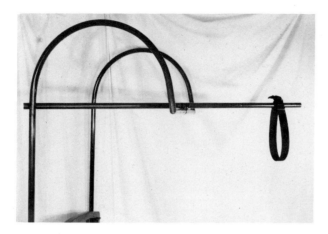

FIGURE 3-4

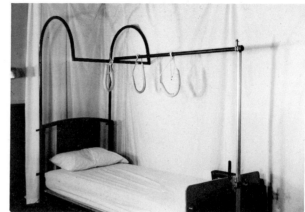

FIGURE 3-5

Two bars, one on either side and eight inches in from the edge of the bed, may be attached to overhead bars at the head and foot of the bed (Fig. 3-6).

An outrigger is a continuation of the overhead bar that projects out over the wheelchair (Fig. 3-7). The end of the projection must be padded to protect people who may inadvertently walk into it.

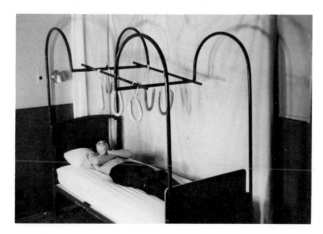

FIGURE 3-6

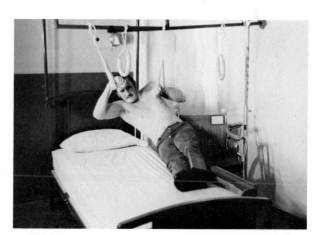

FIGURE 3-7

Floating straps are placed around the overhead bars and left free to slide along the bar. The buckle must be firmly fastened with no projections (Fig. 3-8). Fixed straps are placed around the bar and taped into position (Fig. 3-9).

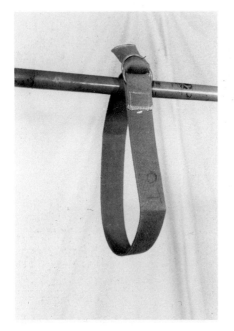

FIGURE 3-8

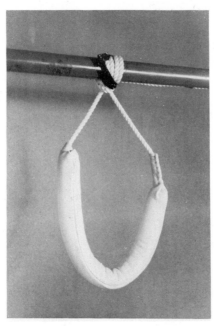

FIGURE 3-9

SELF-POSITIONING IN THE BED

TURNING IN BED

Supine to Prone

Methods of turning can be learned most easily on a gymnastic mat.
Method 1. (Fig. 3-10) The patient tucks one arm under his body palm up, then flings his other arm and shoulder violently across his body. He turns his head sharply in the direction of his arm to add momentum. This twists his upper trunk, and the rest of his body follows until he is prone.

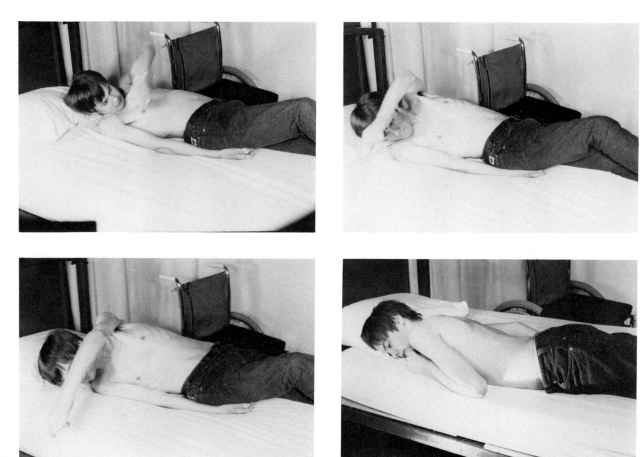

FIGURE 3-10

Method 2.   (Fig. 3-11) The patient sits up, works one extended arm behind him close to his body, pivots on it, and throws himself over the arm onto his face. This can be accomplished more easily if the legs can be crossed first. This is done by leaning forward and inserting an arm under one leg and over the other. Lifting the elbow will lever the leg over.

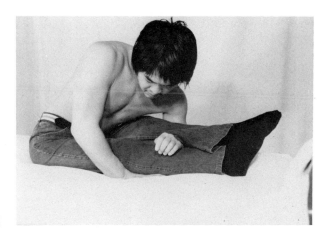
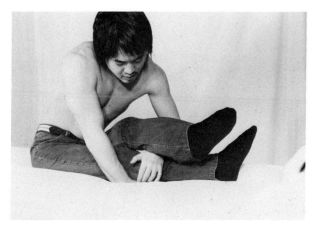

FIGURE 3-11

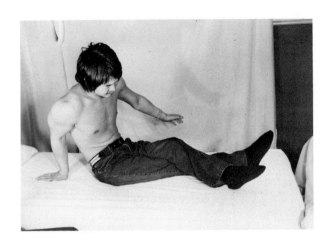

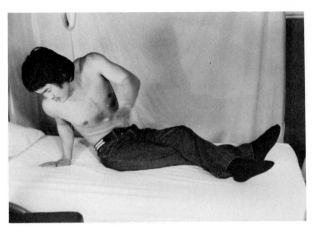

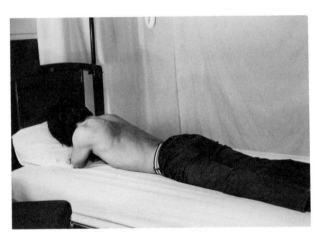

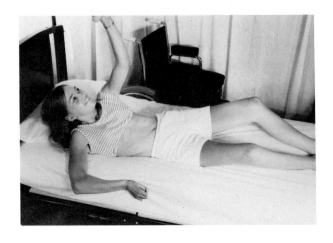

Method 3. (Fig. 3-12) The patient inserts his wrist into an overhead strap and pulls up, enabling him to work his other elbow underneath his upper trunk.

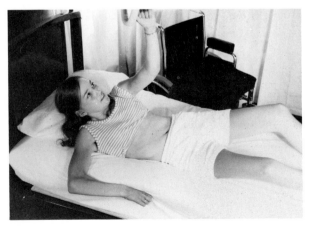

FIGURE 3-12

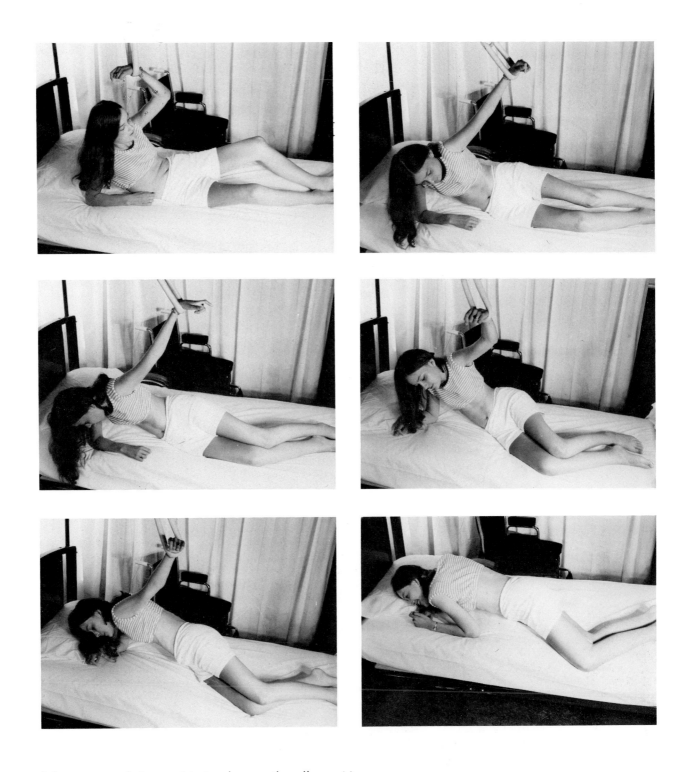

He takes his arm out of the strap and throws his trunk over the elbow. He may have to reach over and hook his wrist through a strap at the side of the bed or use the edge of the mattress to pull himself completely over.

Method 4. (Fig. 3-13) The patient flexes his trunk to one side, using his head and elbows to lever himself over or by pulling on the edge of the bed. The arm on the extended side is swung in behind the back of his head. He reaches vigorously over his trunk with the other arm, thus gaining momentum to roll partially onto his side. He places the hand on the bed, and turns by using the friction of this hand on the bed to pull himself over the flexed arm.

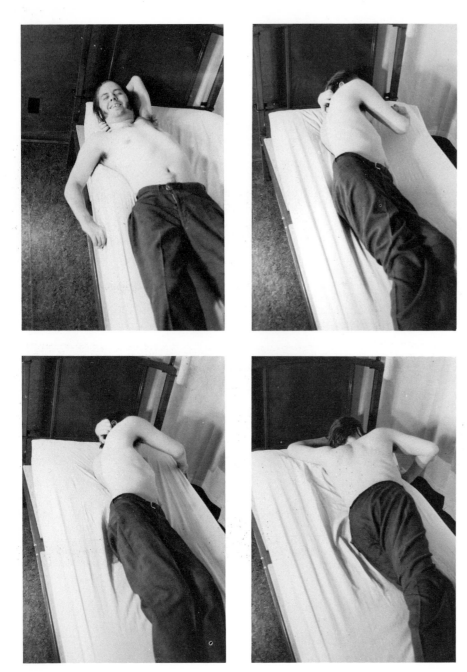

FIGURE 3-13

Prone to Supine, Right to Left (Fig. 3-14)

The patient flexes his trunk to the right. He places his right hand on the bed level with his shoulder, his elbow flexed at 90° above his hand. The left arm is placed under his head. As he pushes with the right hand on the bed, the left arm is worked further under his head until the left elbow points towards the right shoulder. In this position, he can maintain balance. By pushing with the left elbow and flinging the right arm backwards, he will roll over to his left. The patient may, when balanced on the elbow, reach with the right hand for the overhead strap to give additional leverage.

Basically all quadriplegics use this method to turn from prone to supine, although slight variation of hand, arm, and head positions might be noted.

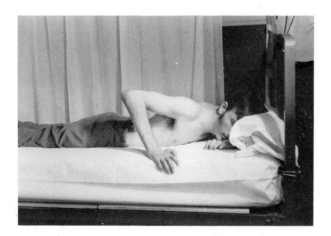 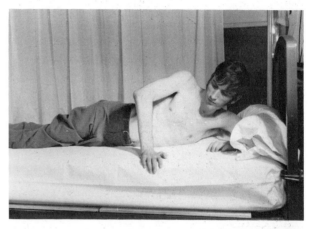

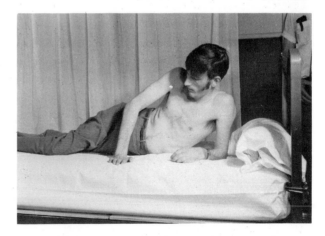

FIGURE 3-14

SITTING UP IN BED

Method 1. (Fig. 3-15) The patient slides his hands palm down under his buttocks and uses his wrist extensors, elbow flexors, and shoulder adductors and flexors to pull himself up onto his elbows. He now leans over one elbow and balances on it while flinging the other arm behind his buttocks and locking the elbow. He balances on the locked arm while flinging the other arm behind and locking it also.

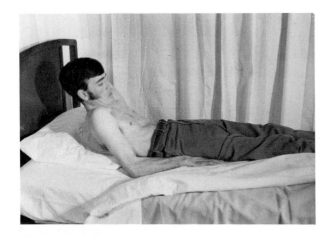

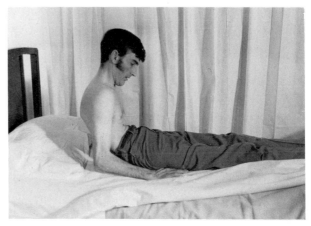

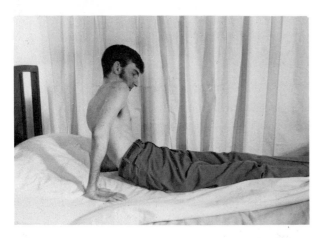

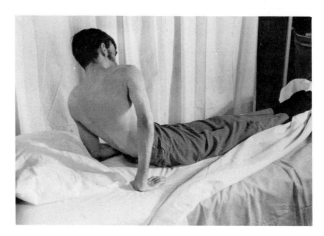

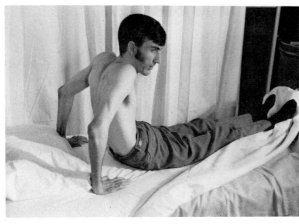

FIGURE 3-15

54

Method 2. (Fig. 3-16) The patient rolls to one side. He places his wrist in an overhead strap, which is just within his reach, and he pulls his head and shoulders off the bed. This allows him to throw his disengaged arm behind him and to lock the elbow. He now removes his arm from the sling and, balancing on the locked arm, he throws his other arm behind him and locks the elbow. By flexing his head and shoulders sharply, a bouncing motion is produced, giving him the opportunity to slide his hands forward on the bed until sitting balance is reached.

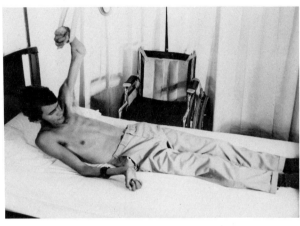
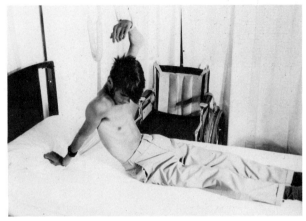

FIGURE 3-16

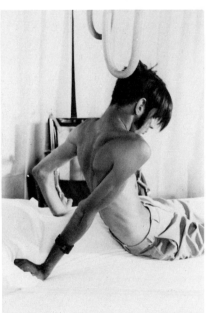
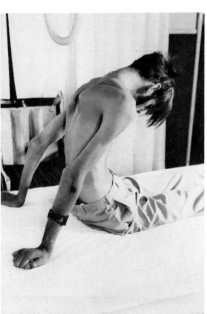

Method 3. (Fig. 3-17) The patient rolls to one side. He places his wrist in an overhead strap, which is just within his reach, and he pulls his head and shoulders off the bed. This allows him to throw his disengaged arm behind him and to lock the elbow. He now removes his arm from the sling and, balancing on the locked arm, he reaches for a fixed sling that has been placed in a more forward

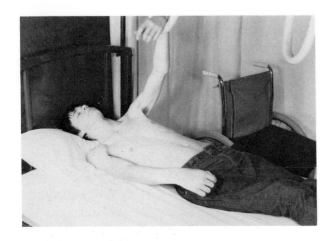
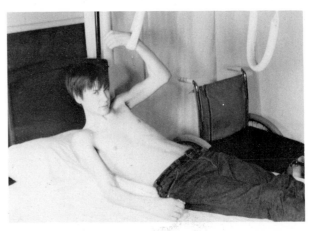
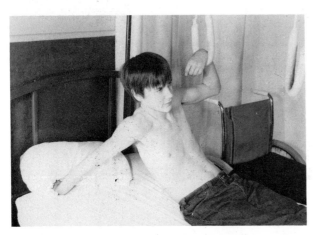
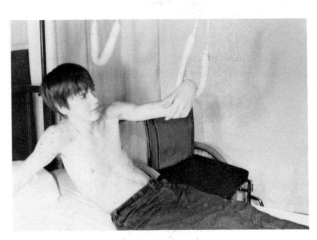
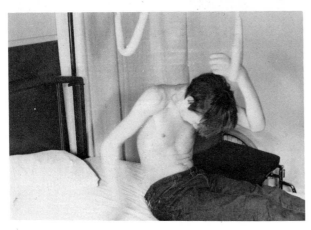

FIGURE 3-17

56

position. He now pulls himself to the upright position. His locked arm is then moved forward towards his buttock and his other arm may be removed from the sling.

Method 4. Two overhead bars are fixed, one at the head and one at the foot of the bed. A rope ladder is attached to the corners of these bars, thus giving maximum stability. The ladder is allowed to hang loosely so that the patient can just reach it (Fig. 3-18A). The smoothly padded rungs should be spaced as far apart as possible within the patient's reach. He reaches forward and hooks his wrist up behind the first rung (Fig. 3-18B). He pulls himself up as far as possible before reaching for the next rung with his other wrist. He repeats this until he reaches sitting balance.

FIGURE 3-18

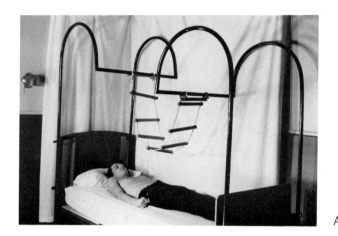

A

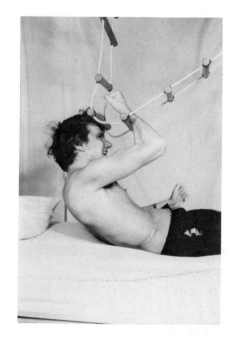

B

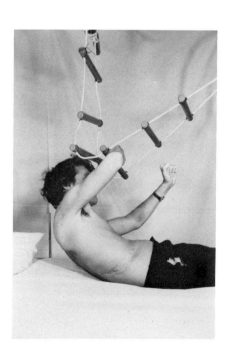

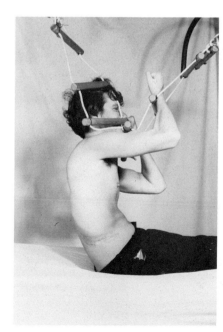

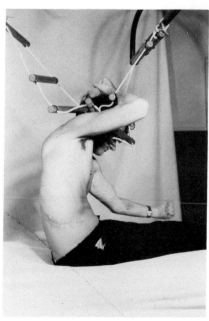

A more permanent arrangement can be made with two balkan beams placed about 8 inches in from the edges of the bed. Fixed and floating straps can be attached to these in the positions predetermined by the rope ladder (Fig. 3-19). This equipment is more stable than the ladder.

A strap may be fixed to the bed frame for insertion of the wrist, giving initial leverage so that an overhead sling may be reached (Fig. 3-20).

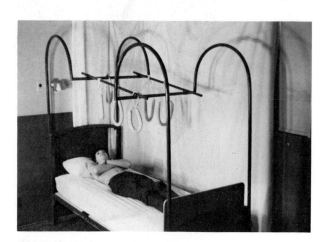

FIGURE 3-19

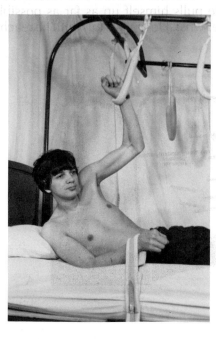

FIGURE 3-20

A bed with an electrically operated gatch may be required. The lever or micro-switch should be operated by the patient if possible (Fig. 3-21). There is psychological benefit in any independence that can be gained, even though by mechanical means.

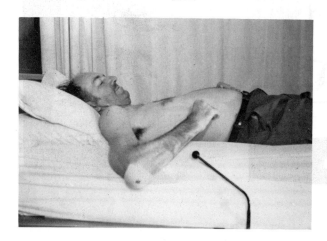

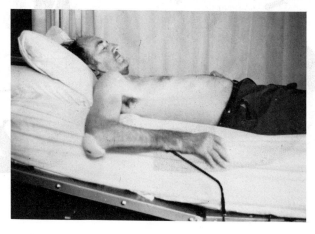

FIGURE 3-21

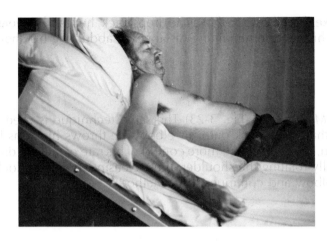 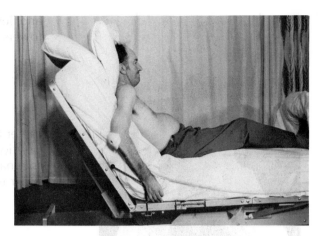

SITTING TO LYING

Method 1. (Fig. 3-22) The patient is in long sitting position with his hands on the bed at midthigh level and the elbows locked. He flexes his head, and pushes his trunk back to just beyond the point of balance. He quickly extends his shoulders

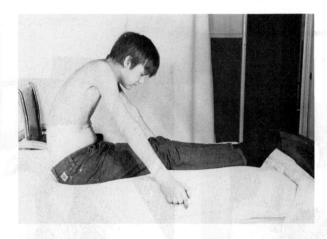 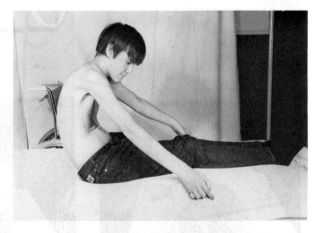

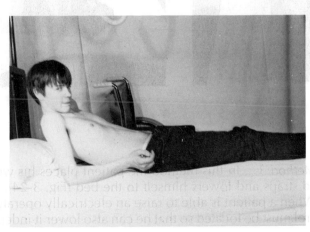 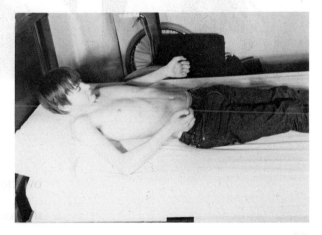

FIGURE 3-22

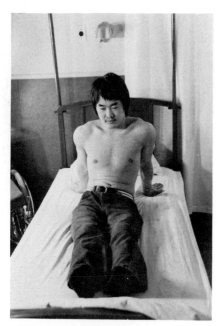

and flexes his elbows so that as he drops back, he rests his weight on his elbows. He lowers himself the remaining distance by abducting his shoulders.

Method 2. (Fig. 3-23) The same technique is used as in Method 1, but rather than drop back onto his elbows he throws his arms back into the locked position, thus giving him more control of his rate of fall. He drops onto an elbow by internally rotating the shoulder, thus releasing the elbow lock. He drops onto the other elbow and continues as in Method 1.

FIGURE 3-23

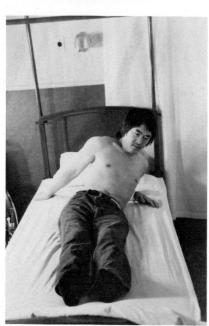 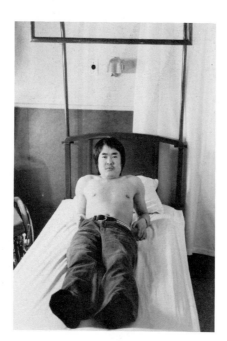 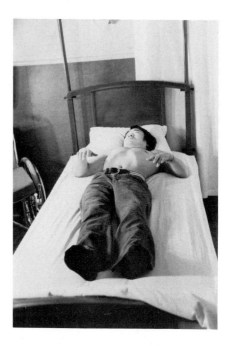

Method 3. In this method the patient places his wrists in suitably placed overhead straps and lowers himself to the bed (Fig. 3-24).

When a patient is able to raise an electrically operated head gatch himself, the control must be located so that he can also lower it independently (Fig. 3-25).

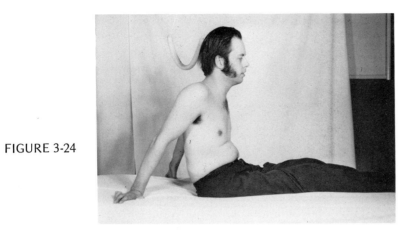

FIGURE 3-24

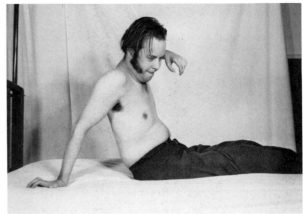

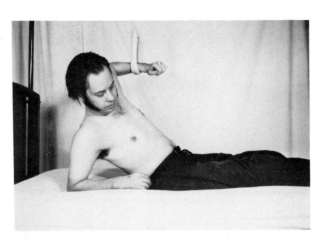

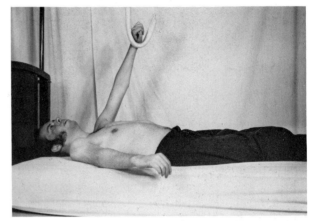

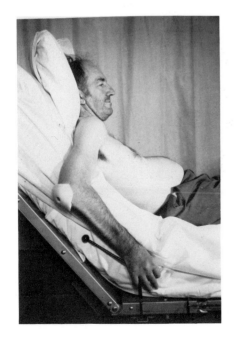

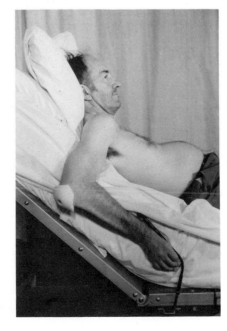

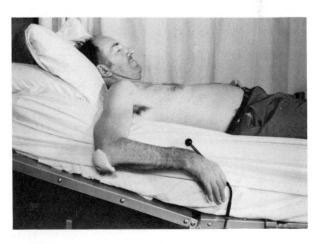

FIGURE 3-25

61

MOVING UP THE BED

Method 1. (Fig. 3-26) The patient sits with his arms locked and his hands on the bed at about midthigh level. As he flexes his head and shoulder sharply, his buttocks are lifted from the bed and moved back.

Method 2. (Fig. 3-27) The patient sits with his arms locked, hands on the bed well behind his buttocks. He moves up the bed by extending his upper trunk over his arms and adducting his shoulders. The patient places his hands further back before he reaches a point where he would lose his balance.

Method 3. For the patient who sits but requires an overhead strap for balance, a twisting method is used (Fig. 3-28). A wrist is placed in the strap, and the other hand is placed on the bed with the elbow locked. The patient leans over the locked arm, twisting his buttocks back and to one side. As he alternates the arm positions and repeats the action, his buttocks move further back and to the middle of the bed again.

FIGURE 3-26

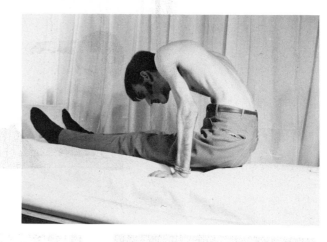

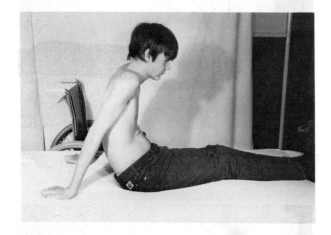

FIGURE 3-27

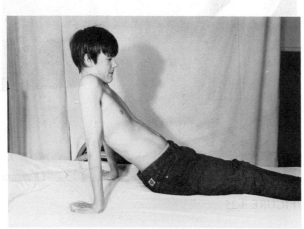

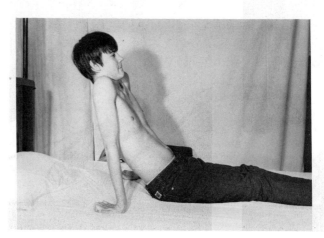

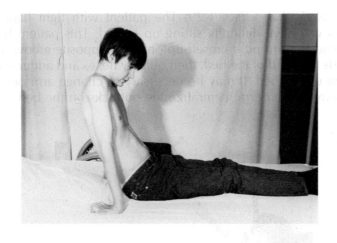
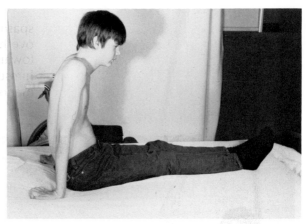

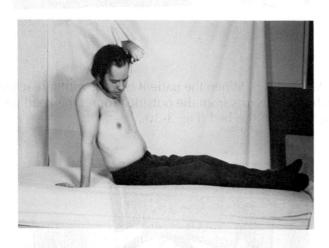
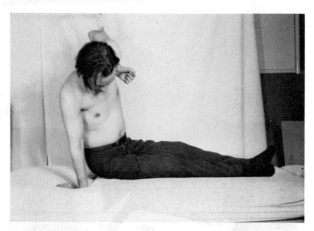

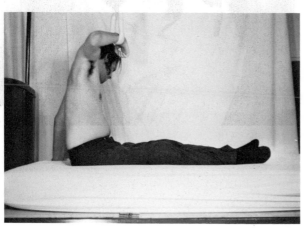
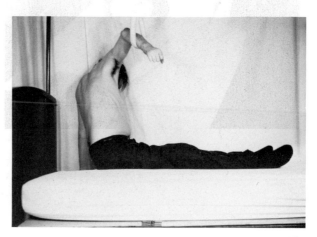

FIGURE 3-28

Method 4. (Fig. 3-29) The patient with tight hamstrings or interfering spasms will have difficulty sitting up in bed. This patient hooks an arm into an overhead strap to pull himself up onto the opposite elbow. He works this elbow towards the head of the bed, then quickly flexes and adducts the shoulder, pulling himself up the bed. It may be necessary to change arm positions and repeat the manoeuvre in order to centralize the buttocks on the bed.

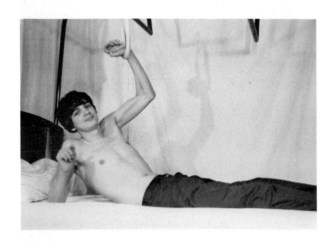 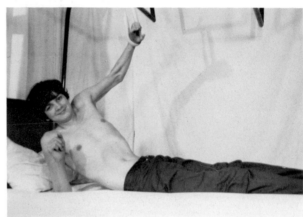

FIGURE 3-29

Method 5. When the patient is lying within reach of the head of the bed, he can hook his wrists from the outside around the head panel of the bed and, by pulling, move up the bed (Fig. 3-30).

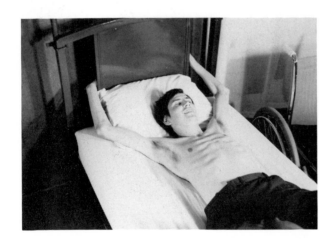 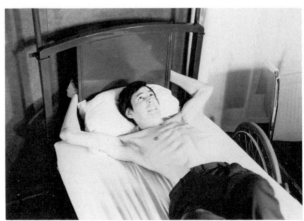

FIGURE 3-30

64

Method 6.   Cribsides or ladders can be used on either or both sides of the bed. After hooking the wrists around the rungs from the outside as far up the bed as possible, the patient will pull himself up the bed (Fig. 3-31). Extremely weak quadriplegics can be taught this method.

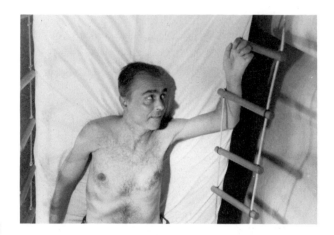
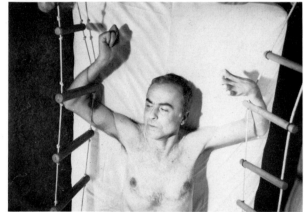
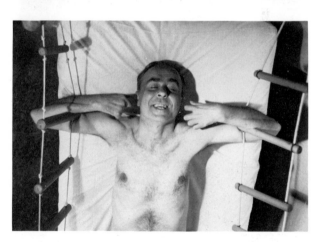

FIGURE 3-31

MOVING DOWN THE BED

Method 1.   (Fig. 3-32) The patient sits with elbows locked and his hands on the bed at midthigh level. He flexes his trunk forward as far as possible and he briskly extends his upper trunk and neck while remaining in the forward position. The resulting bouncing action raises his buttocks and moves him forward.

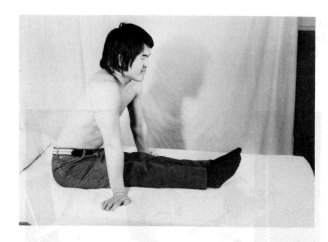

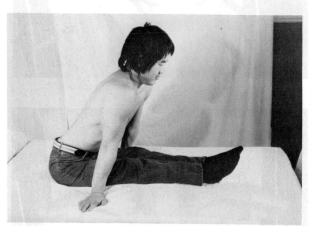

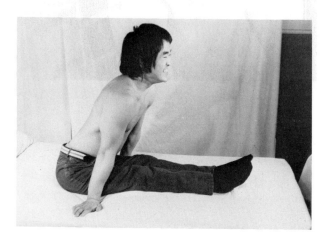

FIGURE 3-32

Method 2. (Fig. 3-33) The patient sits with his arms locked, hands on the bed slightly behind his buttocks. A wriggling motion is produced by extending his upper trunk over his arms and extending his shoulders alternately. Along with this motion the patient leans first on one arm, then the other, thus taking the weight off the buttocks alternately. This will result in the patient sliding down the bed.

Method 3. For the patient who can sit but requires an overhead strap for balance, a twisting method is used (Fig. 3-34). With one wrist in a strap, placed as far forward as possible, he puts the other hand on the bed close to his buttock and locks the elbow. Pulling himself up by the strap, he relieves some of the weight from his buttocks. He depresses and externally rotates the shoulder of the locked arm, producing a pushing motion. The combination of this push on the bed and pull on the strap will move him down the bed.

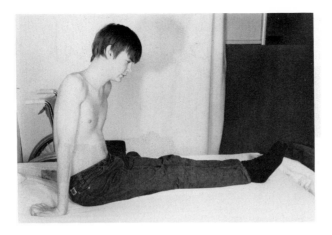
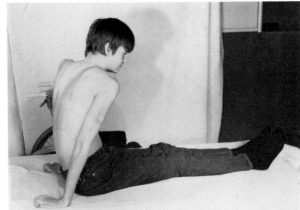

FIGURE 3-33

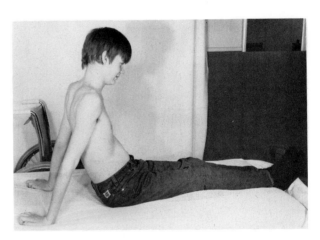

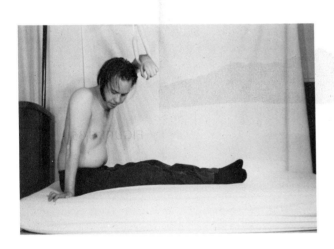

FIGURE 3-34

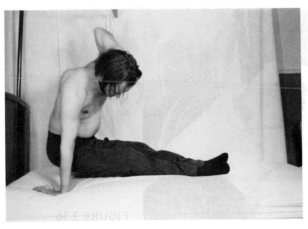
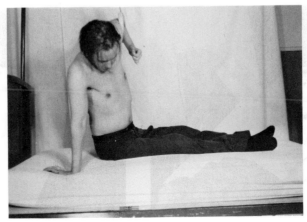

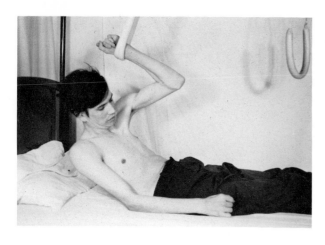
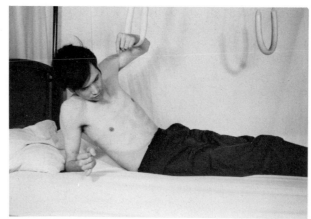
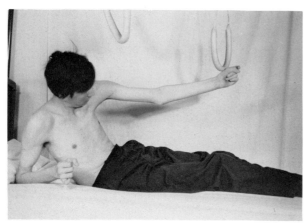
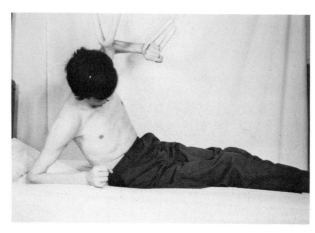

FIGURE 3-35

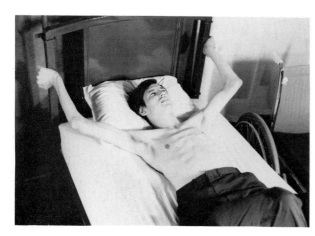
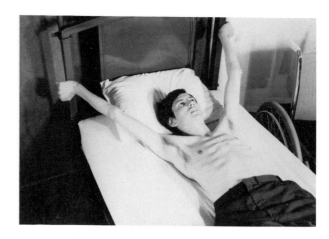

FIGURE 3-36

Method 4. (Fig. 3-35) The patient with tight hamstrings or interfering spasms may not be able to sit up in bed. This patient hooks his arm into an overhead strap, pulling himself onto the opposite elbow. While balancing on the elbow, he reaches for another overhead strap further forward. He moves his elbow as far forward as possible keeping it close to his body. He slides down the bed by pulling with the arm in the strap and extending the other shoulder.

Method 5. When the patient is lying within reach of the head of the bed, he can place the palms of his hands against the head panel in line with his shoulders. He will slide down the bed by pushing (Fig. 3-36). This is a functional push developed through the shoulder girdle, not by active extension of the elbow.

Method 6. The patient with restricted hip flexion may use an overhead rope ladder (Fig. 3-37). When the patient pulls on the ladder, he only partially raises his trunk. Therefore, further pulling will slide him down the bed.

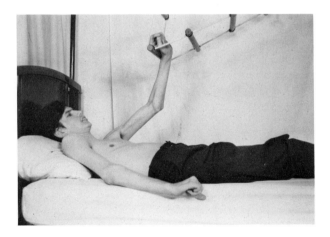

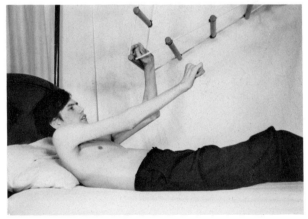

FIGURE 3-37

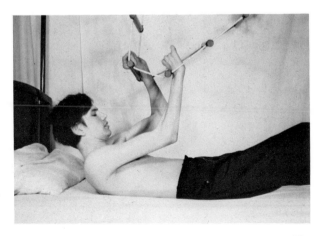

Method 7. Cribsides or rope ladders may be used by a very weak patient. The ladders provide a better angle of pull, because they move close to the patient's trunk as he flexes his elbows (Fig. 3-38).

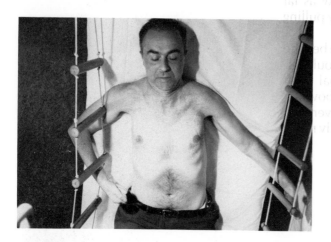
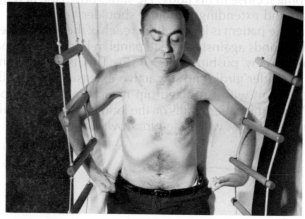
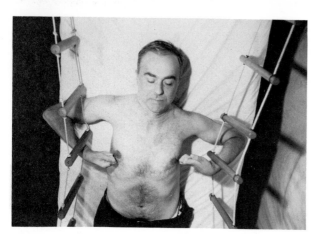
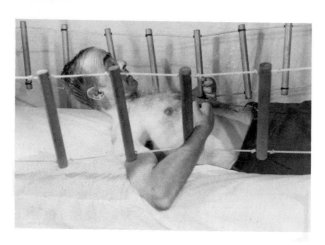

FIGURE 3-38

MOVING ACROSS THE BED

Method 1. (Fig. 3-39) The patient sits with one arm in an overhead strap and pulls strongly to raise his buttocks clear of the bed. He places the other hand on the bed and pushes to swing his buttocks over. He now moves his feet across the bed to straighten himself.

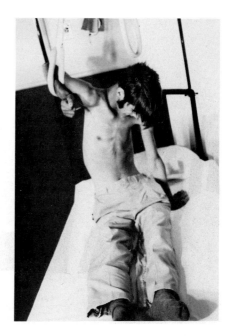

FIGURE 3-39

Method 2. The patient who moves up or down the bed by using locked arms, hands on the bed, will use the same method for moving across the bed (Fig. 3-40). One hand is placed about a foot away from the body and the patient leans over this arm, permitting his other hand to be placed on the bed under the buttock. The patient then does a push up and his body swings from the near to the far arm. He must now move his feet across and, if necessary, repeat the whole action.

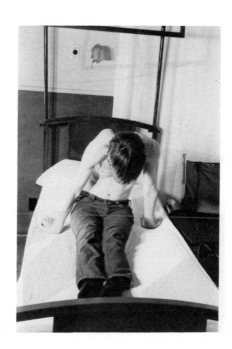 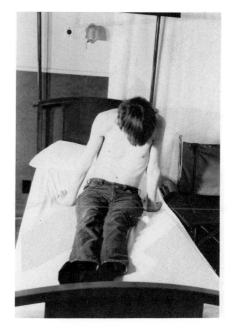

FIGURE 3-40

71

Method 3. (Fig. 3-41) Instead of swinging between his locked arms, the patient may twist his trunk and place both hands on the bed on one side. Throwing his weight over his locked arms, he will push his buttocks away.

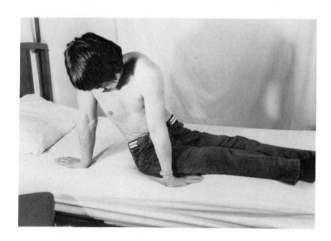 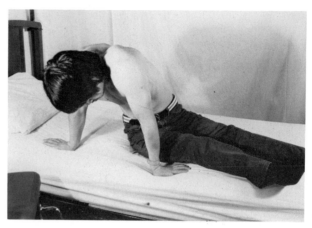

FIGURE 3-41

Method 4. (Fig. 3-42) The patient places a wrist in an overhead strap, slightly forward of and in line with the opposite shoulder. The other elbow is locked with a hand on the bed close to the buttock. A pull on the strap, together with a push on the bed, will move the buttocks over.

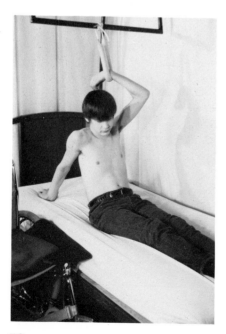 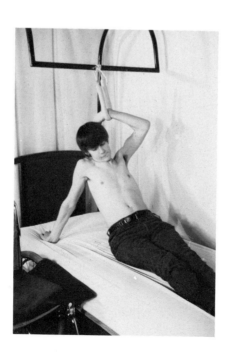

FIGURE 3-42

Method 5. (Fig. 3-43) The patient, who is unable to sit up, lies on his side and pulls himself onto an elbow using an overhead strap. By pushing away with the elbow and pulling on the strap, he moves his buttocks over and down the bed. The amount of flexion of his trunk determines his direction of travel. The greatest sideways travel occurs when the patient is most flexed.

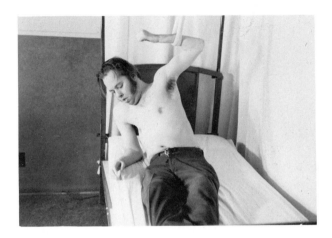 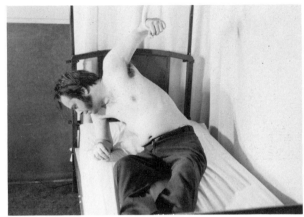

FIGURE 3-43

TRANSFERRING

BRIDGE BOARDS

Bridge boards are usually necessary to facilitate transfer from chair to bed, toilet, shower, bath, or car. Whatever design is used, it should be suitable for as many transfer situations as possible except transfer to car. A different design is used for the latter. An unpadded board may be used only by patients with good skin tone and muscle bulk. A 3/16 inch tempered hardboard is strong and develops a highly polished surface when rubbed with talcum powder. The corners must be rounded, bevelled, and well sanded. Patients who are prone to skin breakdowns should be provided with boards which are padded and nylon covered (See Appendix).

Placing It in Position

Method 1. (Fig. 3-44) The patient slides forward in the chair and removes the chair arm. He places the board on the bed and pulls it under the buttock as far as possible using his wrist over the far side of the board. He then hooks the arm furthest from the bed over the chair arm, and raises the near buttock by pulling his trunk away from the bed. He may now pull the board further under him.

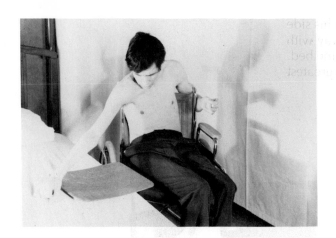
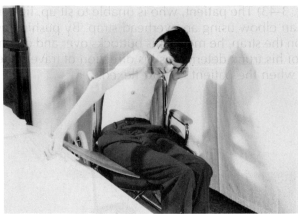

FIGURE 3-44

Method 2. (Fig. 3-45) The patient rests one end of the board on the bed and the other end just on his thigh. By pulling his trunk away from the bed using both arms over the outer chair arm, the board will fall into place as his buttock is raised. Methods 1 and 2 can be used with legs up or down.

Method 3. (Fig. 3-46) The padded board must be placed in position before the legs are lifted onto the bed either before or after sliding forward in the chair. The post on the underside of the board is placed in the arm rest socket and the wheel recess is placed over the wheel. This board leaves no gap between bed and chair and increases the size of the sliding area. (See Appendix for construction and plans.)

FIGURE 3-45

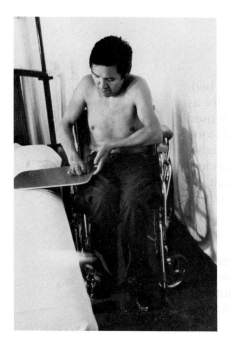
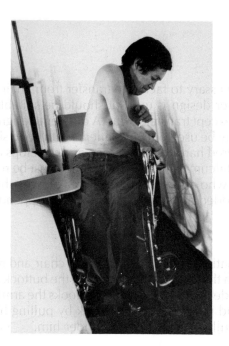
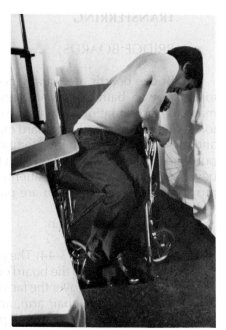

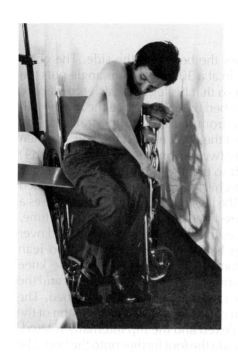

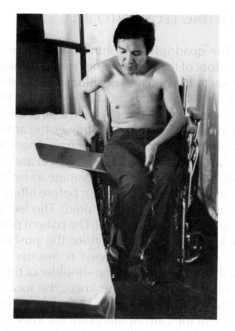

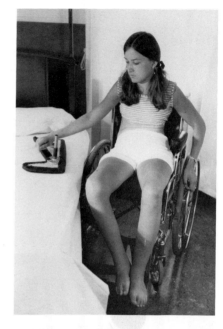

FIGURE 3-46

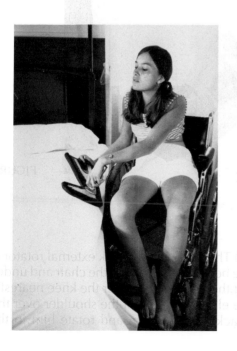

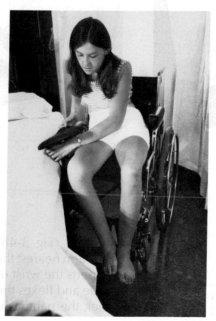

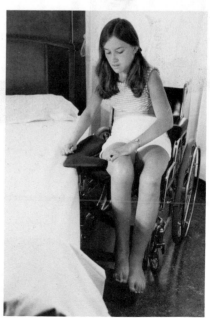

LIFTING LEGS ONTO BED

The quadriplegic commonly approaches the bed from the side. The chair faces the foot of the bed and the front is turned in at a 30° angle. This angle puts the seat closer to the bed and positions the patient so that his legs are easier to lift onto the bed. The wheelchair must be secured to the bed by a hook since the brakes will not stop the front of the chair swinging away from the bed during transfer. The patient locks the brakes and removes the arm of the chair nearest the bed. He then shifts his buttocks forward in the chair. There are two reasons for the manoeuvre: (1) so that the buttocks will clear the wheel and (2) so that the patient has room to rock his trunk back, giving added leverage as he lifts his legs onto the bed. The padded bridge board must be in position before lifting the legs onto the bed. In most cases a leg retainer board will be required. The feet are lifted onto the bed one at a time.

Method 1. (Fig. 3-47) The patient places the arm furthest from the bed over the back of the chair and under the pushing handle. This enables him to lean forward safely. The other wrist is inserted from the lateral side under the knee nearest the bed. By flexing the shoulder of the arm over the back of the chair and the elbow of the arm under the knee, the foot is raised to the level of the bed. The foot is levered onto the bed by external rotation of the shoulder and extension of the wrist against the calf. At this point the knee is flexed and the hip internally rotated; pressure on the knee will extend the knee and slide the foot further onto the bed. The other leg is raised in a similar manner except that the wrist is inserted from the medial side of the knee. When the foot is on the bed, the hip is externally rotated before pressure is applied to extend the knee.

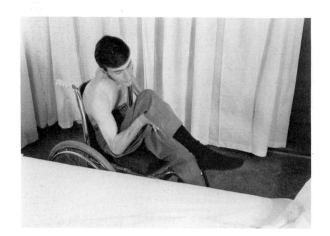 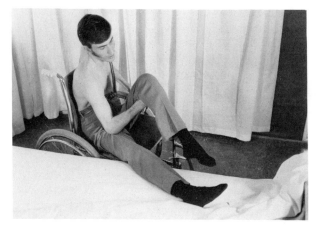

FIGURE 3-47

Method 2. (Fig. 3-48) The patient with weak external rotators of the shoulders places the arm nearest the bed over the back of the chair and under the pushing handle. He inserts the wrist of the other hand under the knee nearest the bed from the medial side and flexes the elbow. Flexion of the shoulder over the back of the chair will rock the patient back, raise his leg, and rotate him in the chair, thus moving his leg towards the bed. Protraction and flexion of both shoulders in a hugging action will swing the foot onto the bed. The knee is straightened as in Method 1. The other leg is raised in a similar manner except that the wrist is inserted from the lateral side of the knee.

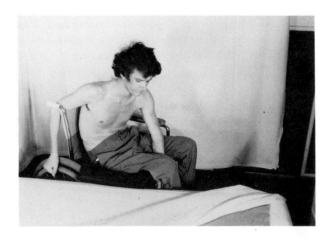
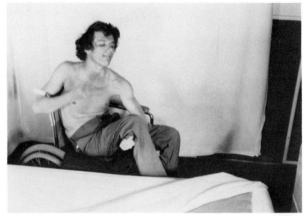
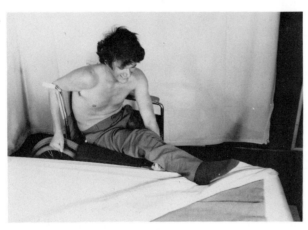
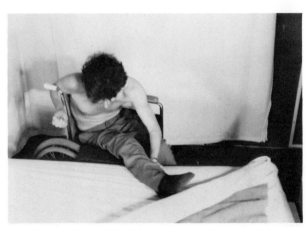

FIGURE 3-48

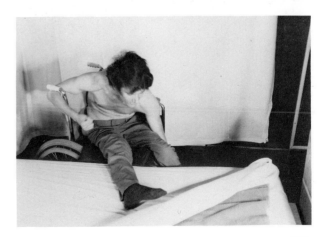

Method 3. The patient may use a loop of rope or webbing to swing his legs to the bed (Fig. 3-49). In this case the foot is moved forward on the footrest so that the instep is free. This is done by raising the foot partially and swinging it forward by extending the wrist against the calf. The patient sits with the arm nearest the bed over the back of the chair and the elbow flexed around the pushing handle. He inserts his other wrist into the loop of webbing and flexes his trunk forward as far as possible to place the loop of the strap over his forefoot. The loop should be as short as possible to allow the greatest lift. The forearm rests on the thigh with the hand on the medial side of the leg so that leverage can be obtained by using the thigh as a fulcrum to extend the knee. The hip is internally rotated permitting the foot to swing over onto the bed. Knee extension and hip rotation occur simultaneously as the patient rocks back using both shoulder flexors and protractors. (Leg position is determined by placing the hand on one or the other side of the knee.)

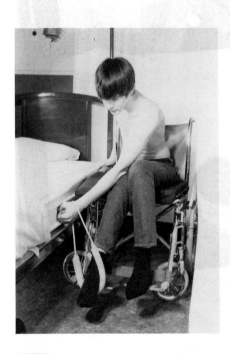 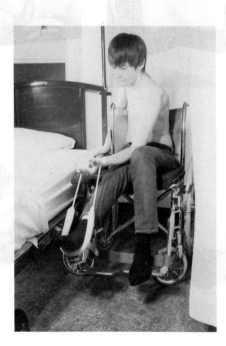 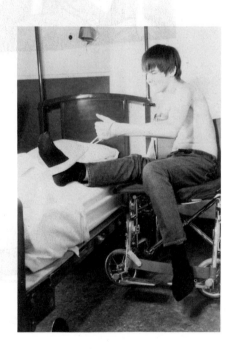

FIGURE 3-49

A figure-of-eight wire-core rope may be necessary to train the patient who cannot lean forward far enough to control the loop (Fig. 3-50).

Method 4. The patient may use a pulley that is attached to a balkan beam at the point above the bed where the foot is to be placed (Fig. 3-51). A rope is sheaved through the pulley and a loop formed at one end to pass over the forefoot. A loop, large enough to enable the patient to insert his wrist is tied at the other end as close to the pulley as possible. As many other loops as are necessary are tied in this tail end of the rope. These merely enable the patient to pull the loop nearest the pulley within reach and so keep the rope taut. A strong pull should elevate the leg and carry it onto the bed.

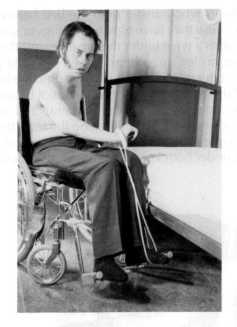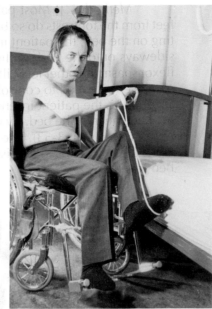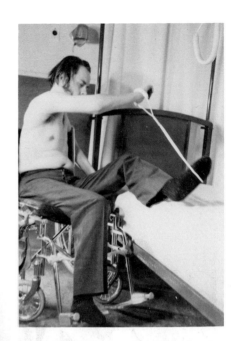

FIGURE 3-50

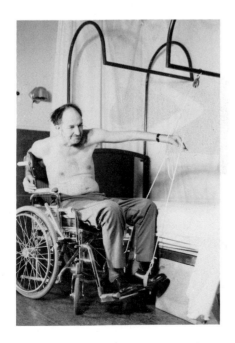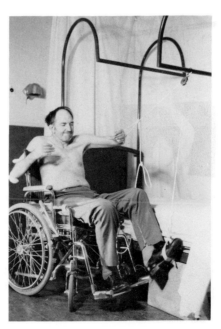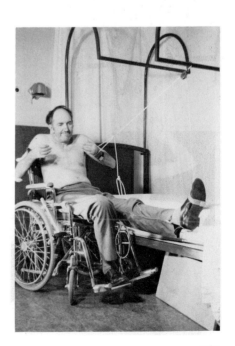

FIGURE 3-51

Method 5. Most patients who transfer onto the bed before moving their feet from the footrests do so because they have tight hamstrings or spasm. When sitting on the bed, the patient inserts a wrist under the knee nearest the bed and rolls sideways onto the bed, pulling his leg up as he rolls (Fig. 3-52). In a patient with flexor spasm the other leg will frequently follow the first leg onto the bed; the patient can be encouraged to control this spasm. When spasm cannot be used to raise the second leg, the patient inserts one wrist in the overhead strap and the other under the knee nearest the bed. By rocking back and pulling on the strap the leg is placed onto the bed (Fig. 3-53). The same procedure is used for the second leg. Some patients are able to insert a wrist under both knees, thereby pulling both legs onto the bed together.

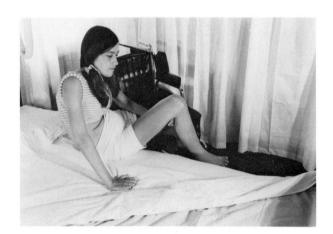
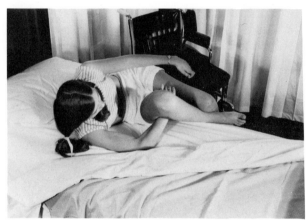

FIGURE 3-52

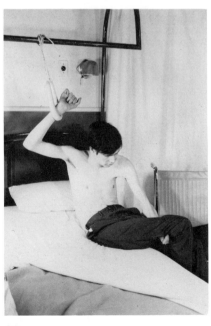
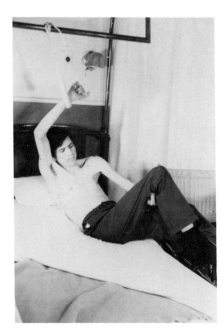
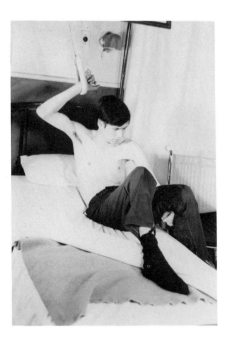

FIGURE 3-53

WHEELCHAIR TO BED TRANSFER

When it is stated in this section that a side approach is used, it indicates that the patient places his chair at a 30° angle to the bed, facing the foot of the bed with his shoulders just behind the level of the overhead bar. When it is stated that the patient prepares to transfer, it signifies these steps: he hooks his chair to the bed, applies his brakes, slides his buttocks forward in the chair, removes the arm rest on the exit side of the chair, and places his bridge board if necessary. The necessity for complete stability of the chair cannot be overemphasized.

Method 1. The patient with a low cervical lesion and excellent balance may accomplish transfer without the use of overhead bars. He uses a side approach and prepares to transfer with his feet on the footrests (Fig. 3-54). He places one hand on the bed and the other close to his buttock, then locks both elbows. He leans forward until he reaches his point of balance, then depresses his shoulder girdle and flexes his shoulders. He swings his buttocks across by abducting and externally rotating the far shoulder while adducting and internally rotating the near shoulder. To gain added momentum and lift, he flexes his neck and turns his head away from the bed. At first he may move only a short distance, in which case a bridge board will be necessary. The bridge board will not be necessary as he gains facility so that one movement takes him over to the bed.

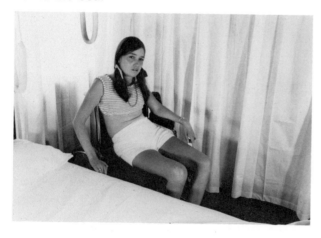
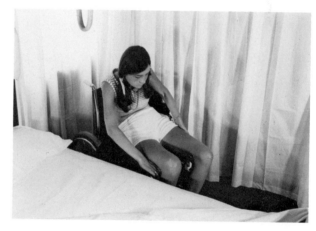
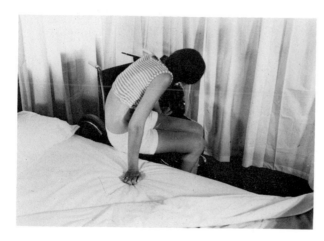
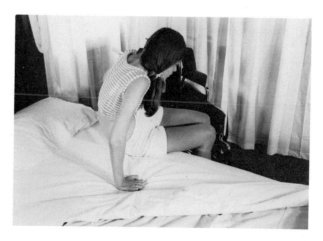

FIGURE 3-54

The more flaccid patient may place his legs on the bed first (Fig. 3-55).

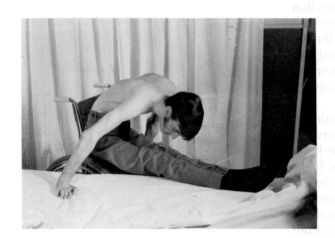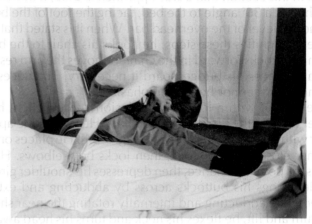

FIGURE 3-55

Method 2. (Fig. 3-56) The patient prepares to transfer using the side approach, in this case from the left of the bed. He places a small cushion in the gap between wheelchair and bed and over the wheel. He now places his right leg on the bed. He picks up the left leg and places the heel over the knee of the right leg. When pressure is exerted on the left knee, it will straighten with the legs crossed. The patient now abducts the left arm and adducts the right arm across his chest at shoulder level. He then swings both arms rapidly across, turning his head, shoulders and upper trunk towards the head of the bed. As he rolls into bed he drops onto his right elbow. The left shoulder is flexed above his head so that his head rests on his forearm. He is now in position to roll over onto his back, using the momentum gained from rolling out of the chair.

Method 3. The patient, who can move on the bed in long sitting by locking his elbows and doing a pushup to shift his buttocks, can use the following method to transfer from wheelchair to bed (Fig. 3-57). He faces the middle of the bed and locks his chair about a foot away from the side of the bed. This leaves room for him to put his feet on the bed and swing his foot rests away. He unlocks his brakes and wheels his chair forward until the chair seat is against the mattress. Automatic spring locks will secure the wheelchair to the bed frame (see Appendix). He slides his buttocks forward in the wheelchair and then leans forward and locks his elbows. He shifts his buttocks forward until he is almost on the bed before levering his legs over towards the foot of the bed. He now shifts sideways to the centre of the bed and levers his legs over again if necessary.

82

FIGURE 3-56

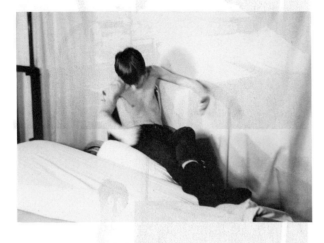
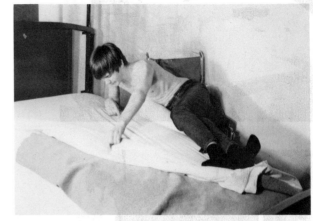
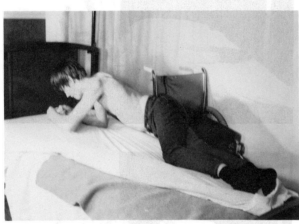
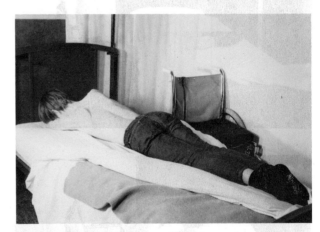
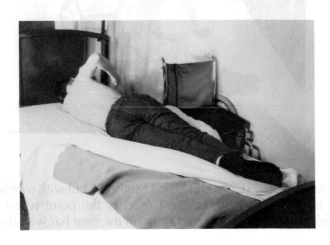
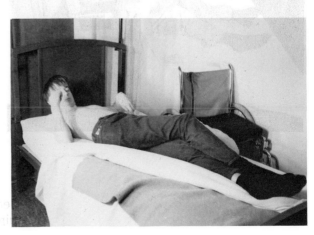

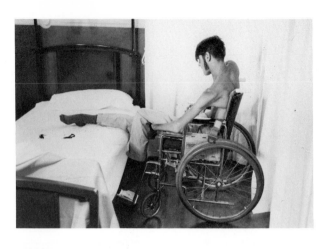
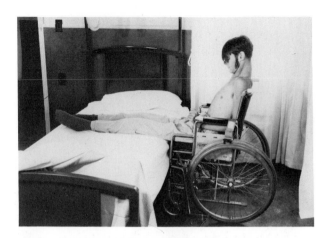
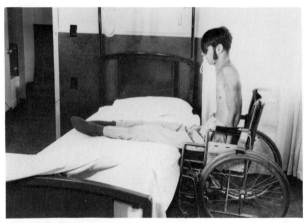
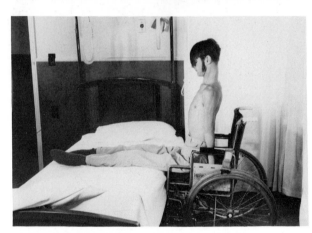
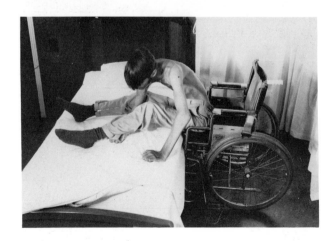
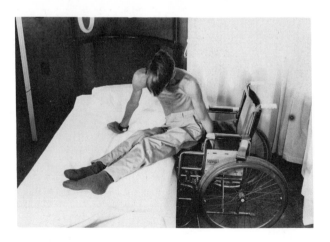

FIGURE 3-57

Method 4. (Fig. 3-58) Using Method 3 but with overhead bars as described earlier in this chapter, the patient reaches the point where a pushup would be required. He reaches for a fixed strap on the near bar with the arm nearest the foot of the bed. He levers his feet towards the foot of the bed, using the free arm. He now reaches for a fixed strap on the far bar with his free arm, and pulls up with both arms, lifting his buttocks up and over onto the bed.

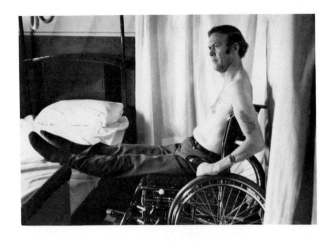

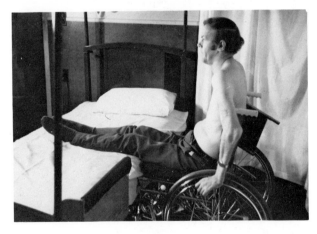

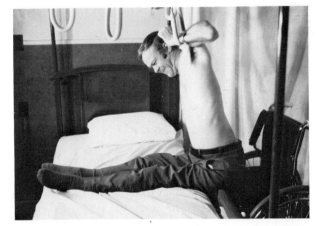

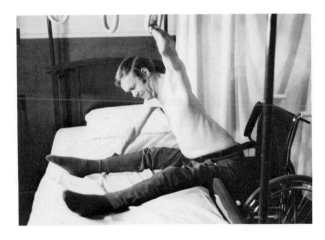

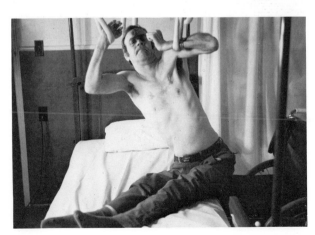

FIGURE 3-58

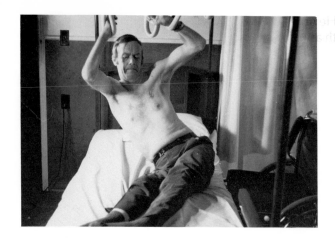
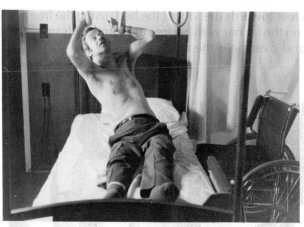

Method 5. (Fig. 3-59) The patient prepares to transfer, using the side approach, and places his legs on the bed. He uses one overhead bar with one floating strap adjusted so that he can insert his wrist into it when sitting. He puts the

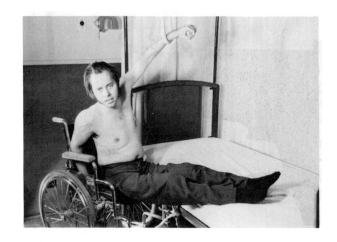
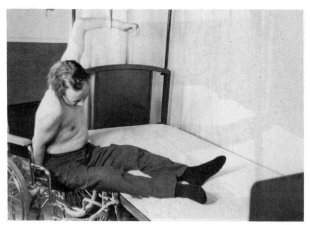

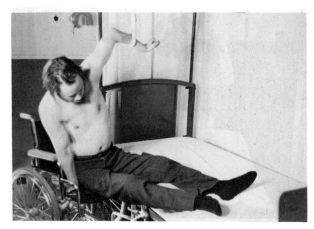
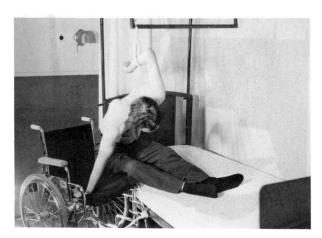

FIGURE 3-59

arm nearest the bed through the strap. The other hand, wrist extended, can be placed against the far tire behind the chair back, or against the arm of the chair. The patient then leans his trunk away from the bed to gain the fullest mechanical advantage. By strongly contracting his elbow flexors and shoulder adductors bilaterally, he will develop a pushing action with his hand on the wheelchair and a pulling action with his arm in the strap. This will move him from the chair to the edge of the bed. At this stage, he must move the floating strap further away from himself along the bar. His other hand is moved to either the seat of the chair or the wheel nearest the bed. A repetition of the bilateral pull will place him well on the bed.

Method 6. (Fig. 3-60) The patient uses the same equipment and the same method for initiating the move as in Method 5. He reaches the edge of the bed and places the arm furthest from the bed in the strap. He places the other hand on the bed with the wrist extended, while he moves the strap further over. He rolls himself by pulling on the strap, dropping onto his elbow, and twisting his body towards the bed. He is now on the bed in side lying and can remove his arm from the strap.

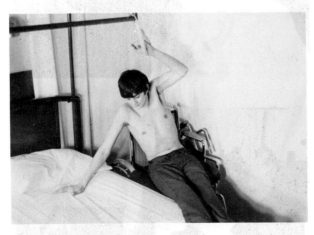
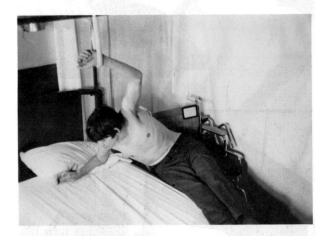
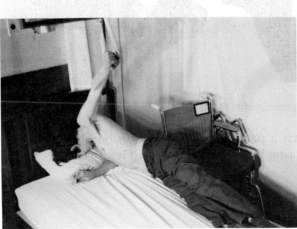
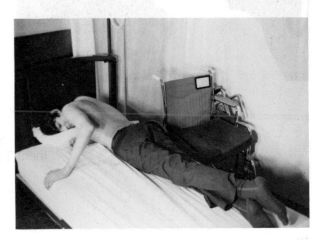

FIGURE 3-60

Method 7. The patient who uses a side approach and is unable to make use of trunk torsion because of flaccidity, uses an overhead bar with several fixed straps at intervals along the bar (Fig. 3-61). He prepares for transfer in the usual way and places his feet on the bed but, instead of leaning away from the bed, he leans towards it. He gains no mechanical advantage from this position and must rely solely upon muscle strength. He inserts the wrist nearest the bed into the second strap to pull his trunk over. This enables him to reach the first strap with the other arm. He pulls himself as far as possible towards the bed. He now moves his wrists into straps further along the bar to give him fresh purchase to pull and so continues until he is on the bed.

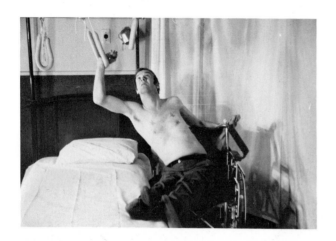
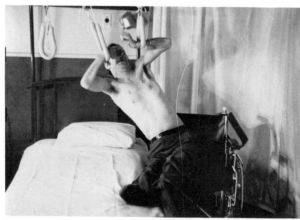
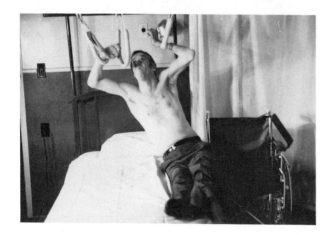
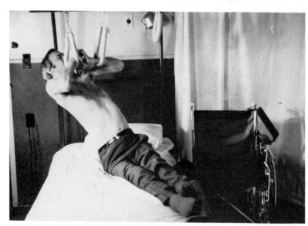

FIGURE 3-61

Such a patient may require the outrigger (described in "Bed and Equipment") during the learning process (Fig. 3-62).

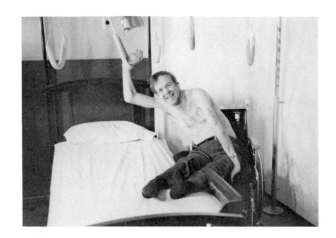 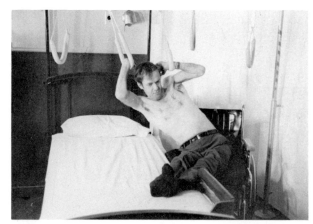

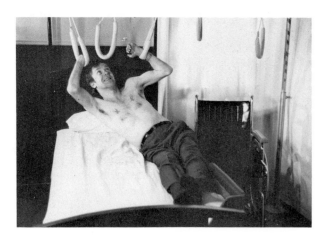 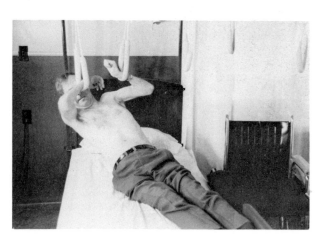

FIGURE 3-62

Method 8.   A practical and permanent method of transfer can be accomplished through the back of the chair with the chair positioned at the foot of the bed. This method is very useful as a demonstration to the patient of his ability to move independently. It is also useful as a strengthening exercise to enable the patient to use another transfer method utilizing less equipment at a later date. For this method of transfer three overhead bars are required (Fig. 3-63A), one at the head of the bed and two at the foot facing in opposite directions. In the place of the footboard, a special end is made to support the two overhead bars and permit entry. A box is made and padded with 1 inch foam rubber and is nylon covered. This fills the gap at the end of the mattress and projects to the seat of the chair (Fig. 3-63B). Two eye bolts are fastened to the uprights of the overhead bars at the level of the wheelchair arms. Hooks are made out of 3/16 inch welding rod. These hooks are hung from the eyebolts and are dropped into holes drilled in the top back of the wheelchair arms; these hooks lock the chair to the bed. The chair must be equipped with a detachable back. A horizontal rope ladder is fastened to the foot and head at each side of the bed. The bottom of these ladders should be about 4 inches above the mattress to permit the patient to place his wrists underneath. The rungs should be about 10 inches apart, although this distance may have to be modified. Another rope ladder is attached to the bar that projects over the chair. The other end is tied to the other bar at the foot and is looped downwards so that the patient can reach it when lying.

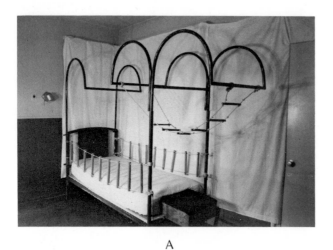

A

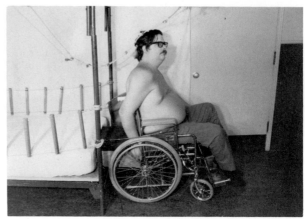

FIGURE 3-63

B

To transfer (Fig. 3-64), the patient first locks the chair in position and removes the back. He then lowers his trunk to the bed, usually using the rope ladder looped at the foot of the bed. The patient reaches up the bed to put a wrist under each ladder and behind a rung. By adducting his shoulder and flexing his elbows, he will move up the bed. This process is repeated until he reaches the desired position. When the patient is learning this process, he will be greatly assisted if his knees are extended for him.

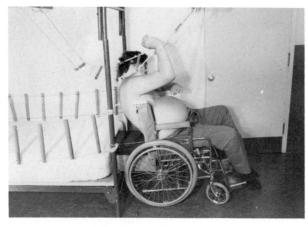

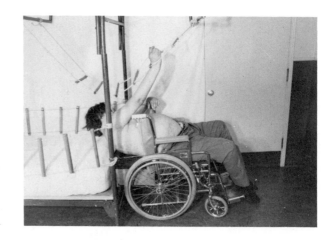

FIGURE 3-64

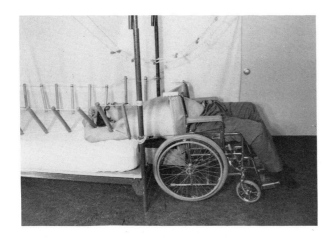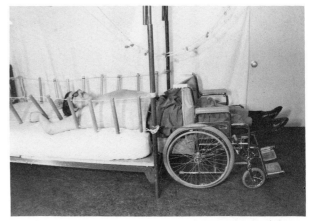

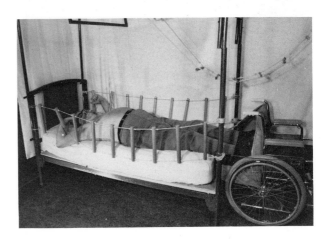

The patient reverses the process to get out of bed (Fig. 3-65), reaching down as far as possible and pulling on the ladder rungs. When his feet are on the footrests of the chair, he reaches for the overhead ladder and pulls himself to the sitting position. The chair back is fastened and the locks are removed.

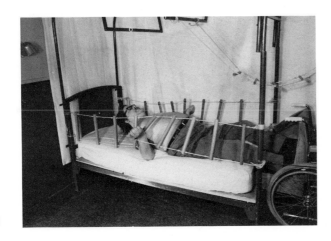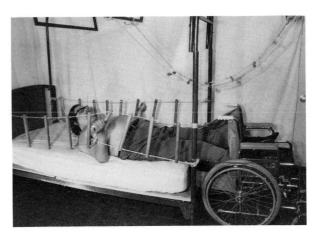

FIGURE 3-65

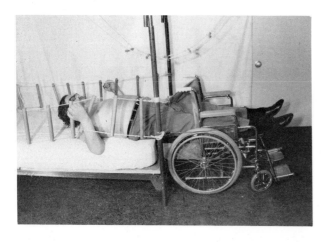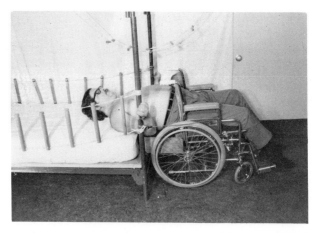

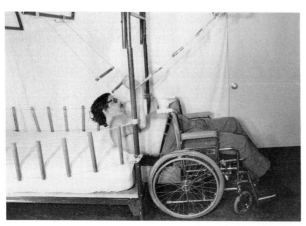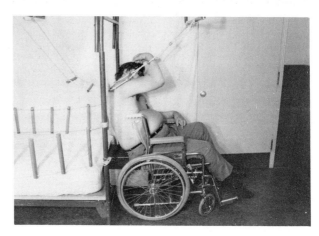

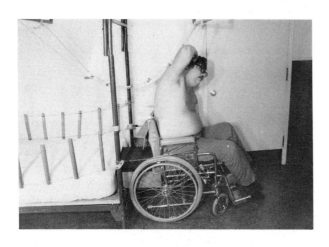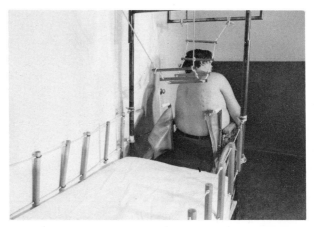

LOWERING FEET TO FOOTRESTS FROM BED

If the patient has tight hamstrings, he will have to put his legs down onto the footrests before transferring from bed to chair. Many patients without tight hamstrings manage better also with legs down. There are several methods of moving the legs from the bed. The patient must first be taught the correct position of his body in relation to the chair, so that his feet will make contact with the footrests each time.

Method 1. (Fig. 3-66) The patient with flaccid lower extremities, sits up and hooks the wrist furthest from the chair into an overhead strap. He then leans forward, placing his wrist under the knee nearest the chair. He inserts the wrist from the lateral side of the leg. Pulling bilaterally he will rock to the upright position, bringing the knee up to his chest. By outwardly rotating his shoulders, he will place the foot over the edge of the bed, then lower it to the footrest. The other leg is lowered, using the same method except that the wrist is inserted from the medial side of the leg.

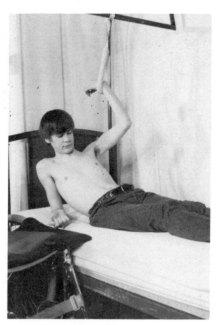

FIGURE 3-66

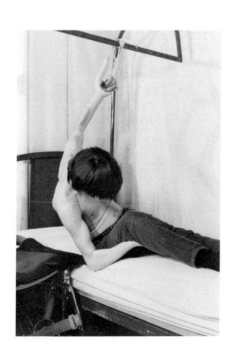
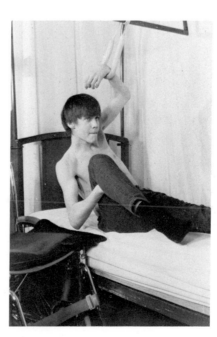
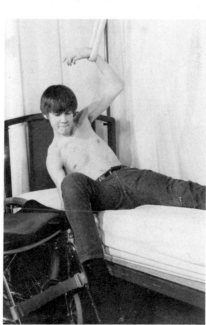

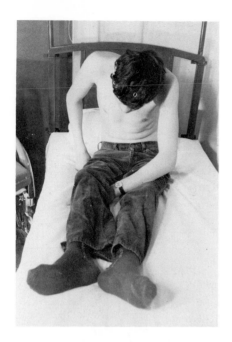

Method 2. (Fig. 3-67) From the long sitting position, the patient leans forward. He maintains balance by using an overhead strap for one arm, by resting on one elbow, or by relying on the normal tension of his hip extensors to hold his position. By inserting a hand under a leg and raising his elbow, the lever action will move his leg over until the heel slides off the bed and to the footrest. Alternatively a bridge board may be used as a lever. The board is slipped under the leg and raised by inserting a wrist under it. The leg will slide down the board.

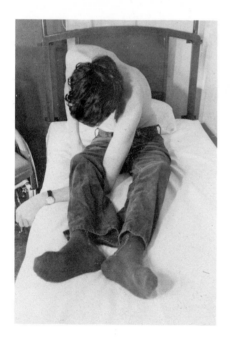
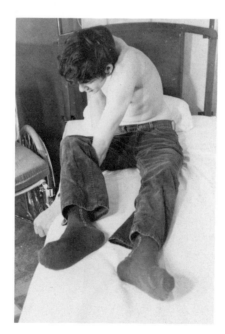
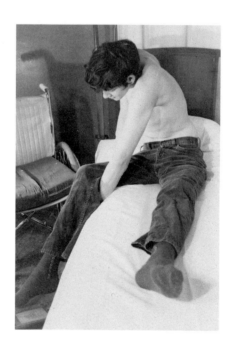

FIGURE 3-67

Method 3. (Fig. 3-68) Leaning away from the chair on one elbow, the patient reaches down and hooks his wrist behind his knee. He pulls his knee up as far as possible so that he will be able to pull his foot towards his buttocks. He then pushes on the knee, extending the leg. This may have to be repeated to move the leg over the edge of the bed. The other leg is managed similarly.

94

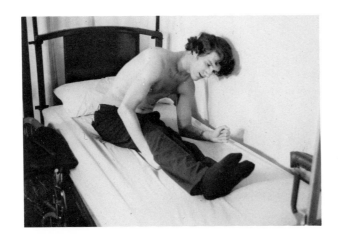
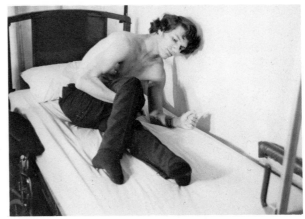

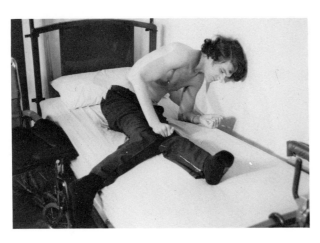
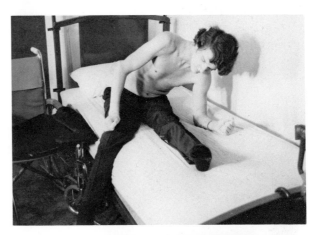

FIGURE 3-68

Method 4. (Fig. 3-69) The patient with some rigidity of trunk and hip may side flex his trunk away from his chair so that his legs will swivel towards the footrests.

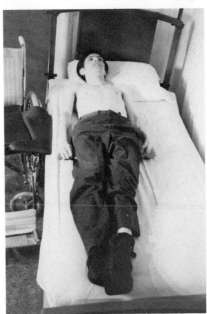

FIGURE 3-69

95

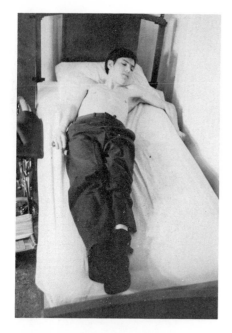
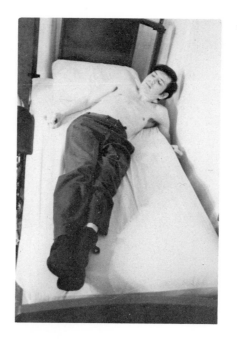
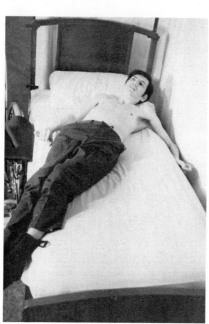
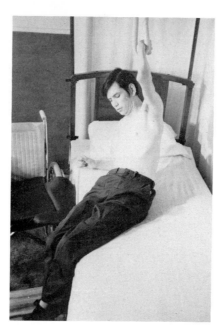

BED TO CHAIR TRANSFER

The patient is in long sitting at the side of the bed, forward of the rear wheels of the chair. If a bridge board is used, it is positioned at this time. The feet may be lowered to the footrests either during transfer or when the patient is in the chair.

Method 1. The patient who is able to transfer onto the bed without the use of an overhead bar will use the same pushup method to transfer back onto the chair (Fig. 3-70). He may lower his feet to the footrests either before or after transferring. The hand nearest the chair may be placed on the chair seat or on the armrest. The patient leans forward until he reaches his point of balance; then he depresses his shoulder girdle to raise his buttocks from the bed. He flexes his neck sharply and turns his head away from the chair to give him extra momentum as he lifts himself over into the seat.

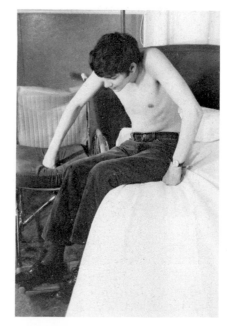

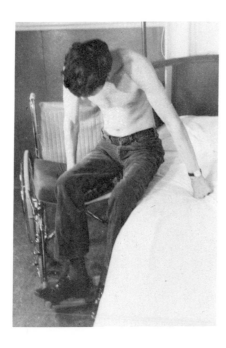
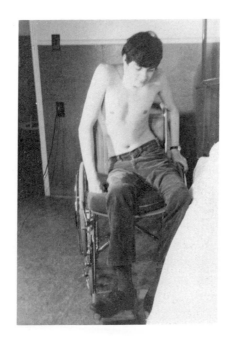
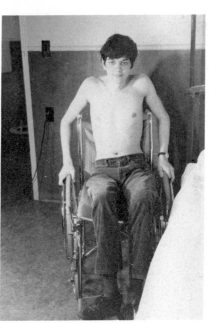

FIGURE 3-70

Method 2. (Fig. 3-71) The patient places the wrist furthest from the wheelchair in an overhead floating strap. He places the other hand on the wheelchair seat and locks the elbow. He pulls up on the strap so that the buttocks are raised from the bed. Adduction and flexion of the other shoulder will pull him into the wheelchair seat. He then moves his buttocks back into the chair.

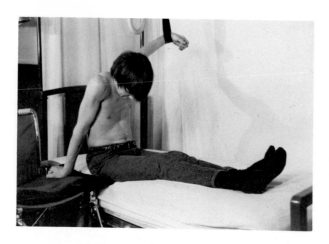

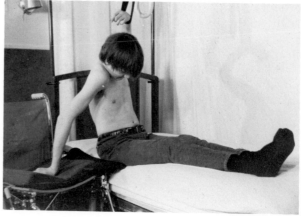

FIGURE 3-71

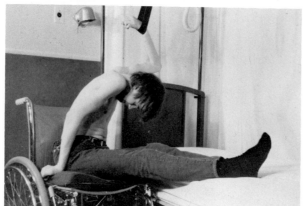

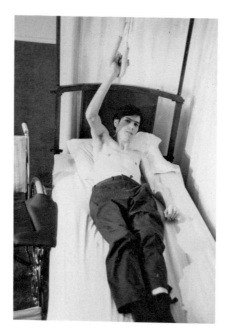

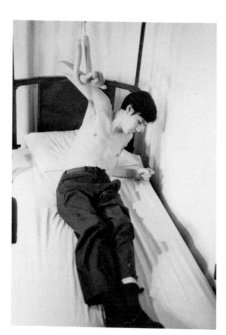

FIGURE 3-72

98

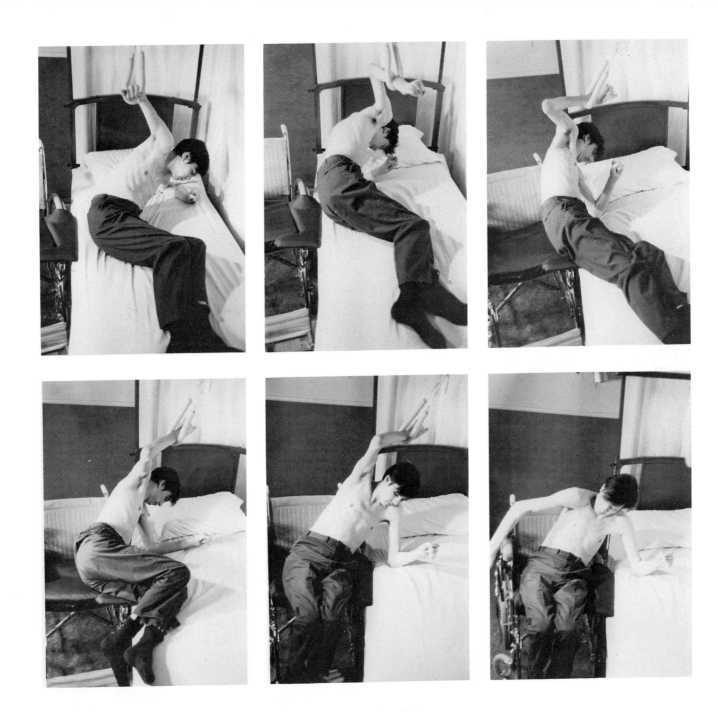

Method 3. (Fig. 3-72) The patient sits up and puts the wrist nearest the chair into an overhead strap. The other hand is placed on the bed behind him with the elbow locked. (If unable to straighten his arm he can lean on his elbow.) The patient then leans forward over the locked arm. This, in conjunction with a pull on the strap, will move the buttocks towards the chair. It may be necessary to repeat this procedure to move onto the wheelchair seat. At this point, the patient must lean forward and move back into the chair.

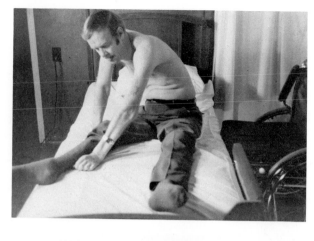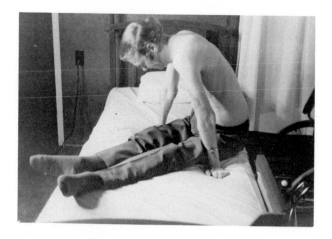

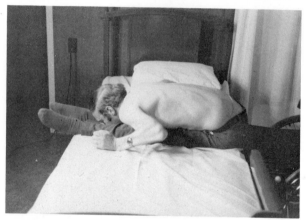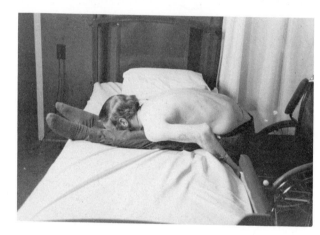

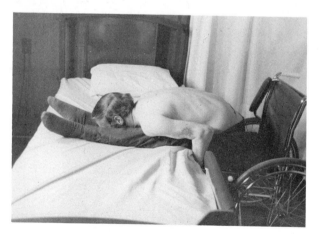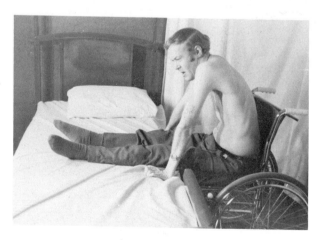

FIGURE 3-73

Method 4.   The patient who uses a front approach to transfer onto the bed will reverse the method to transfer back (Fig. 3-73). He positions himself so that he faces away from the chair. He allows his trunk to flex forward and reaches behind to hook his extended wrists over the edge of the mattress. Using his elbow flexors, he pulls his buttocks back onto the seat of the chair. He now releases the locks on the chair and wheels back far enough to swing the footrests back and lower his feet. The patient who uses this method of exit but another method of entry must learn to reposition his chair while on the bed.

Method 5.   In this method, the patient uses an outrigger (described in "Bed and Equipment") and a padded nylon covered bridge board (Fig. 3-74). He sits up with both wrists in floating overhead straps and moves them towards the chair as far as possible. As he pulls bilaterally his buttocks are raised and slide over towards the chair seat. This manoeuvre can be repeated until the patient is seated in the chair.

FIGURE 3-74

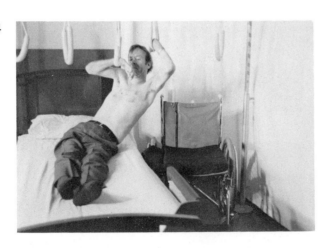
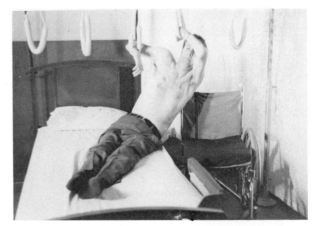
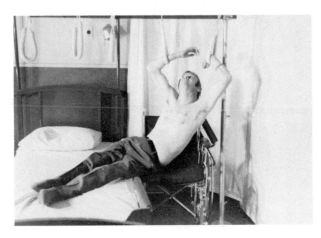
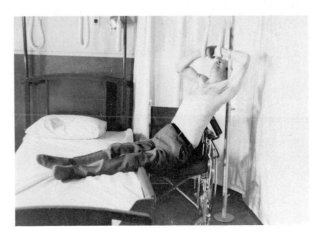

BEDMAKING TO PERMIT HANDLING OF THE COVERS

When the patient is adept at transferring himself into bed, it is time for him to put his skill into practical use. This is accomplished when he can complete the task of going to bed by pulling up the bed covers.

The bed must be made so that it permits easy entry. It should be made in the normal way except that covers are tucked in on one side only. The top corner is rolled diagonally across the bed from the untucked side. This will leave the bed unobstructed from the top corner of the footboard to the top of the tucked in side of the bed. After he has transferred to the bed, the patient can very easily use his wrist to unroll the bed clothes and cover himself (Fig. 3-75).

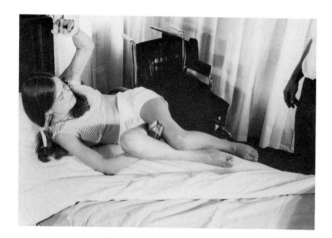
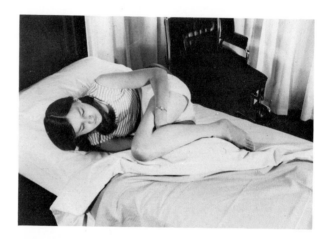
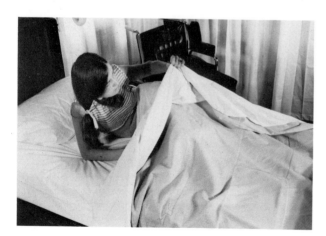
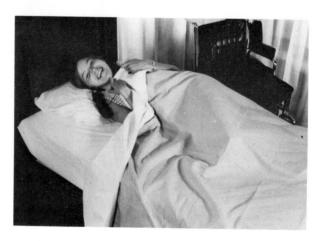

FIGURE 3-75

102

4

Toilet Transfers

VARIETIES OF RAISED TOILET SEATS

A raised toilet seat (Fig. 4-1) should be the height of the compressed wheelchair cushion.

Toilet seats can be constructed with a small hole so that the patient does not sink down too far. The small hole also prevents spreading of the buttocks, thus helping to prevent natal cleft tears. Toilets with modification in height are for the patient who slides one way easily but has difficulty sliding in the other direction.

A flat seat (Fig 4-2) facilitates sliding.

A padded toilet seat (Fig. 4-3) protects the skin of the emaciated or decubitus-prone patient. This is covered with a soft fabric-backed plastic material with a smooth surface.

A projection, incorporated with the seat, acts as a sliding board (Fig. 4-4).

A delta wing toilet seat (see Appendix) provides the maximum in stability and in surface area for convenient placement of hands (Fig. 4-5). For these reasons the seat is extremely useful in early training. The seat has a minimum size keyhole opening. Because the patient does not sink down into this hole, he does not have to lift to slide off the seat. If the patient's knees should abduct they will be retained by the shape of the seat front. The rubber-tipped post is placed into the chair arm socket. The chair is then turned towards the toilet so that the post catches behind a lip on the underedge of the wing, locking the chair to the toilet seat. The leg is screwed into a floor flange on the underside of the toilet seat on the side away from the wheelchair. This is reversible so that transfers may be practised from either side or, if it is used permanently, it may be used in different situations. (This seat was developed by John Borthwick, R.G., of G. F. Strong Rehabilitation Centre, Vancouver, British Columbia.)

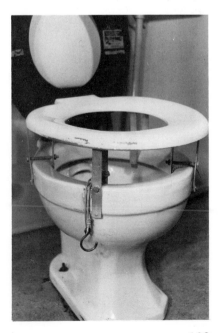

FIGURE 4-1

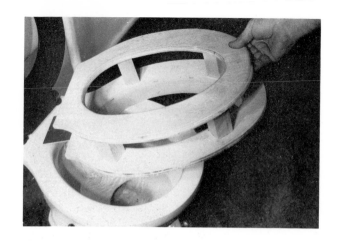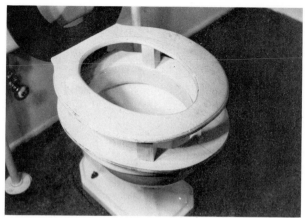

FIGURE 4-2

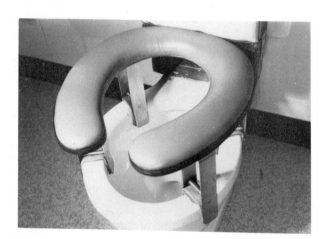

FIGURE 4-3

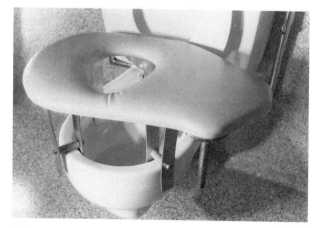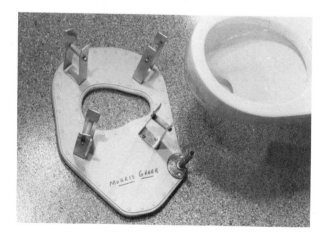

FIGURE 4-4

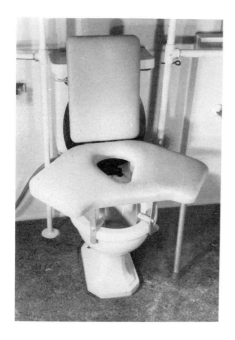

FIGURE 4-5

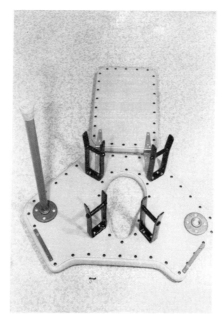

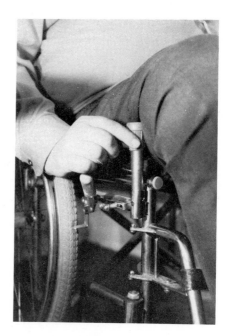

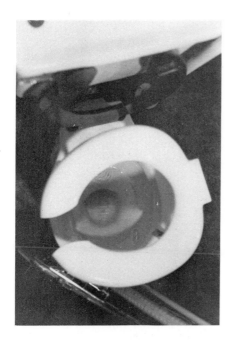

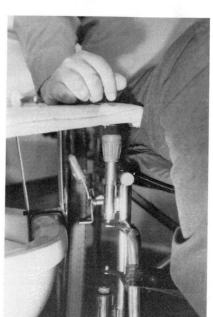

FIGURE 4-6

A raised toilet seat may be placed at an angle on the toilet bowl to accommodate a wide angle approach (Fig. 4-6).

ADDITIONAL EQUIPMENT

A footstool will compensate for the added height of the raised toilet seat. The footstool should have nonskid material such as suction cups underneath to stabilize it. A reversible footstool (Fig. 4-7A) is useful in training patients with different height requirements. A swivel footstool (Fig. 4-7B) stabilizes the feet under the strap and allows the feet to pivot as the patient transfers.

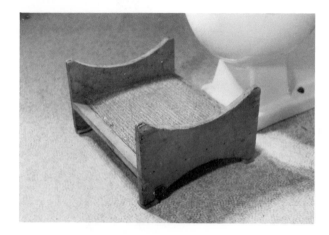

FIGURE 4-7

A

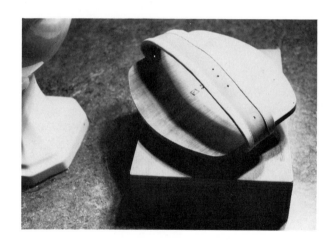

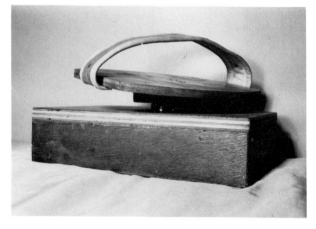

B

A padded backrest (Fig. 4-8) assists in posturing the patient and adds to his security and comfort, a prerequisite in bowel training.

A grab bar alongside the toilet at approximately 33 inches from the floor is necessary for stability during transfer and bowel training. A table can be substituted for a grab bar for some patients, providing room for equipment. The grab bar may be attached to the wall or may be a swing-away bar with the height adjustable as shown in Figure 4-9 (see Appendix).

Fixed or floating straps on an overhead bar frequently are necessary. The bar may be fixed or adjustable (Fig. 4-10).

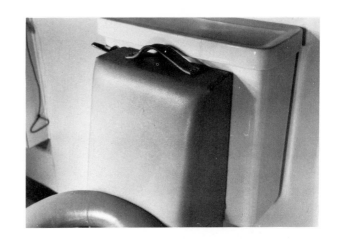

FIGURE 4-8

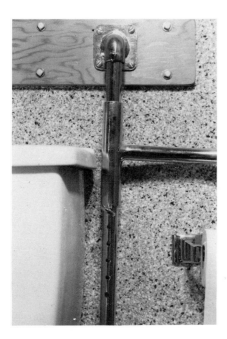

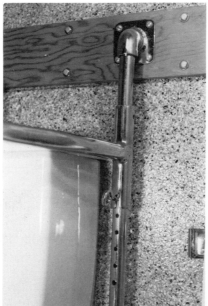

FIGURE 4-9

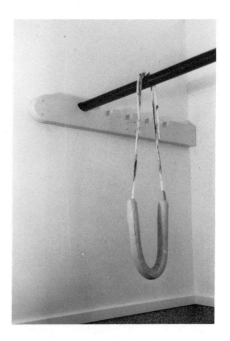

FIGURE 4-10

A rope, strap, or chain, attached to the toilet seat, has a hook to secure the wheelchair to the toilet (Fig. 4-11).

A padded sliding board with a post and flange may be made, so that it can be used for transfer to either side (Fig. 4-12) (see Appendix).

The cutaway cushion and chairseat may be used with either a swing-away back or with a back with a zipper on either side opening halfway up the back from the bottom. This is for use with a semitransfer through the chair back and the cutout

107

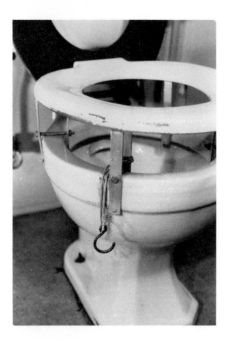

FIGURE 4-11

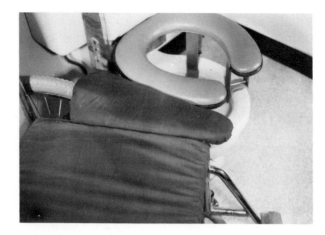

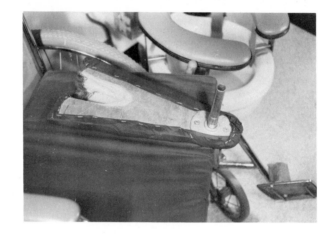

FIGURE 4-12

FIGURE 4-13

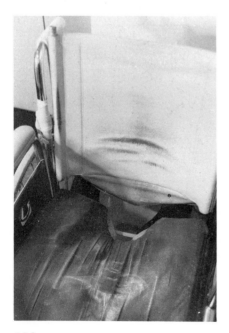

seat will not always be necessary. The U-shaped cutaway in the wheelchair seat must be closed at the top of the "U" with a strong washable (plastic-covered) reinforcement strip to prevent the back of the chair seat from sagging (Fig. 4-13).

TRANSFERRING

WHEELCHAIR TO TOILET

Slacks must be worn by the patient until he becomes proficient at transferring onto the toilet. A bowel regime should be established before the patient starts learning toilet transfers, so that he uses the toilet before dressing in the morning or after undressing at night. This eliminates extra transfers onto the bed for taking off and putting on slacks and underwear.

To get into position for any of the side transfers the patient places the footstool in position and then backs his chair alongside the toilet. He swings the front of the chair in against the toilet bowl, angling the chair at about 35°. He locks the brakes and, if necessary, hooks the front frame of the chair to the toilet bowl. After sliding his buttocks forward in the chair clear of the front of the wheel, he removes the chair arm. The raised toilet seat should be level with the compressed wheelchair cushion.

A footstool will generally be needed to compensate for the extra height of the toilet seat, but the tall patient may not require one. The placing of the feet depends upon the balance, type of spasm, flaccidity, and build of the patient. Experimentation may be required to arrive at the optimum position for an individual. The feet may be moved at any stage of a transfer. The foot positions may be one of the following: both feet on the footrests, both feet on the footrest near the toilet, one foot on a footrest and one on the footstool, or both feet on the footstool.

Method 1. (Fig. 4-14) The patient places one or both feet on the footrest near the toilet and/or one or both on the footstool. He places one hand on the grab bar or a table on the far side of the toilet and the other hand on the cushion close to his buttock. He leans forward, so placing his centre of gravity more over his knees. He internally rotates the arm on the bar enabling him to use the strong elbow and shoulder flexors to lift him and help the other arm to rotate him on to the toilet. He now positions his legs for maximum comfort and stability.

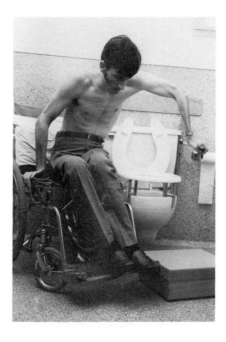
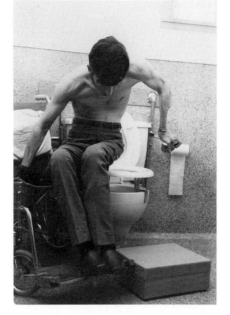

FIGURE 4-14

Method 2. (Fig. 4-15) The patient places one hand close to his buttock and the other hand on the toilet seat. He locks his elbows and leans forward until he reaches a point of balance. A pushup with both arms causes his buttocks to swing towards the toilet. At first the patient may move for only a short distance but as balance and strength improve the transfer will be accomplished in only one or two moves.

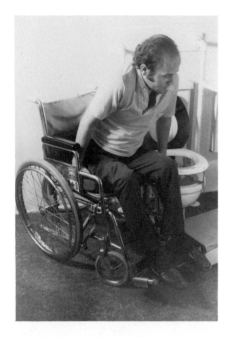
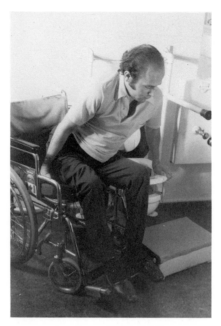
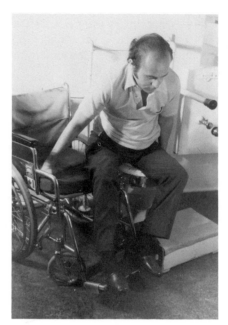

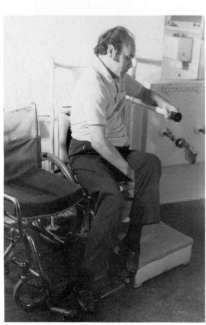
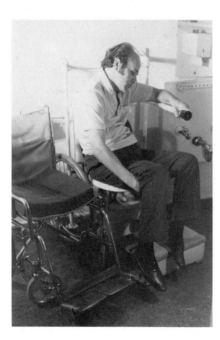

FIGURE 4-15

Method 3. (Fig. 4-16) In this technique the patient moves forward in the chair and turns away from the toilet. He places one hand against the front of the chair arm and the other on the cushion against the back of the chair arm. He locks both arms and leans forward pushing himself backwards onto the toilet seat. He picks up the leg nearest the toilet and lifts the foot onto the footstool; this leaves the other hand at the back of the chair, a position that helps him twist to face forward. This action is completed when the other leg is lifted over onto the footrest. Either arm may be used to lift the second leg over, but a greater degree of twist is developed if the arm near the wheelchair is used.

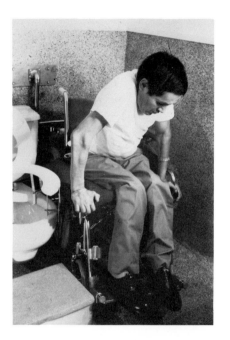
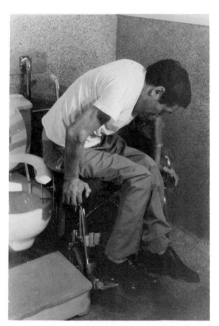
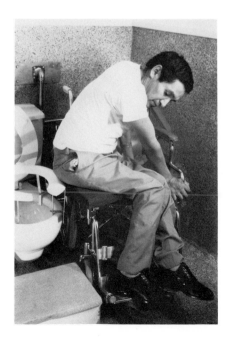
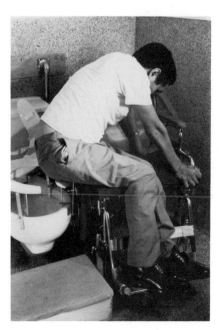
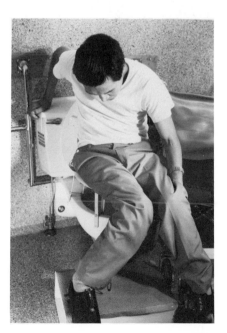

FIGURE 4-16

Method 4. (Fig. 4-17) The patient moves forward in the chair and places the wrist nearest the toilet in a floating overhead strap. He may now lift one or both feet across onto the footstool. He locks the other arm with the hand close to his buttock and leans over it away from the toilet. By pulling with the arm in the strap and pushing with the locked arm he moves part of the way onto the toilet. He shifts the floating strap away from him as far as possible and repeats the action until he is on the toilet. He now positions his feet.

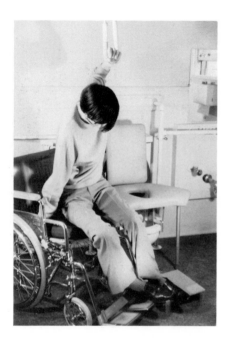
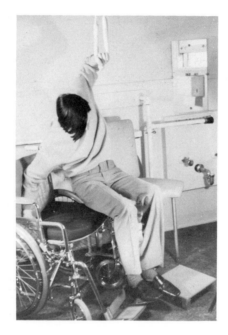
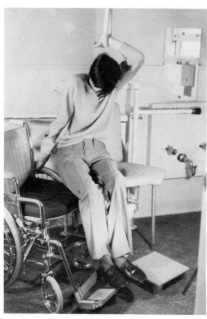
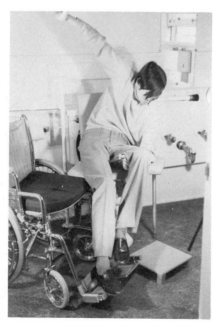

FIGURE 4-17

Method 5. (Fig. 4-18) The patient moves forward in the chair and places his feet on the footstool. He puts his wrist in an overhead strap fixed in position half way between the toilet and the chair. (If necessary two straps may be used in this transfer—one directly over the toilet to assist in getting onto the toilet and one over the chair to assist in getting onto the chair.) The other hand is placed on the far side of the toilet seat with the shoulder internally rotated. Leaning well forward to place some of his weight over his feet he adducts his shoulders and flexes his elbows strongly to lift and swing onto the toilet.

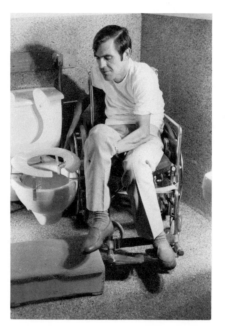
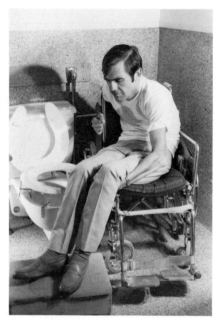
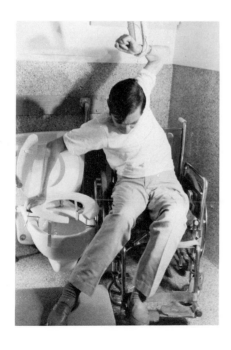
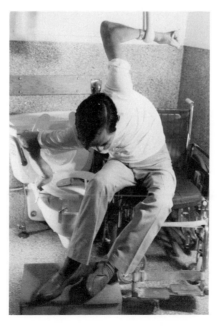
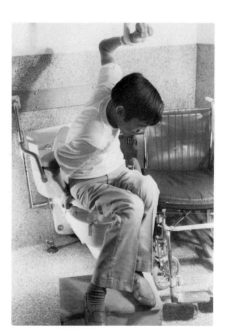

FIGURE 4-18

Method 6. (Fig. 4-19) The patient positions his feet and places both forearms in an overhead fixed strap positioned directly over the toilet seat. By pulling strongly with both arms he lifts himself and swings onto the toilet seat. Care must be taken to ensure that the wheel does not graze the buttocks while the patient is learning this transfer.

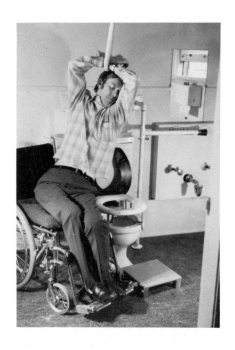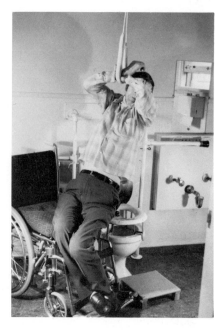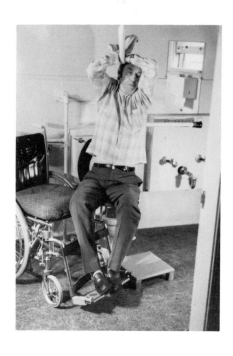

FIGURE 4-19

Method 7. The forward approach is a practical transfer method for a patient who is sufficiently flaccid to allow the knees to abduct without pressure and may be used permanently or occasionally where space is restricted (Fig. 4-20). Sometimes it is advisable to cut off part of each side of the toilet seat and pad the seat; this eliminates the need for extreme abduction. In this technique the patient approaches the toilet from the front and lifts his feet to the outside of the footrests enabling him to wheel up to the toilet so that his cushion is butted to the toilet seat.

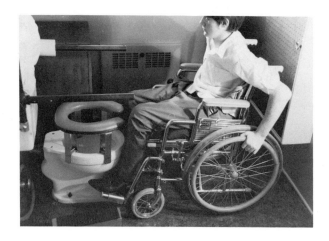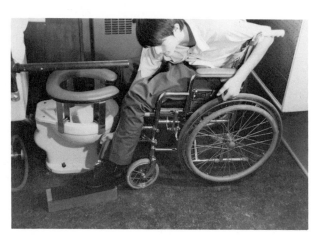

FIGURE 4-20

114

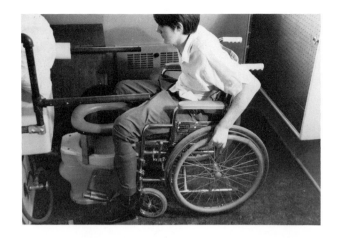
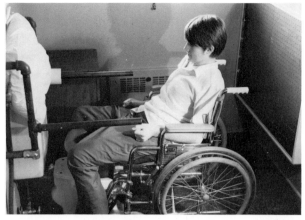

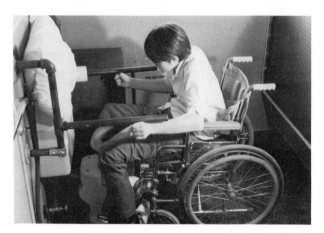
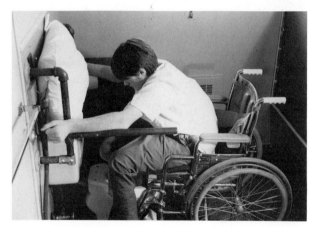

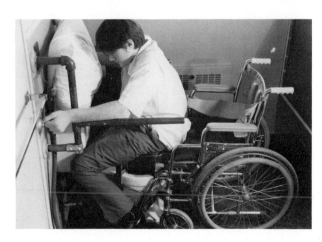
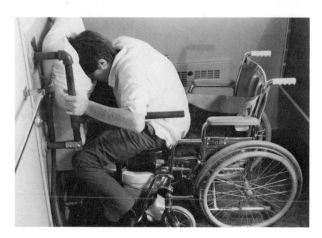

He applied his brakes and slides forward in his chair. He now reaches forward to hook his wrists around the grab bars to pull himself onto the toilet, the grab bars may be provided with knobs to prevent slipping. He may reposition his feet and rest his head on a pillow which has been placed on the water tank. This provides comfort and balance and leaves one or both hands free.

Method 8.   A swivel back chair may be used in a rear approach to the toilet (Fig. 4-21). The patient backs the chair over the toilet and places his feet on the midcalf straps. Leaning forward he pushes with the thumb web against the front upright of the chair arm. The patient's buttocks will slide out of the back of the chair, the swivel back allowing him room as it tips forward. Obesity, tight hamstrings, and spasticity preclude the use of this method.   A cut out in cushion and seat may be necessary for the patient who is unable to slide far enough out of the chair (Fig. 4-13). Women who are bladder trained and who urinate frequently may use this method of transfer because of facility and the short time required. These women may find it more convenient to wear a shirt but no panties. In this case the swivel back must have an extension flap at the base.

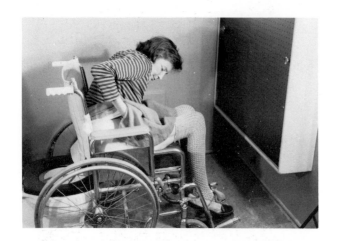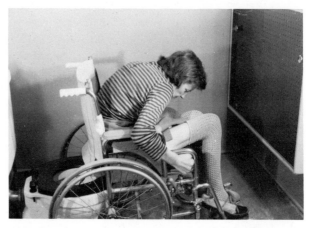

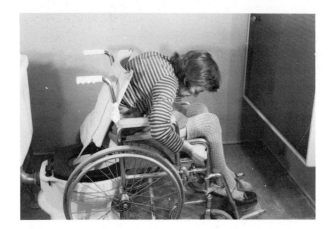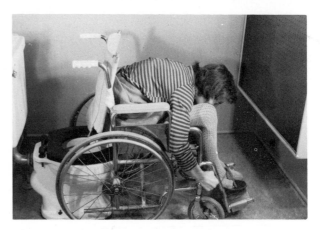

FIGURE 4-21

Method 9.   A rear approach transfer may be a practical transfer and of particular use in a restricted area (Fig. 4-22). Any tightness in the hamstrings will preclude the use of this method. The patient backs over the toilet until the crossbar of the wheelchair touches and locks the brakes. He opens the detachable back and flips it out of the way. He lifts his feet onto a strap half way up the leg rest and leans forward to push himself onto the toilet seat using the wheel or the front upright of the wheelchair arms. Most patients will require a raised toilet seat and a back rest, but the raised toilet seat will be lower than usual since the back of the wheelchair seat is lower than the front.

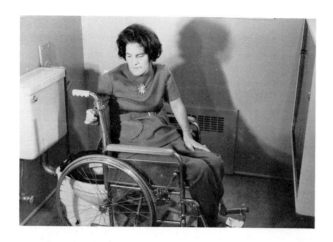 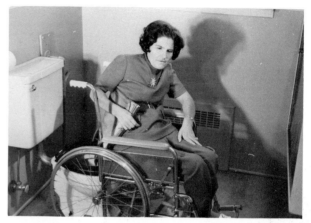

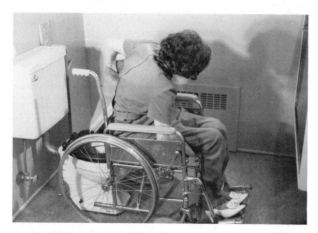 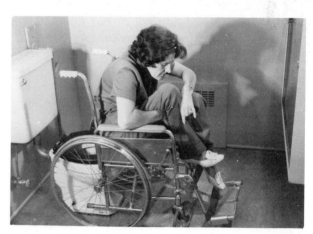

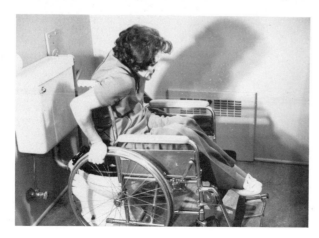 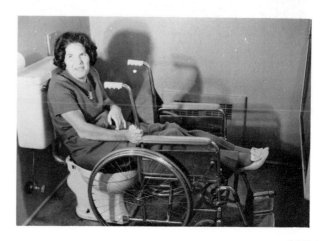

FIGURE 4-22

TOILET TO WHEELCHAIR

Method 1. (Fig. 4-23) The patient places one hand on the wheelchair cushion on the far side and one hand on the grab bar or table beside him. He leans forward towards the wheelchair and pushes up to lift and swivel over onto the wheelchair seat.

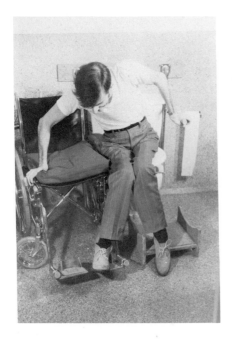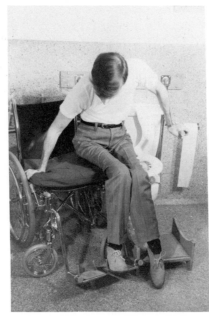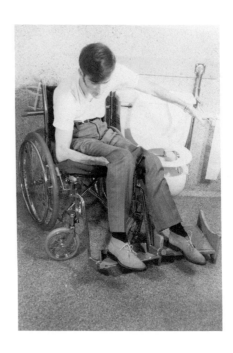

FIGURE 4-23

Method 2. (Fig. 4-24) The patient places one hand on the toilet seat by his buttock and the other on the wheelchair cushion. He locks his elbows and leans forward until he reaches his point of balance. If he now does a pushup his buttocks will swing towards the wheelchair seat. This pendulum action will be increased if he ducks his head and shoulders away from the wheelchair. The action may be repeated as many time as necessary until he is in the wheelchair. This method is more successful with a patient who is of stocky build rather than one with a concertina spine.

Method 3. (Fig. 4-25) The patient puts the wrist nearest the wheelchair into a floating overhead strap, or a fixed strap over the wheelchair, and repositions his feet. He places the other hand on the toilet seat close to his buttock and locks the arm. Leaning forward and over the locked arm he lifts with the arm in the overhead strap and pushes with the arm on the toilet seat. This shifts him toward the chair or onto it. It may be necessary to flick a floating strap closer to the wheelchair and repeat the manoeuvre.

118

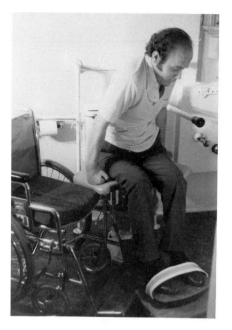
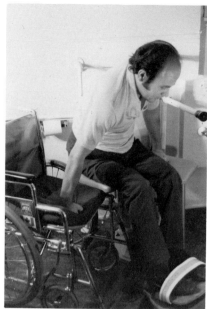
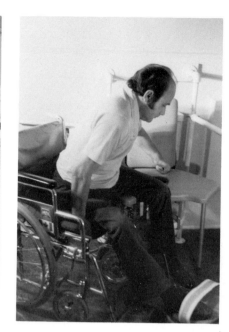

FIGURE 4-24

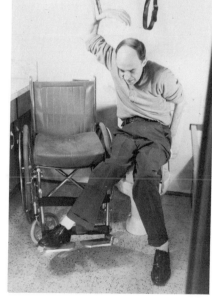
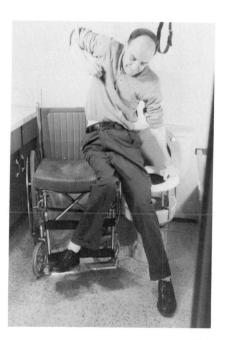

FIGURE 4-25

119

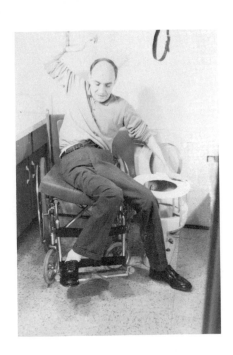
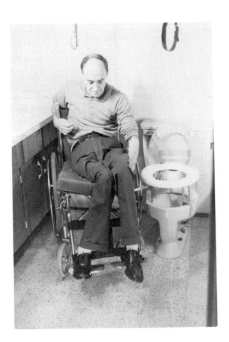

Method 4. (Fig. 4-26) The patient places his feet in position and then inserts both arms into the strap, which is in a fixed position over the wheelchair seat. He lifts with both arms and swings into the chair. This transfer requires careful placement of the feet to prevent the patient being shifted too far forward; precise timing in lowering to sitting is necessary to prevent a return pendulum action.

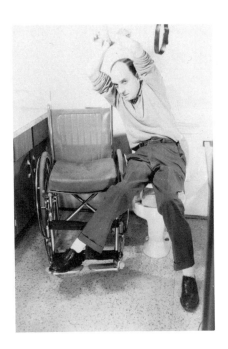
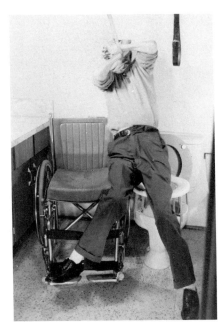

FIGURE 4-26

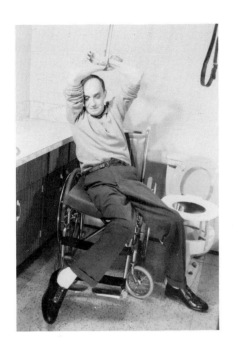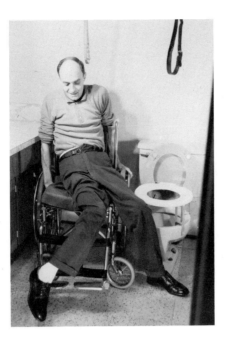

Method 5. (Fig. 4-27) The patient places one foot on the wheelchair footrest and places the wrist furthest from the chair in the floating overhead strap. He now places the other hand on the wheelchair cushion and locks the elbow. As he elevates himself by pulling on the strap and pushing with the hand on the cushion, he swings toward the wheelchair. It may be necessary to repeat this action several times, moving the floating strap over towards the chair each time.

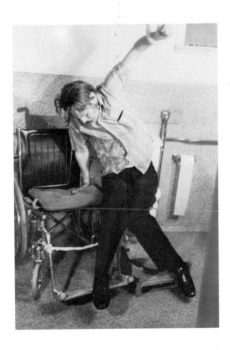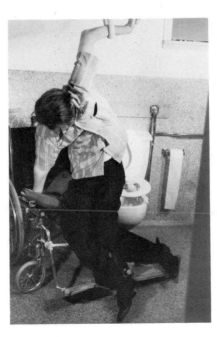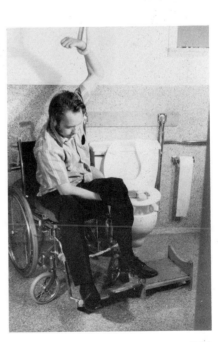

FIGURE 4-27

Method 6. (Fig. 4-28) To move from the toilet to the wheelchair from a forward position, the patient remains in his forward position and pushes together or alternately with his hands against the wall, water tank, or grab bars. To develop this push he must internally rotate his shoulders, so raising his elbows. Since his trunk is flexed he can use a hugging action which pushes his buttock onto the chair.

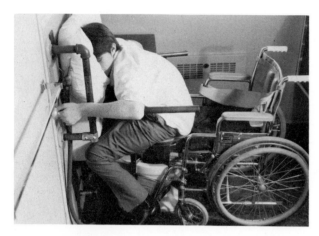
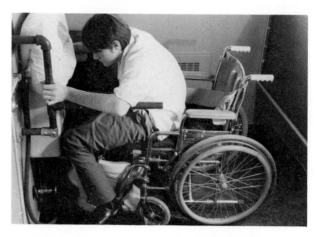
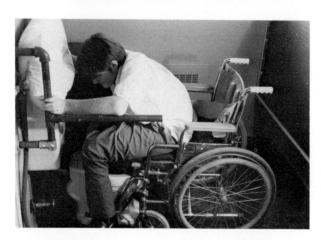
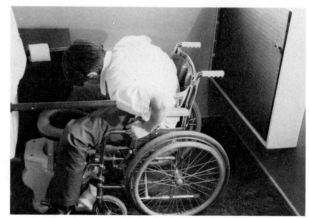
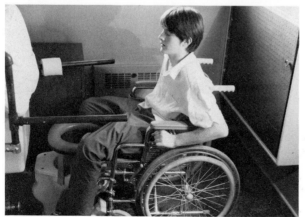

FIGURE 4-28

Method 7. (Fig. 4-29) The patient lowers his feet from the heel strap to the footrests. Leaning well forward he places his elbows against the chair cushion and uses shoulder extension to pull himself well forward in the chair before sitting up.

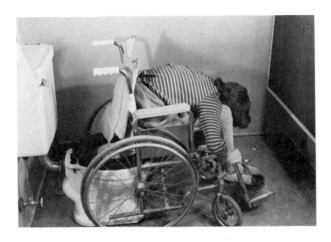 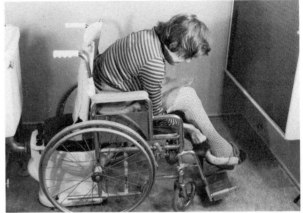

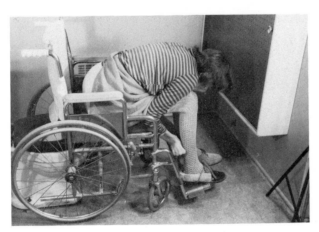 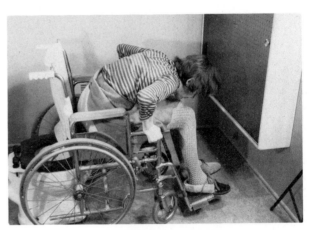

FIGURE 4-29

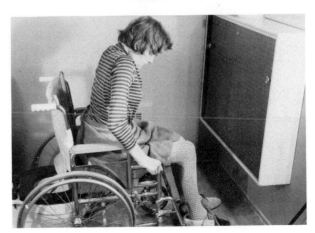

Method 8. (Fig. 4-30) The patient is sitting on the toilet seat with his legs resting through the open back of the wheelchair on the wheelchair cushion. He reaches forward to hook his arms around the chair back uprights. Forward sliding is initiated by the patient's pulling with his arms and throwing his head forward sharply. The forward movement is assisted by the progressive weight of the lower

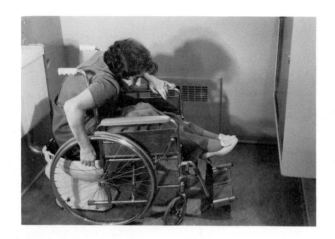
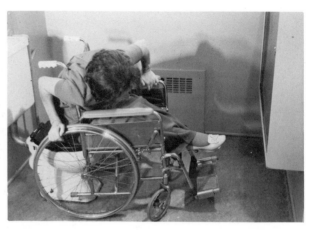
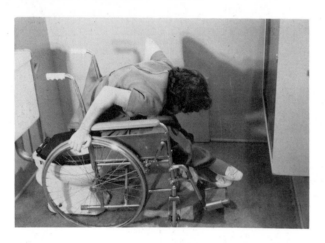
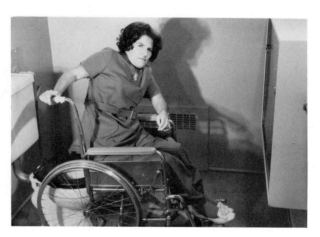

FIGURE 4-30

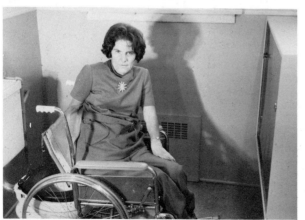

legs as the feet near the footrests. Additional forward movement may be gained by pushing on the wheels or against the cushion or armrests while the trunk stays well flexed forward. An alternate or simultaneous movement may be used to push the patient well forward since adequate room must be left to fasten the chair back (Fig. 4-31). The gutter on the side of the wheelchair back should be positioned against the back upright at the bottom and pushed into place. The safety pin is pushed through the hole far enough to allow the locking dog to drop into the locked position. For convenience, the safety pin is fastened to the wheelchair.

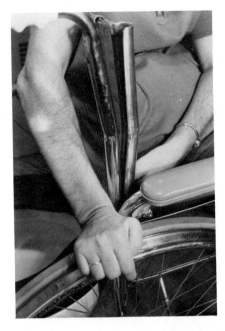 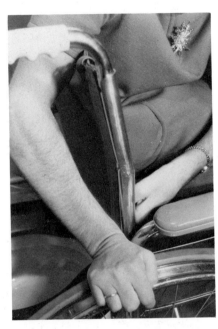

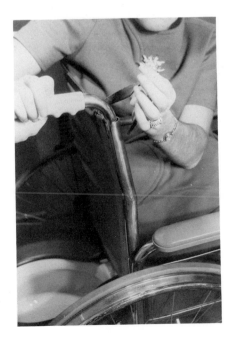 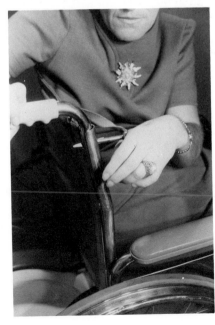 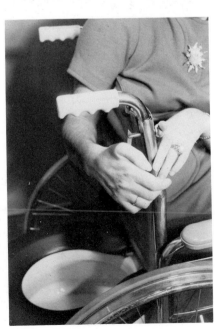

FIGURE 4-31

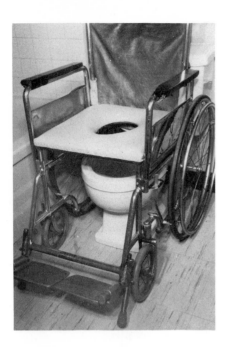

FIGURE 4-32

WHEELCHAIR COMMODE

A commode may be used when the bathroom is too small to place a wheelchair alongside the toilet in a conventional transferring position, when the patient is unable to transfer conveniently to the toilet, or when skin problems make fewer transfers desirable.

A commode with drive wheels at the rear and removable arms, brakes, and footrests is the choice for a patient who is able to transfer from bed to chair. This may also serve as a shower chair, which may be used directly after the toilet to save transfers, to save energy, and to prevent skin problems. The level of the commode seat should be raised to the height of the wheelchair seat plus the height of the compressed cushion. For some patients it is advisable to make a seat with a hole of smaller circumference and an open front to facilitate digital stimulation (see Chapter 7, Bowel Management).

The commode may be made by converting an old wheelchair (Fig. 4-32). The centre cross bars are removed and a length of tubing is welded across the front of the chair at the junction of the front upright and the bottom bar. Additional stability is gained from the wooden padded seat which attaches to the original seat rails. Because the cross bars are removed the commode can be backed directly over the toilet. If the commode must be transported the seat may be made with four bolts used as posts to drop into holes in the seat rails. The bottom cross bar may be attached with clamps or made to be collapsible. Anti-tipping legs may be installed at the front of the commode.

BED TO COMMODE TRANSFERS

This transfer is made from bed to commode, not from chair to commode, and is made in the same manner as a bed to chair transfer.

Method 1. The transfer may be made to the opposite side of the bed from the usual chair transfer. The brakes must be applied and the castors turned forwards. If necessary the commode may be locked to the bed.

Method 2. The wheelchair may be pushed out of the way and the commode put in its place. This requires good reaching ability or a long stick with a shepherds crook to retrieve the needed chair and apply the brakes.

Method 3. The commode may be placed further down on the same side of the bed as the wheelchair facing the bed. In this case the patient must be able to swivel and back out of the bed.

Method 4. The commode may be placed on the same side of the bed as the wheelchair or at the foot of the bed, but facing in the opposite direction to the wheelchair. The patient must be able to completely reverse positions in bed before transferring.

Method 5. Only a very small patient will be able to position the commode chair further down the bed but facing in the same direction as the wheelchair.

5
Bathing

Cleanliness is particularly important for the quadriplegic patient in order to prevent skin problems and unpleasant odors. Despite the efficiency of the patient, occasional drops of urine may escape during changing or emptying urine collecting apparatus. The patient may become accustomed to this smell and, therefore, be oblivious to the effect on others. A convenient time for the daily skin inspection is after bathing and before dressing. A mirror may be adapted so that it can be firmly held. The areas that must be inspected are the skin over the spinous processes of the back, the trochanters, the iliac crests, the sacrum, and the ischial tuberosities. Special care must be taken to check the natal cleft. The knees, the malleoli, heels, soles, and toes must be checked. Toenails should be trimmed regularly and checked to see that they do not become ingrown. Elbows must also be checked for abrasions. Early detection of a skin problem often can save weeks of treatment, weeks which would have caused time loss at work and would have interfered with social activities.

EQUIPMENT

A shower hose permits thorough washing and rinsing. The water *must* be turned on and tested before being directed at any anaesthetic part of the patient's body. Particular care must be taken if there is no mixing valve, and the water must be allowed to run for an adequate length of time to ensure a steady temperature. Ideally the water temperature should be checked at the tap before directing the water through the shower head.

The telephone-type handle of a flexible metal shower hose (Fig. 5-1) may be adapted if necessary by building up the handle, by attaching a velcro-D-ring strap, or by attaching a look handle. The cheaper rubber hose and shower head can also be used, but they generally do not endure.

Taps may be adapted if necessary by rivetting, brazing, or gluing a lever arm to them (Fig. 5-2A). Ideally a long lever tap may be purchased to replace an unsuitable tap (Fig. 5-2B).

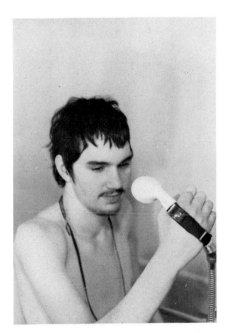

FIGURE 5-1

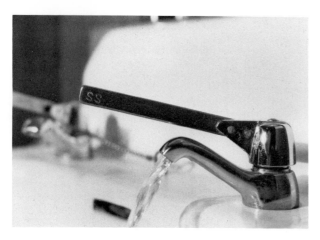
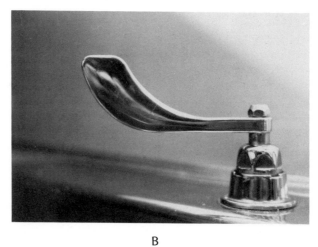

A   B   FIGURE 5-2

Bath mitts are made of towelling sewn around three sides. The wrist may be loose or closed with velcro. The soap may be slipped in with the hand for washing and removed for rinsing. Soap may be drilled to take a length of cord so that it can be hung around the neck, so remaining within reach (Fig. 5-3). A bath brush may be adapted so that it can be firmly held to enable the patient to reach the back and extremities (Fig. 5-4).

FIGURE 5-3   FIGURE 5-4

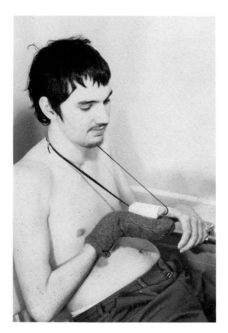
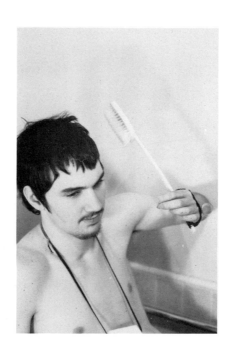

Shampoo should be placed in an easy-to-reach position. The dispenser may be adapted if necessary, or a small amount placed in a tin lid or equivalent. Screw top bottles (preferably plastic bottles) may be loosely fastened and, if necessary, a lever such as a tongue depressor taped to the cap (Fig. 5-5).

A spray bottle may be placed in a box made to fit with a lid hinged to the top so that it acts as a lever to depress the valve (Fig. 5-6). A 2-inch-diameter hole may be made on the hinged side so that the spray can be directed through it. An adaptation may be made quickly by taping two tongue depressors together end to end. One is then taped to the spray can with the hinge level with the valve (Fig. 5-7).

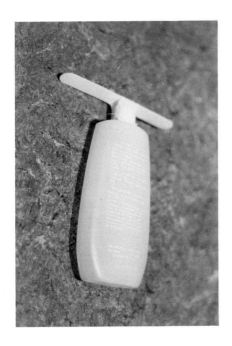

FIGURE 5-5

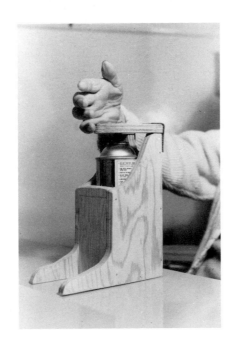

FIGURE 5-6

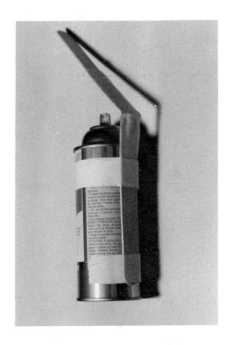

FIGURE 5-7

Commercially available handles can be attached to any spray can and often are easy for a quadriplegic patient to handle (Fig. 5-8).

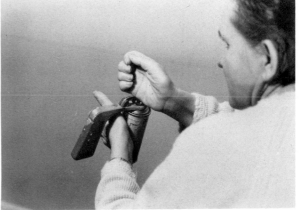

FIGURE 5-8

The mirror for daily skin inspection may require an adapted handle (Fig. 5-9). Frequently shampoo brushes are manufactured with a loop handle, making them ideal as hair brushes or shampoo brushes for many patients.

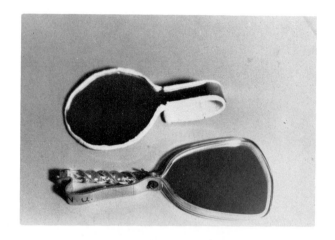

FIGURE 5-9

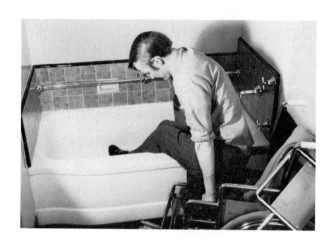
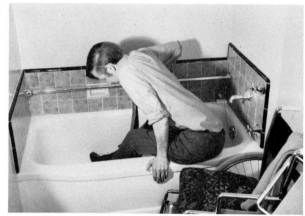
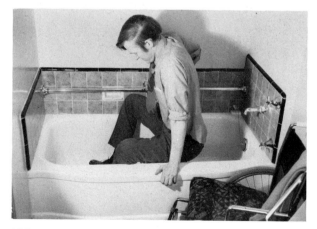
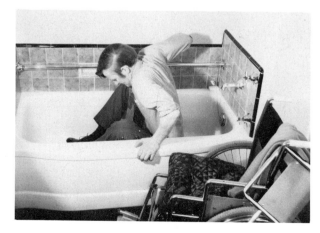

FIGURE 5-10

BATHTUB TRANSFER

A quadriplegic patient who can get from the floor to his chair will probably be able to get into the tub and out. A grab bar is firmly fastened to the far wall of the bathtub, far enough from the wall to permit a hand to grip it. The height must be worked out for the individual; it is usually 6 inches above the tub rim.

In the technique for getting into the tub (Fig. 5-10) the patient may approach the bathtub with his chair at a 30° angle to the tub or he may use a front approach with both footrests swung away. He slides forward in the chair, lifts both feet into the tub, and slides to the edge of the bathtub before reaching for the grab bar. He places both feet on the bottom of the tub to take part of his weight but makes sure that his feet point towards the foot of the tub so that they will not buckle under him as he lowers himself.

To get out of the tub the patient brings his knees up against his chest and leans forward, lifting himself up and then over to the bathtub edge (Fig. 5-11). This requires skill, balance, and a good deal of strength. When a patient is learning this skill, a helper can slip a towel around his waist or chest as a stand-in belt which can be controlled with one hand.

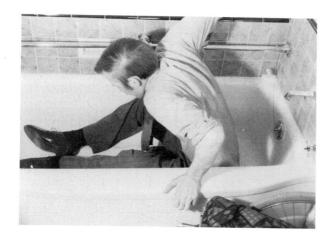

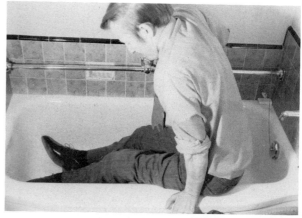

FIGURE 5-11

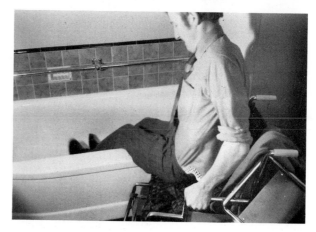

131

THE WHEEL-IN SHOWER (Fig. 5-12)

By far the most convenient situation is to have a shower area large enough to accommodate a wheelchair. The floor of the shower should be recessed for drainage, levelled to the regular floor by duckboards close enough together so that the wheels will ride over them, or made of a perforated metal sheet. A second wheelchair is the best choice for a wheel-in shower. It must be equipped with brakes, footrests, and removable arms. A waterproof cushion should be provided to bring the chair seat up to bed level.

A commode wheelchair may be used for showering. A convenient time to shower is immediately after toiletting, for this ensures cleanliness and saves transfers. A stainless steel wheelchair will not deteriorate when used as a shower chair. An older wheelchair may be used as a shower chair, but it must have regular maintenance to prevent rusting. The upholstery should be waterproof.

If a patient is unable to procure an alternate chair for showering, the regular chair must be used, but it should be protected with a plastic sheet and extra attention must be given to maintenance. A wheelchair cushion may be protected with plastic and covered with towelling or an air cushion may be used.

FIGURE 5-12

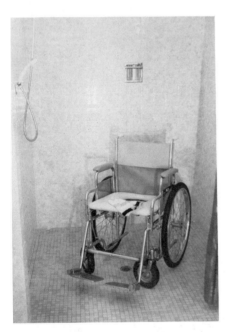

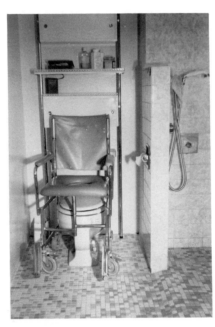

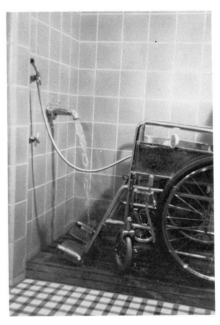

A, Large wheel-in shower with minimal slope to drain.

B, Adjoining toilet and shower.

C, Shower with duckboard flooring.

The patient should undress in bed and then transfer to the shower chair, returning to the bed to dress after he has finished showering. The taps and mixing valve of the shower must be within easy reach. In addition, the patient must be able to test the water temperature with a sensitive part of his body. To be able to do this, the water should run through a tap before the patient turns the shower lever on. Washing aids should be within reach.

132

THE BATHSEAT SHOWER

The bathseat extends from the wall to a point 5 inches beyond the outer edge of the bathtub. A separation is left between the back and the seat to allow free drainage (Fig. 5-13). The back is attached to the seat with strong angle irons leaning back at about 108°. Both back and seat are padded with ¾-inch foam and covered with a smooth naugahyde. The upholstery is grooved just inside the edge of the bathtub rim for drainage. The seat must be raised to the height of the compressed wheelchair cushion by means of wooden blocks or nonferrous legs. The legs are designed to prevent the bathseat from moving outwards.

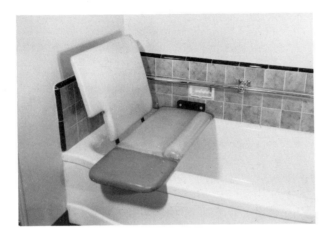
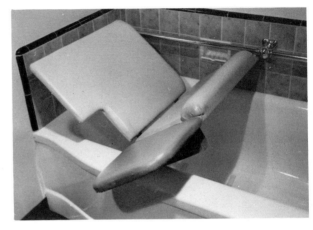

FIGURE 5-13

The bathseat may be stablized on the wall by means of blocks or bars just above the seat. This prevents the bathseat from tipping forward, back, or sideways. If it is not possible to attach equipment to the wall, a bar may be bolted to the bottom of the legs to run along the rim of the tub to prevent forward or backward tipping (Fig. 5-14A). The part of the bathseat which protrudes beyond the tub (Fig. 5-14B) may be hinged so that it swings up out of the way (Fig. 5-14C).

A

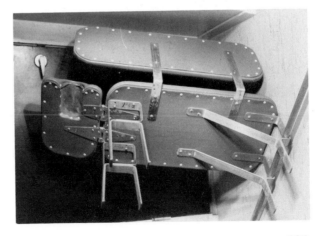

FIGURE 5-14

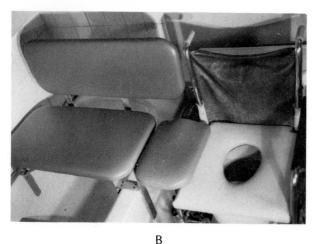

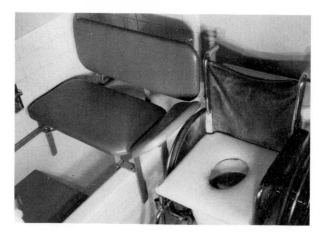

B   C

If necessary the seat may have a padded cut-out on the hinged section to fit over the wheel of a commode or a wheelchair. It may be made with a raised and padded front edge so that the patient does not slide forward. A small toilet seat hole in the bathseat may facilitate perineal washing. The upholstered back normally reaches the outside edge of the tub, but it may be extended to the upright of the wheelchair back although it interferes with the shower curtain, which must be tucked around it. (A damp towel will hold the bottom of the curtain down on the seat.)

An overhead strap may be used not only for transfer but also so that the patient can lean and manoeuvre to wash underneath himself on the bathseat. A grab bar may run the length of the bath. This must be far enough from the wall to allow a hand to be inserted and at elbow height when the patient is sitting on the seat. The taps should be lever type for easy turning and must be within reach. As the seat may be moved forward or back this is easy to ensure. The taps may be behind the seat or in front, depending upon the balance and reach of the patient and the layout of the bathroom. A telephone type shower on a hose is required.

TRANSFERRING TO BATHSEAT

Frequently the patient will use the same methods and overhead equipment in this transfer as in his bed transfer. For this reason the overhead equipment and methods of moving are not described. The main difference between a bed transfer and a bathseat transfer is in the positioning of the legs and the use of the side of the bathtub to assist in the transfer. It is advisable for the patient to learn the method of transfer wearing his slacks to provide skin protection and ease of sliding. When the patient has progressed to a wet run, talcum powder may be used to make the dry seat slippery. He may place a damp facecloth for any nonslip hand positions.

Method 1. (Fig. 5-15) The patient lifts one leg into the bathtub and leaves the other on the footrest near the bathtub. This wide base gives him stability. The leg inside the bathtub will tend to pull his buttocks towards the bathtub until the foot

134

makes contact with the bottom. He must now pivot his shoulders towards the chair until the knee is stopped against the side of the tub. Further effort to pivot will lever him onto the bath seat with minimum effort because the knee creates a fulcrum against the bathtub side. As soon as the leg on the outside of the tub prevents further progress, it is lifted in.

FIGURE 5-15

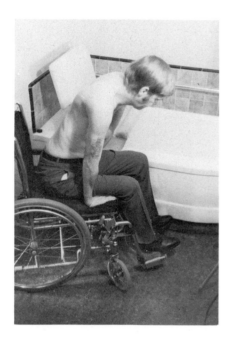
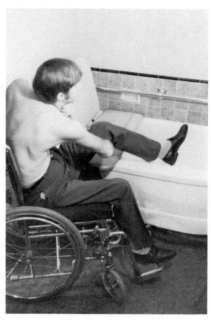
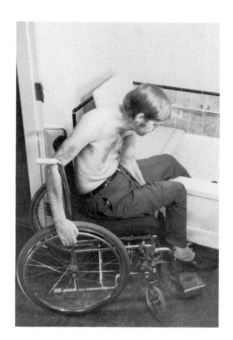
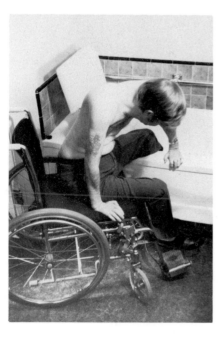
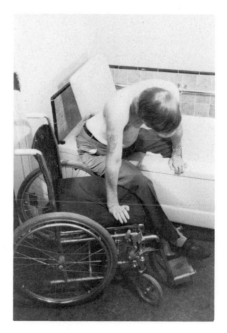
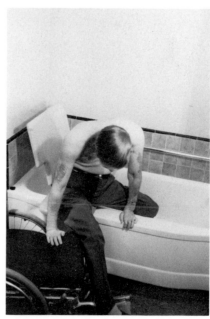

135

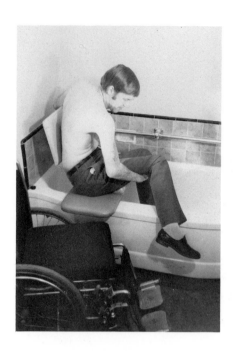
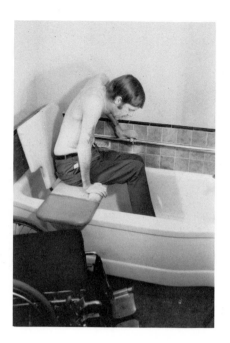

Method 2. (Fig. 5-16) Both legs may be lifted into the bathtub first to provide additional help, because the extra weight of the legs will pull the patient onto the bath seat more easily although he sacrifices some stability. As in the first method the knees become a fulcrum against the side of the tub after the feet have reached the bottom of the bathtub. The shorter patient may require a footrest inside the bathtub to prevent the weight of his legs pulling him forward off the bathseat and

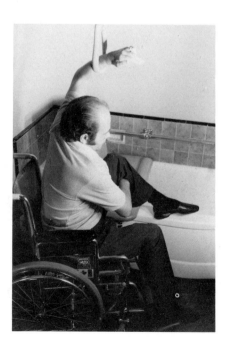
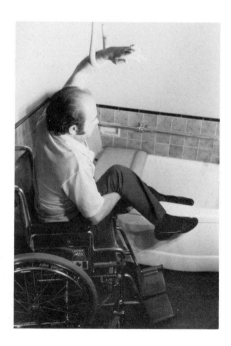

FIGURE 5-16

136

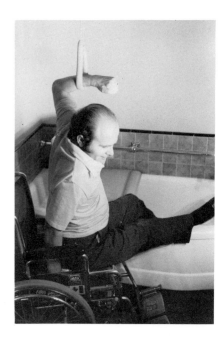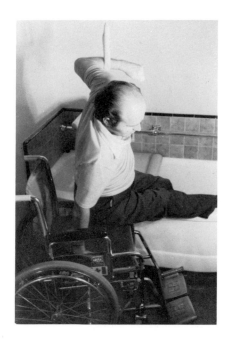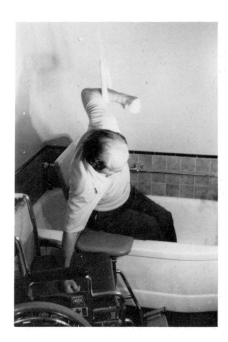

to provide a secure sitting position. It is not recommended that the patient leave both legs on the footrests of the wheelchair while moving onto the bathseat because he loses stability and leverage and could push the chair away unless it is locked to the bathseat.

   Method 3.   (Fig. 5-17) The patient turns his wheelchair at a right angle to the bathtub in line with the bathseat. He locks his chair about a foot from the bathseat, leaving him room to lift his legs and place them on the seat. He swings the footrests away to allow him to wheel forward and bring his cushion into contact with the lip of the bathseat. He shifts forward until his feet nearly touch the far wall. He then lowers his legs and moves further onto the seat. Although the patient gains little leverage from the side of the bathtub, this method provides great security and stability, particularly for the patient with flaccid lower extremities.

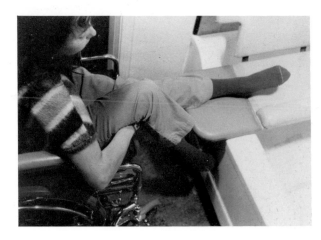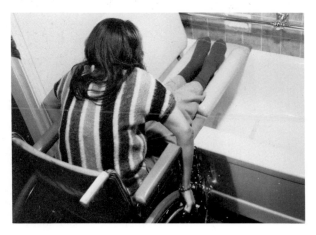

FIGURE 5-17

137

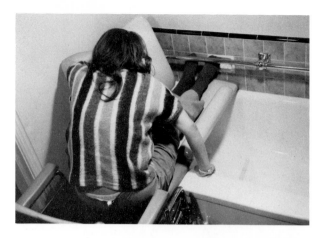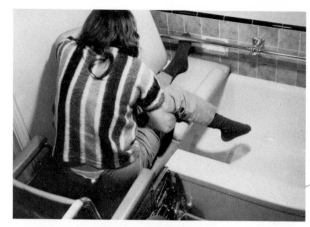

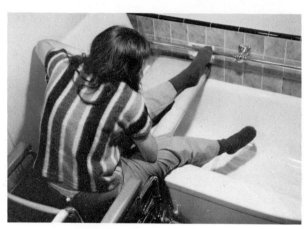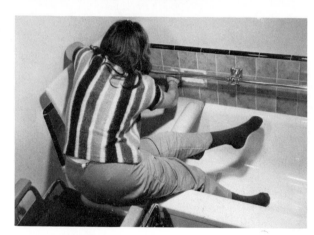

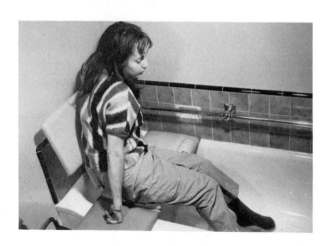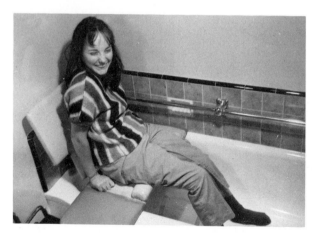

TRANSFERRING FROM BATHSEAT TO CHAIR

When the patient is ready to transfer from the bathseat to chair he spreads a flannelette sheet over his chair to absorb all moisture, particularly from the perineal area which would be difficult to dry otherwise.

FIGURE 5-18

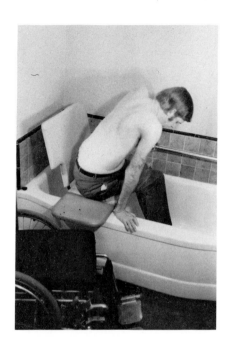
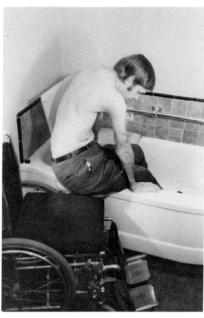
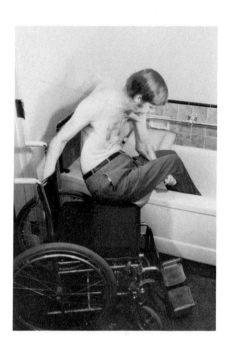

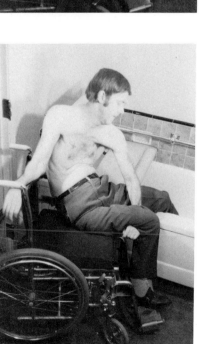
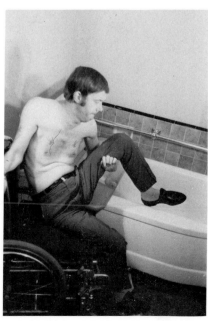

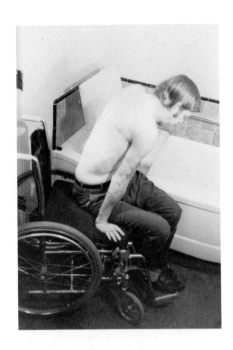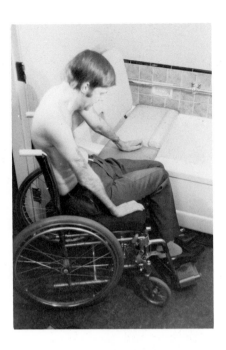

Method 1. (Fig. 5-18) The patient who must lean forward in order to move back will leave both legs in the bathtub for stability. Since a good deal of his weight is taken through his legs when he leans forward, the effort used to move back is lessened. He moves back until his legs meet the side of the bathtub; at this point he may lift one leg out and move back further before lifting the second leg out or he may lift both legs out. If the patient lifts both legs out, his buttocks will twist towards the chair. If he then turns his trunk towards the bathtub, his knees will act as a fulcrum against the side of the bathtub and help to pivot him into the chair.

Method 2. (Fig. 5-19) An alternative method is to leave both legs in the bathtub and, by continuing to move back, the legs straighten and slide onto the bathtub rim. They are lowered when the patient is back in his chair. This method is suitable for the patient with flaccid legs, who is able to maintain stability while he leans forward but is unable to lift the legs out in this position.

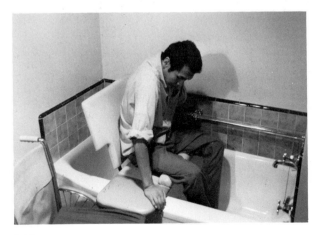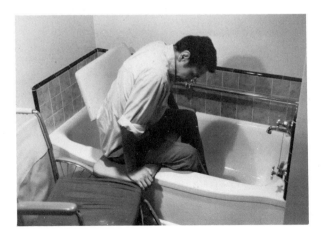

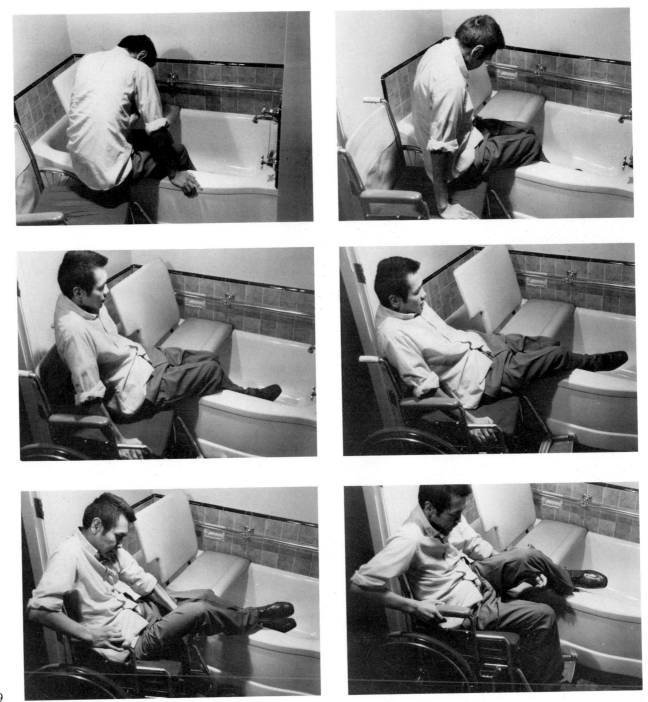

FIGURE 5-19

Method 3. (Fig. 5-20) Lifting both feet out of the bathtub first provides a pulling action, which helps to move the patient towards the chair. As he turns away from the chair, the knees become a fulcrum against the bathtub so that further movement will pivot him into the chair.

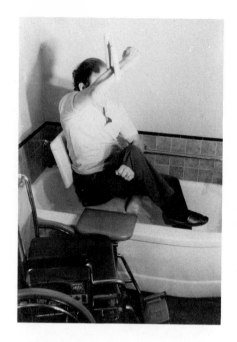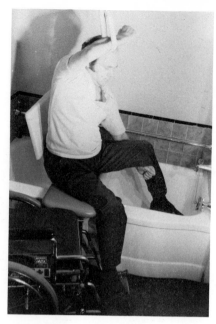

FIGURE 5-20

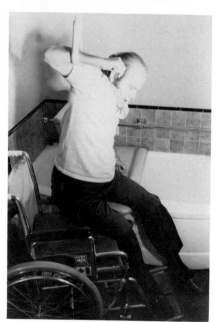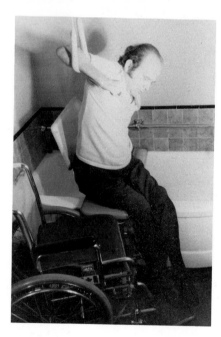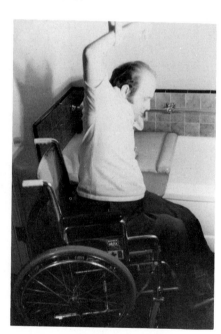

Method 4. (Fig. 5-21) The patient shifts along the bathseat and turns his back towards the chair. He lifts his legs onto the seat and moves further back

towards the chair. When lifting his legs he may place his feet against the wall with his knees flexed. This will assist him to move back. When he is seated in the chair he unlocks the brakes, wheels back far enough to swing the footrests into position, and lowers his legs.

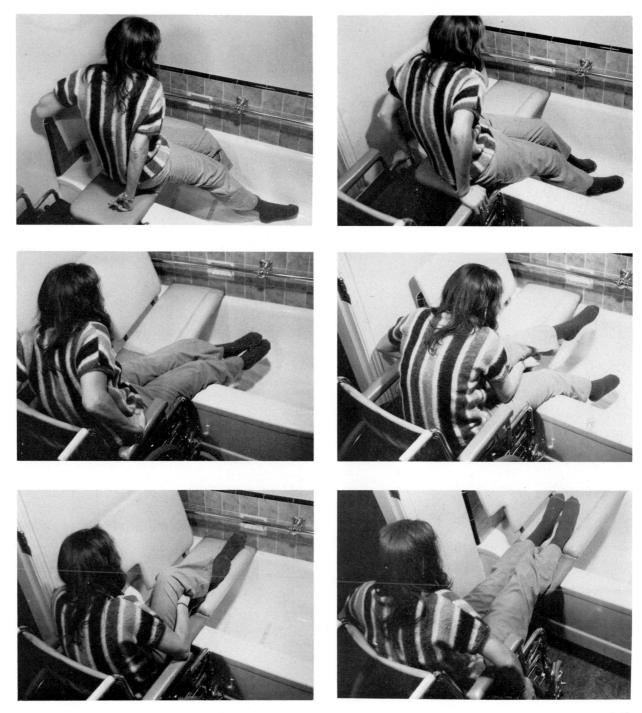

FIGURE 5-21

143

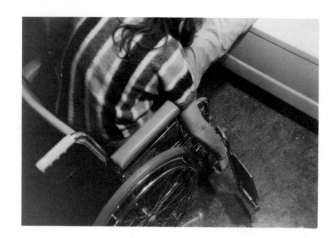

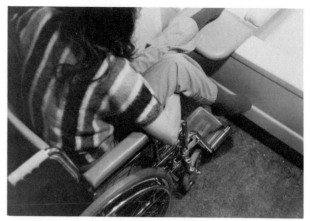

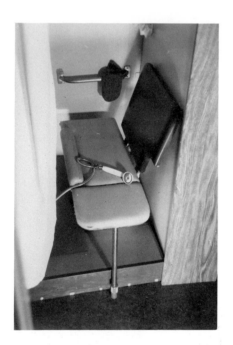

CABINET SHOWER

A bathseat, as previously described, adapted for use in a commercially available cabinet shower, must protrude through the doorway of the shower providing a bridge board from the wheelchair into the shower (Fig. 5-22). The shower seat must be provided with legs to bring it to the correct height.

DAILY WASH

If the patient can approach the basin so that his knees are underneath, the bottom of the basin and the drain pipe must be insulated. A side approach may be necessary for some patients because of bathroom design. In both cases the patient must be able to reach the taps; the taps should be lever type or adapted to the patient's needs. The patient should fill the basin with water and check the temperature rather than leave the tap running. Soap and washcloth must be within reach. The washcloth or bath mitt may be wrung out by squeezing between the heels of the hands or pressed against the wash basin.

All areas should be washed except the buttock area. The feet may be washed with the leg resting on the opposite knee, with the feet on the footrests, or with the feet on a footstool of convenient height. The patient dries himself as thoroughly as possible using a towel, a dry bath mitt, or a towel with a pocket sewn into the ends. He then transfers onto a flannelette sheet on the bed. This will absorb any further moisture. He washes buttocks and perineum on the bed as described in Chapter 7. The daily skin check must not be overlooked on completion of this routine.

FIGURE 5-22

6
Dressing and Undressing

The quadriplegic patient should clothe his upper half while sitting in the wheelchair because this position provides better balance than does long sitting on the bed. Feet can remain on the bed or on the footrests of the wheelchair, depending on the ability of the patient to stabilize himself. The order of dressing must be worked out in order to eliminate unnecessary manoeuvering. For instance, if the patient goes to the toilet in the morning, he should dress his upper body in the chair, go to the bathroom, and then dress his lower body. If he has his legs in position to put his pants over his feet but uses another position to pull them over his buttocks, he should put both underpants and pants on over his feet before changing the position.

EQUIPMENT

A loop may be sewn onto a garment to enable the patient to pull by hooking a thumb or finger into it. The loop should be sewn so that it remains open (Fig. 6-1). Loops should match the material as closely as possible for better cosmesis.

FIGURE 6-1.

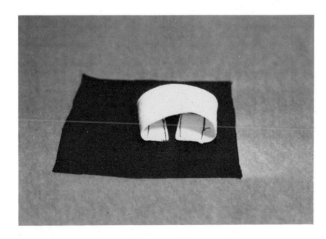
A, Centre loop

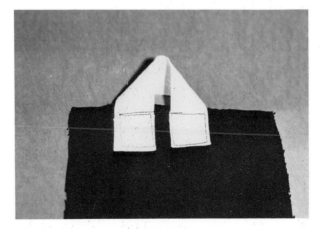
B, Edge loop.

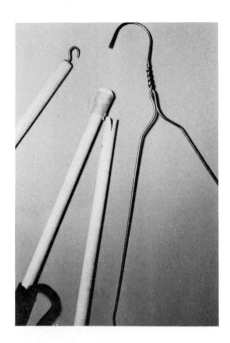

A dressing stick may be useful for the patient who lacks range, strength, or balance to reach extremities (Fig. 6-2). The length must be adjusted to the individual, but being as short as possible. The handle may have to be adapted so that it can be firmly held. Sticks for pulling require a hook; sticks for pushing require a V cut or a padded nonslip end. A wire coat hanger, pulled so that it is elongated, may often suffice as a temporary but effective pulling stick. Usually dressing sticks are used only in the early stages of training.

SHIRTS AND BLOUSES

PUTTING ON

Shirts should have large armholes and loose cuffs. Women will be unable to manage blouses with back openings. Strong material is necessary, particularly while the patient is learning to dress. Sport shirts worn outside the pants are easiest to put on for general wear as they eliminate tucking in.

The method chosen depends upon the patient's ability to balance and the time spent on fastening the shirt. The reach-round-the-back method will be used by the patient with excellent balance and good shoulder musculature. The methods employing a throwing action require fair balance and practice. Although a buttoned shirt must be larger and can be harder to put on and take off, this may be compensated for by the time saved in fastening and unfastening.

Method 1. The very low-lesion patient may be able to put a shirt on in a normal fashion, slipping one arm into a sleeve and reaching behind his back with the other arm to the second sleeve.

Method 2. (Fig. 6-3) The patient pushes the sleeve of the shirt completely into position on the arm and shoulder, using tenodesis or a thumb of the other hand hooked into the material. He leans forward to allow the shirt to fall behind the shoulder, working it as far round his back as possible. He reaches behind his neck and hooks thumb or fingers into the collar to pull the shirt further round the back. Leaning forward and balancing with an elbow on the knee or a hand against the front arm upright of the wheelchair, he reaches down behind his back to put the hand into the other armhole and straightens the arm, shaking the sleeve on. He now sits up to arrange the collar and front of the shirt.

FIGURE 6-2

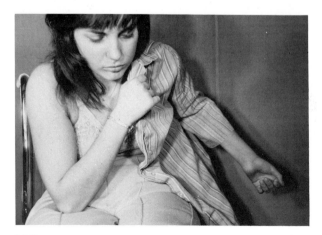

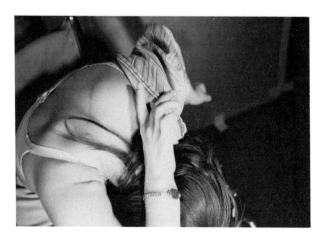

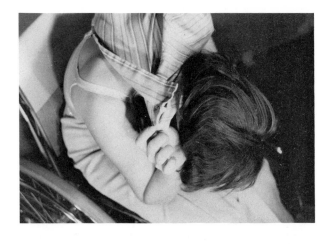
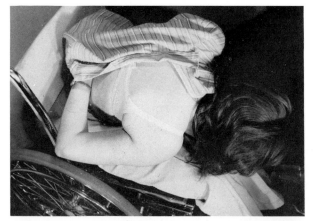
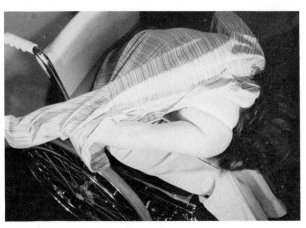
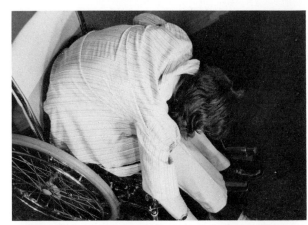

FIGURE 6-3

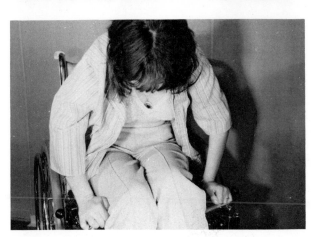

Method 3. (Fig. 6-4) The patient places the back of the shirt on his knees with collar towards him and the front of the shirt opened out. He inserts his arms into the sleeves until the armholes are above the elbows and his hands are free. Placing his hands under the bulk of the shirt across his chest he pushes the shirt away from his chest and flings it up and over his ducked head. At the moment that the shirt

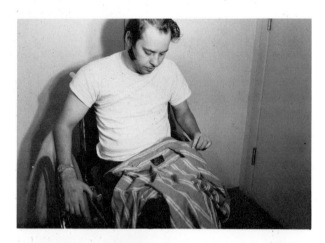

FIGURE 6-4

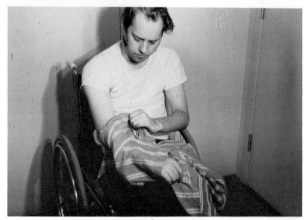
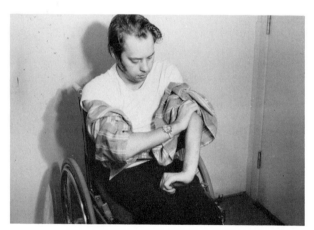

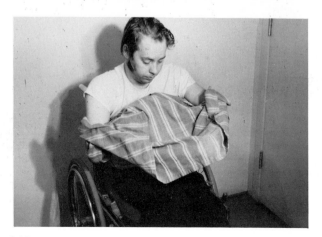
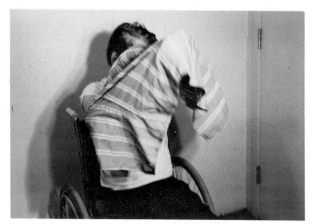

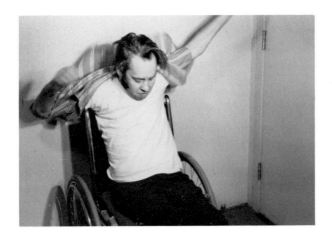
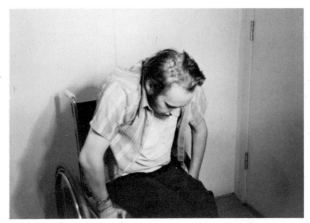

reaches the back of the neck, the arms straighten, allowing the shirt to drop into position on the shoulders. He leans forward to allow the back of the shirt to slip down between his trunk and the chair back.

Method 4.　(Fig. 6-5) In this method the patient places the shirt on his knees with the front down and the collar facing him. He crosses his arms to insert his hands into the armholes. He throws his arms up to flip the shirt over his head uncrossing his arms as he does so. Uncrossing the arms adds momentum and flares the shirt out in a smooth flow to drop in place over the back as he straightens his arms. He leans forward and wiggles his trunk to let the shirt drop down his back.

FIGURE 6-5

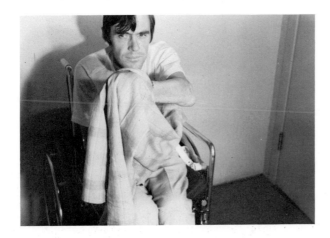
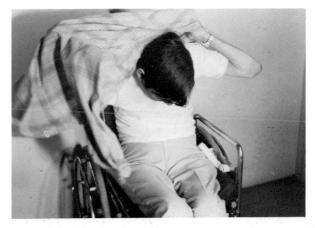

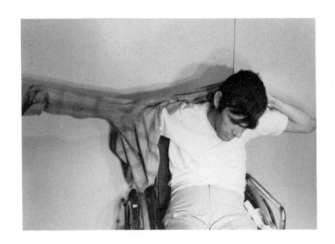 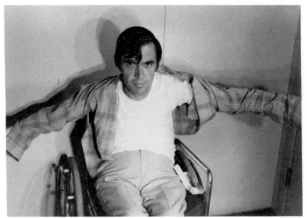

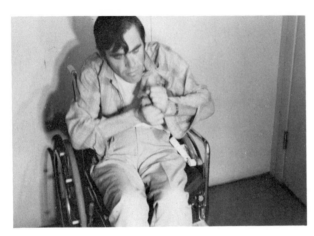

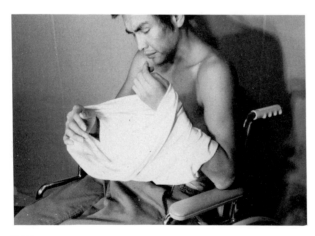 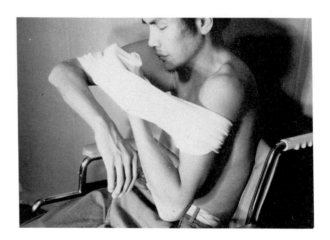

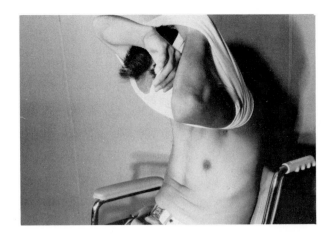
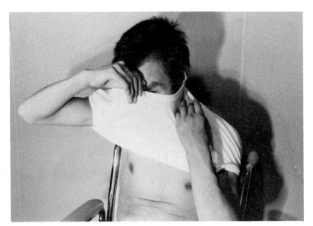
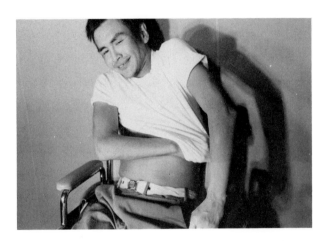

FIGURE 6-6

Method 5. (Fig. 6-6) The patient places the buttoned shirt or T-shirt on his knees inside out and front down with the collar facing him. He inserts his arms until the armholes are above his elbows. He bunches the back of the shirt on his hand and thumb web. He throws his arms up and back so that the collar slips over his head. As he drops his arms down again, the collar is pulled down over his head and he slips his hand inside to pull the shirt into position.

This method may also be used when the shirt is right side out. In this case the shirt is placed front down and with the collar away from the patient. If the shirt has long sleeves this is the easier method.

Method 6. (Fig. 6-7) The patient places the buttoned shirt or T-shirt front down on his knees with the collar facing away from him. He puts his arms into the sleeves and abducting and externally rotating his straight arms, he pushes his hands through the cuffs. He then puts both or one thumb into the collar opening and bunches the back of the shirt onto his thumb web. He can push the shirt onto the crown of his head by pushing up and ducking his head. He forces the shirt to the back of his neck by alternately flexing and extending his neck and then moving his arms down and back. He now leans forward to let the shirt drop down his back.

151

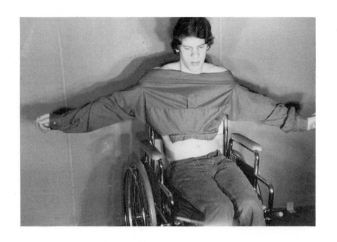
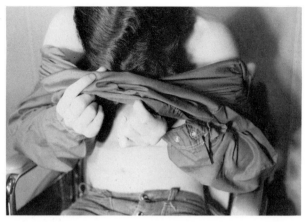
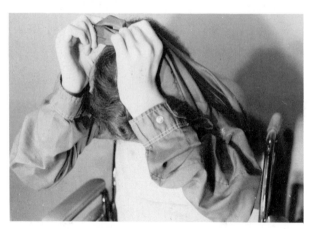
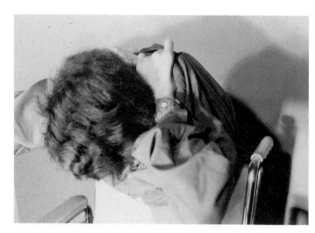
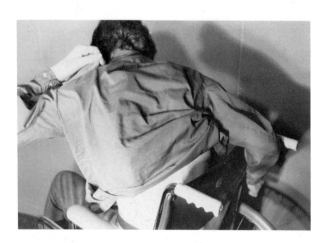
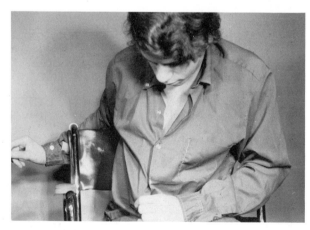

FIGURE 6-7

Method 7. (Fig. 6-8) The dressing stick may be used if the patient lacks range or strength to push the shirt over his head with his hands. In this case he places the shirt on his knees with the collar towards him. He inserts his arms using hands or teeth to pull until the armholes are above his elbows. He now straps the dressing stick to his hand using a velcro D-ring or loop and puts the end under the bulk of the shirt. He works the shirt over his head, flexing and extending his neck while maintaining the pushing action with the dressing stick until the shirt reaches the back of his neck. If necessary balance may be maintained by hooking an arm around the back of the chair. The shirt will drop down the back when the patient leans forward. He can then hook a thumb into the facing to arrange the front of the shirt.

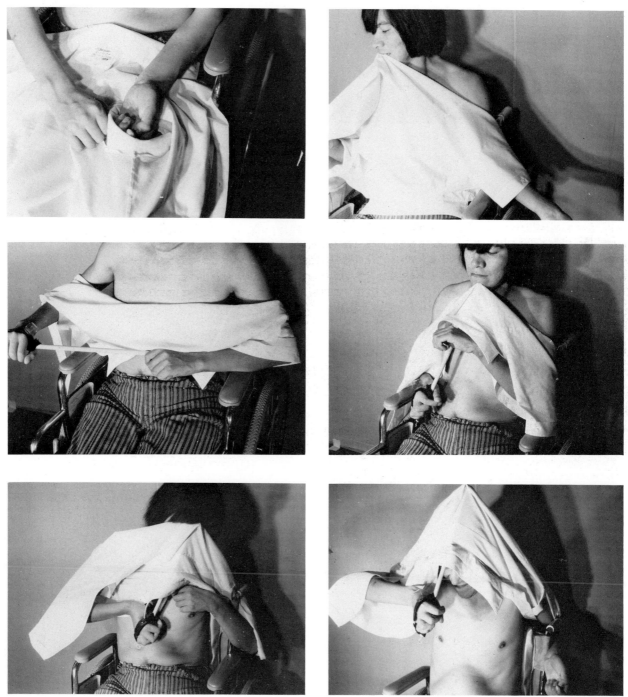

FIGURE 6-8

153

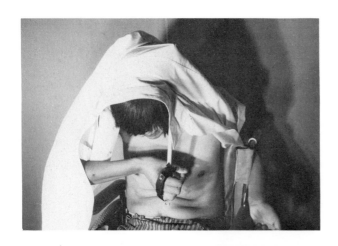

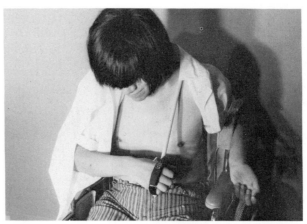

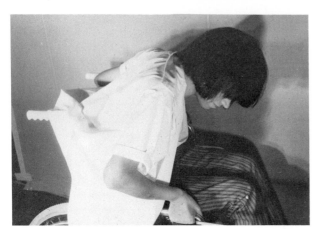

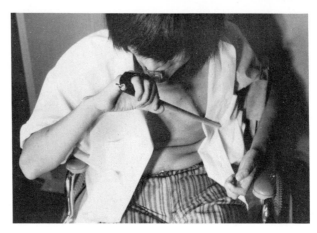

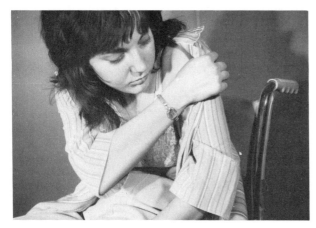

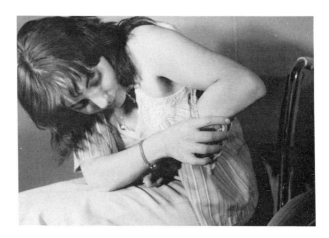

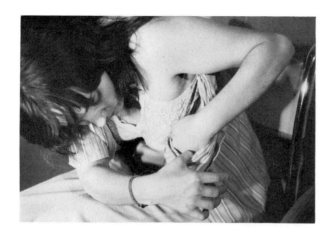 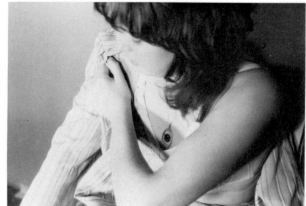

FIGURE 6-9

REMOVING

Method 1. (Fig. 6-9) The shirt must be unbuttoned and opened out. The thumb on the dominant side is inserted under the shirt near the opposite shoulder and pushes the material off the shoulder and down the arm past the elbow. The shoulder is shrugged to assist in this manoeuver. When the elbow is flexed and the shoulder is extended, the sleeve will slide down the arm until it can be shaken off the hand. The bulk of the shirt is thrown behind the chair, and the sleeve is pushed off the other arm in a similar manner.

Method 2. (Fig. 6-10) This method may be used with shirts with roomy armholes, T-shirts, or sweaters. The patient puts his hand inside the shirt and pulls the armhole down to slip it over the flexed elbow and pulls his arm out of the sleeve. He takes the other sleeve off in a similar manner. He pulls the shirt from his head by bunching the front of the shirt round his hands and pulling up and forwards.

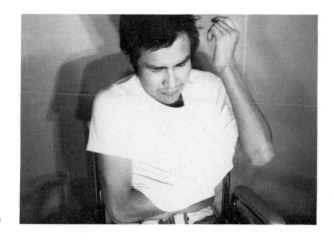 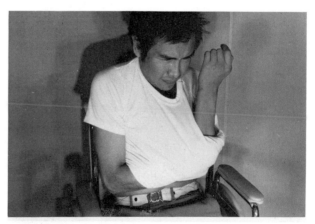

FIGURE 6-10

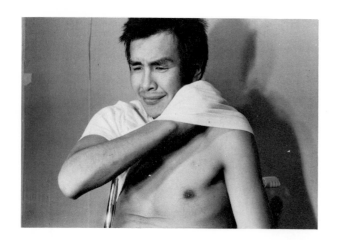

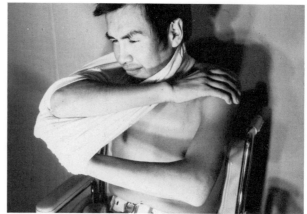

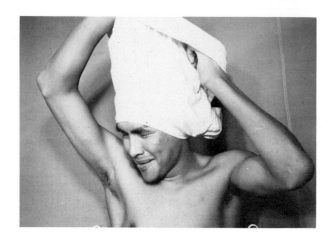

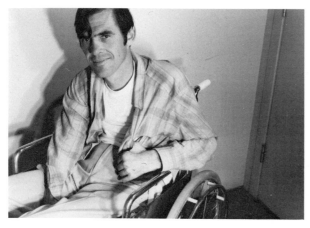

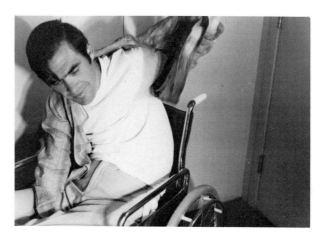

FIGURE 6-11

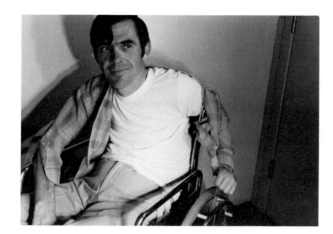
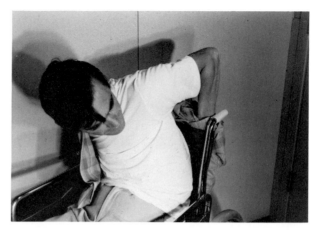

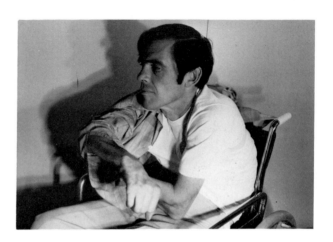

Method 3. (Fig. 6-11) The shirt is unbuttoned, and the thumb is hooked into the facing on the lower part of the shirt front. He flings this arm over the back of the chair and catches the armhole of the shirt on the pushing handle of the wheelchair. By leaning forward and lifting the elbow, he removes his arm from the sleeve. As he pushes the remaining sleeve off, a forward bouncing action of the trunk may be necessary to release the shirt back from between his trunk and the wheelchair.

Method 4. (Fig. 6-12) The patient pushes the front of the buttoned shirt or T-shirt up until it is bunched across his chest at armpit level. He inserts his thumb or thumbs under the material so that the front of the shirt rests on his thumb web. He then pushes it over his head, flexing and extending his neck to work the material to the back of his neck. He places one arm over the back of the chair and hooks the armhole of the shirt onto the pushing handle of the wheelchair. By leaning forwards, he pulls the sleeve down the arm until it is below the elbow. The sleeve can then be shaken off this arm. The other sleeve is easily removed by hooking the free hand into the armhole and pulling it downwards.

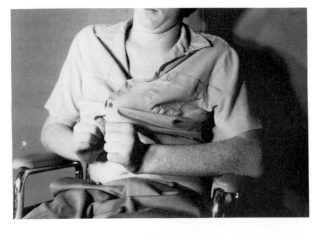 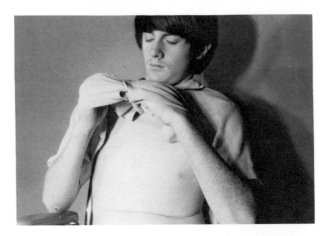

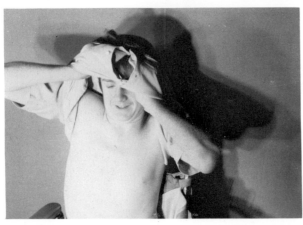 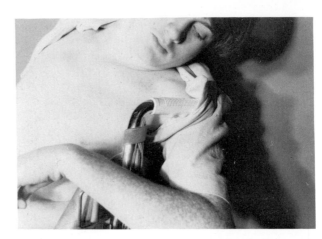

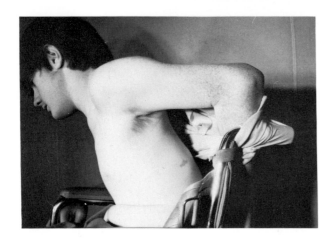 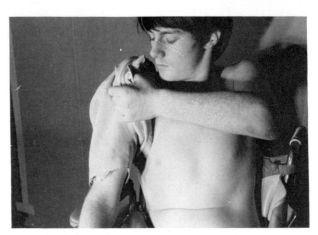

FIGURE 6-12

158

Method 5. (Fig. 6-13) This method may be used with a buttoned shirt or with a pullover. The patient hooks one arm behind the pushing handle of the wheelchair for stability. He reaches behind his neck with the other hand, and hooks under the collar with his thumb. A loop across the inside collar back, sewn so that it remains open, may be required during the learning process. The patient ducks his head and pulls forward while allowing his trunk to swing slightly forward to release the back of the shirt. He maintains his pull on the collar while alternately flexing and extending his neck. He continues this until the shirt is pulled over his head. It is now simple to pull the sleeves off by using his hands or teeth.

FIGURE 6-13

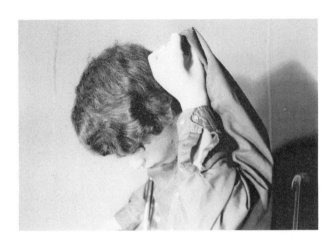
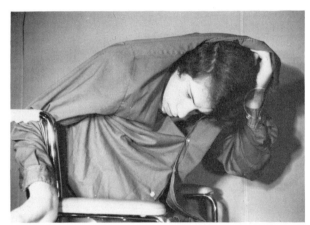
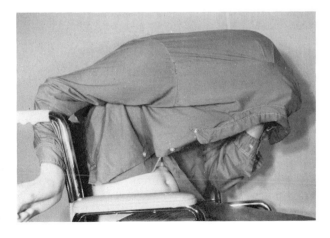
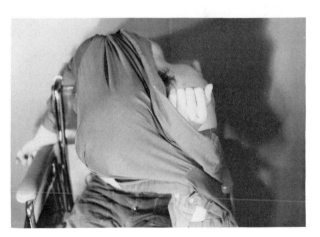

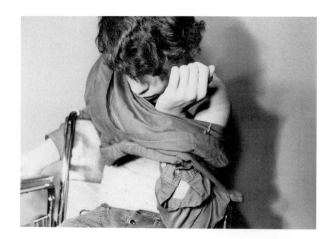

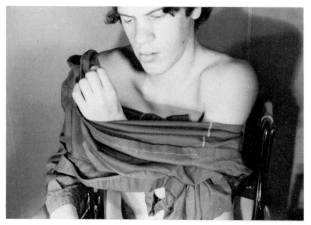

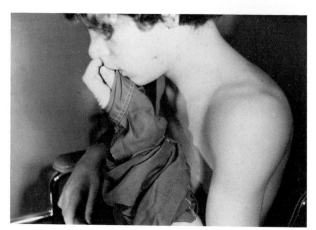

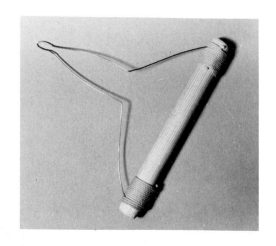

FASTENING

Buttonholes should be vertical and large enough to permit easy insertion of the button. A flat button is easiest to manage, particularly if it has a sewn shank.

Equipment

Very simple aids to dressing may be easily made. Several types of buttonhooks are described here.

A 4½-inch length of a ½-inch hardwood dowel and about 11 inches of 12 gauge music wire are used in this hook. The wire should be bent to shape and the ends inserted through holes drilled near the end of the dowel and bent back (Fig. 6-14). Whipping of the bent ends serves two purposes—both covering the sharp ends and preventing them from moving. The design permits the throat of the buttonhook to accommodate any size of buttonhole without strain. The handle may require adaptation for a firm hold.

A length of ¼-inch hardwood dowel and about 7 inches of 12 gauge music wire are required for a second type of hook. Two holes are drilled down at

FIGURE 6-14

160

opposite obtuse angles from the centre of the dowel, so that the drill breaks through the sides about ¾-inch down. The wire is bent to shape and the ends inserted into the holes. After bending the ends upwards, the wire and dowel may be covered with whipping. The handle may require adaptation (Fig. 6-15A). The angle may be varied if required (Fig. 6-15B).

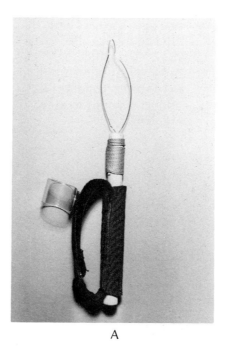

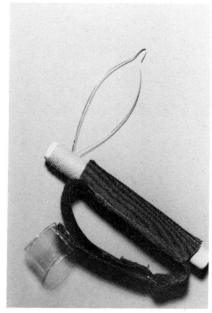

FIGURE 6-15

A

B

A 5-inch length of ½-inch 14 gauge stainless steel or tempered aluminum is cut. Ten inches will be required if it is to be bent into a loop handle. The tip is ground to half the gauge, and a ¼-inch hole is drilled in the centre leaving ⅛-inch of material at the end. A cut ⅛-inch wide is made from the edge to the hole, and all edges are smoothed. The handle may be bent into a loop to fit the hand, or otherwise adapted for a firm hold (Fig. 6-16).

One-inch velcro squares may be substituted for buttons (Fig. 6-17). The top velcro is invisibly sewn and the button is resewn in the buttonhole so that the shirt appears to be buttoned.

Open-ended zippers such as those on jackets are very hard to start and may require velcro strips as a substitute.

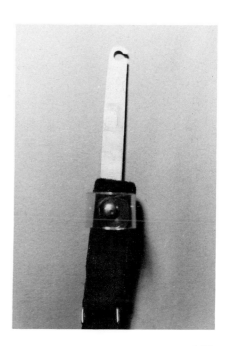

FIGURE 6-16

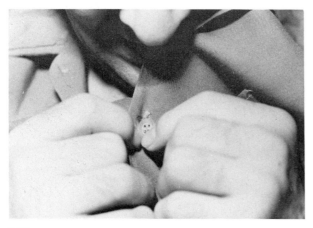

FIGURE 6-17

Procedures

The shirt button may be held, using tenodesis or remaining finger function, and worked through a buttonhole held in the same manner (Fig. 6-18A). Teeth may be used to hold the facing taut while buttoning (Fig. 6-18B). Many Western style shirts have press studs instead of buttons. These may be easier for some patients to manage. The heel of the hand may be pressed against a rigid thumb, chest wall, or the heel of the other hand (Fig. 6-18C).

The patient who can control his arm best when it is by his side, making it possible for him to pull in a horizontal plane, will use the hook shown in Fig. 6-19A. The handle may require adaption for a firm hold. The patient who can abduct his arms to reach the higher buttons may prefer the buttonhook shown in Fig. 6-19B.

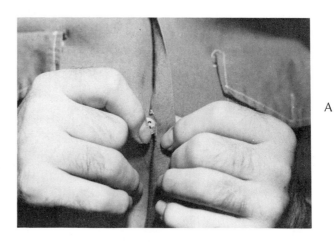

A

FIGURE 6-18

B

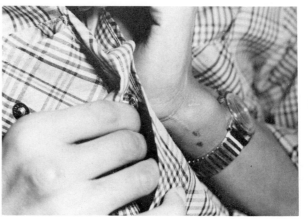

C

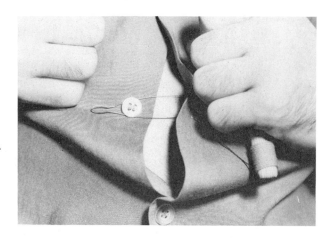
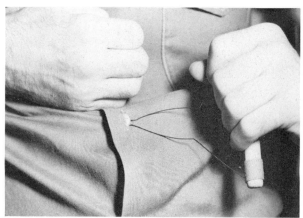

A

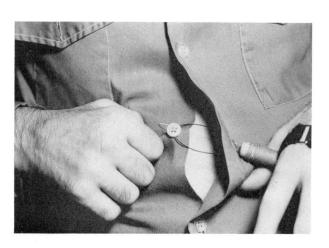
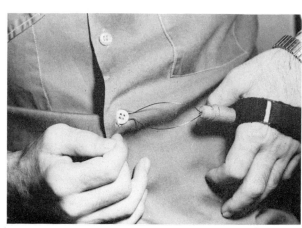

B

FIGURE 6-19

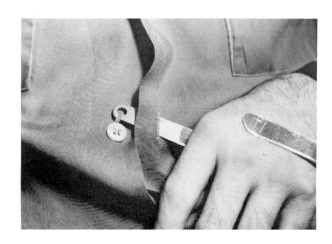
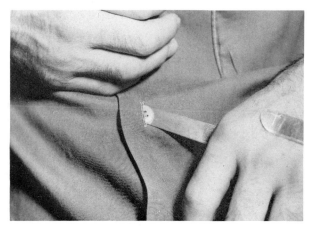

FIGURE 6-20

163

The stainless steel or aluminum buttonhook is not as easy to use as the wire buttonhooks for buttoning but is easier to use for unbuttoning (Fig. 6-20). Velcro squares may be pressed together by using tenodesis, the heels of the hands, or a rigid finger (Fig. 6-21).

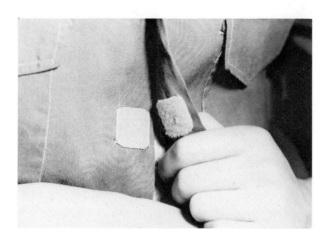 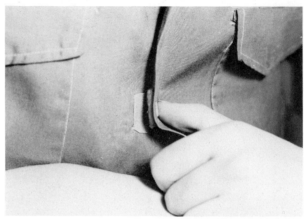

FIGURE 6-21

Cuff Buttons

Cuff buttons are more difficult to manage than shirt front buttons because only one hand and the teeth are available for fastening and unfastening. The simplest method is having a cuff loose enough to permit the hand to pass through without unfastening. If it is not loose enough, the button may be moved closer to the edge or may be sewn with an elastic shank to permit the cuff to expand. If cuff links are used they may be replaced with a cuff link made of two buttons sewn with an elastic shank between them.

The cuff may be fastened by using a buttonhook in one hand while the teeth are used to pull the buttonhole over the button. A velcro fastening may also be used on the cuff.

UNFASTENING

In one technique, a thumb or finger is inserted into the shirt front opening under the button and holds the button in position while the other hand pulls the buttonhole down over it (Fig. 6-22A). Another means is to insert a thumb or finger into the shirt front opening and hold the buttonhole firm while the button is pushed out with a finger or fingernail of the other hand (Fig 6-22B).

If the buttonhole is quite loose, it may be worked over the button with one thumb behind the facing (Fig. 6-23A). Additionally, a thumbnail may be used to lift one side of the button, forcing the other side down through the buttonhole (Fig. 6-23B). The teeth may be used to hold the facing taut while the button is undone (Fig. 6-23C).

164

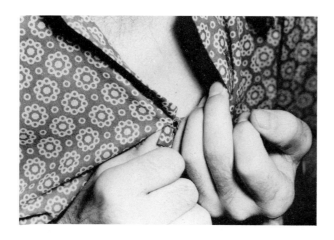

FIGURE 6-22

A

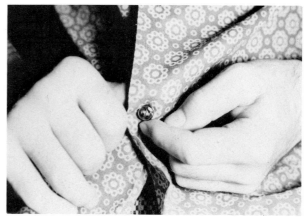

B

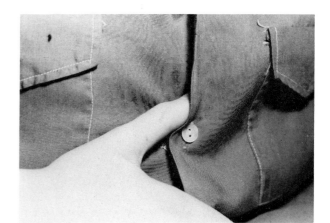

A

FIGURE 6-23

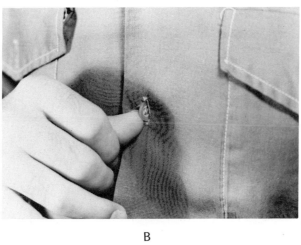

B

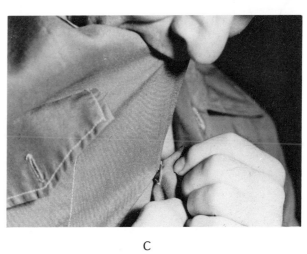

C

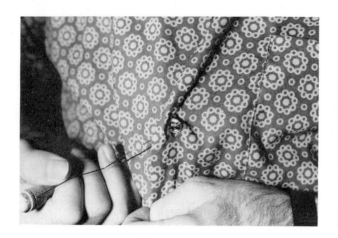

FIGURE 6-24

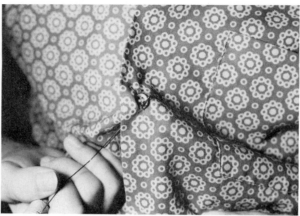

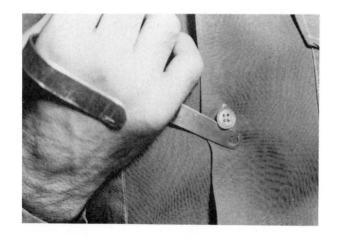

FIGURE 6-25

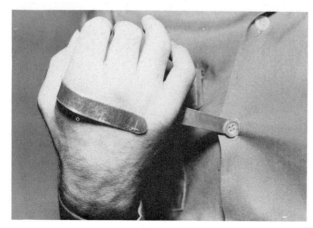

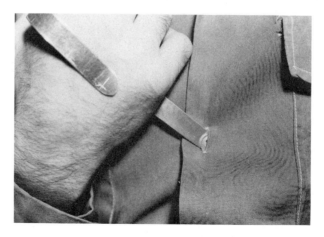

If a buttonhook is used, it is pushed into the buttonhole and then turned so that it lies half over the button. This lifts the buttonhole on one side and permits the button to slide out (Fig. 6–24). If a patient has more difficulty unbuttoning than buttoning, the stainless steel or aluminum hook should be used (Fig. 6–25).

Press studs are very simple to pull apart with the thumb or a finger (Fig. 6-26). Velcro squares may be pulled apart easily with thumb or fingers (Fig. 6-27). The velcro should be closed before laundering or lint will accumulate preventing closure.

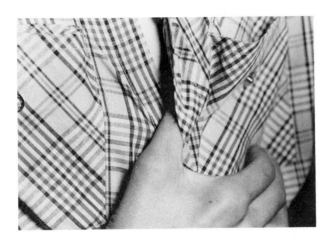 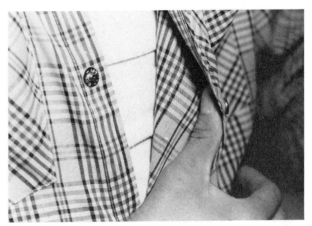

FIGURE 6-26

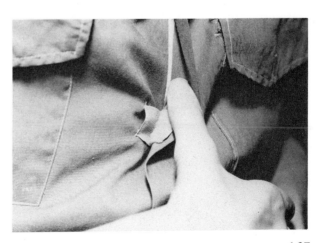

FIGURE 6-27

BRASSIERES

Brassieres should have a narrow band and should be a fairly loose fit for easier fastening. Back-hooked brassieres will always be fastened in front and then turned to the back. An advantage of this brassiere is the small number of hooks necessary for a good fit. Front-hooked brassieres may be used by preference or because the patient is unable to turn a conventional brassiere fastening to the back. Difficulty in turning the brassiere may be aggravated by the excessive perspiration that sometimes occurs in quadriplegics, especially in the early stages of rehabilitation. A brassiere that hooks in the front is usually fastened around the waist before positioning the straps because the waist is usually the smallest section of the torso in circumference and vision is less obscured. Stretch brassieres are difficult for most patients to manage because, if the brassieres are not fairly tight, small women find they slide up during activity. Larger women may have trouble positioning this type of brassiere.

ADAPTATIONS

A large hook such as a pant's hook may be substituted for normal hooks (Fig. 6-28A). This hook must be used only in a front-hooking brassiere because it will create a pressure area on the back when the patient leans against the chair. Loops may be sewn to the brassiere under the hooks and eyes so that the thumbs can be inserted (Fig. 6-28B). The hooks may need to be opened a little. A loop may be sewn or temporarily tied to one of the loops, long enough so that it may be hooked over the chair arm.

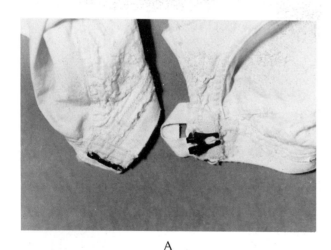

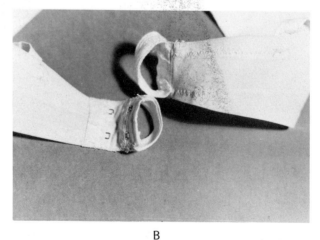

A   B

FIGURE 6-28

A front-hooked brassiere may be adapted, or a brassiere with a hooked back may be converted to a front-hooked brassiere, by cutting and binding the seam between the cups. The band is fastened with a velcro D-ring, the hook velcro facing out, and a thumb loop is attached near the free end (Fig. 6-29A). The upper part may be fastened with large or small hooks with thumb loops under the hooks and under the eyes. A velcro D-ring fastening is easy to align and is a firm fastening. It should not be used at the back because of the probability of creating a pressure area. A velcro closure with no D-ring is not a reliable fastening for a brassiere. A length of elastic may be inserted into the brassiere shoulder straps to enable the patient to push them onto her shoulders and to assist in keeping them in place.

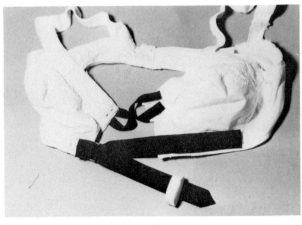

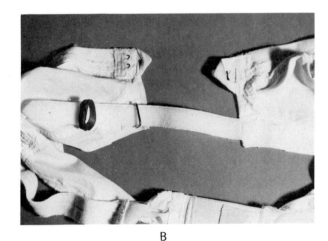

FIGURE 6-29

A   B

PUTTING ON

Method 1. (Fig. 6-30) The patient places the brassiere on her knee with the top towards her and the outside up. She hooks thumb or fingers of one hand into the strap on that side and leans forward maintaining balance with the other arm. She now pushes the brassiere around her back as far as possible. She changes arms and leaning forward again she reaches behind her back for the released strap. When there is lack of sensation or position sense in the hand, this may take practice and she may have to observe movement in the part of the brassiere which remains at the front, indicating that she has caught the loose end. Care must be taken not to pull the strap too far around.

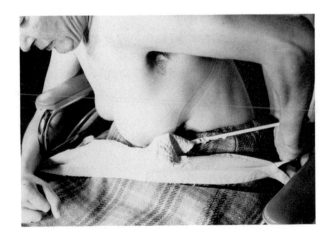

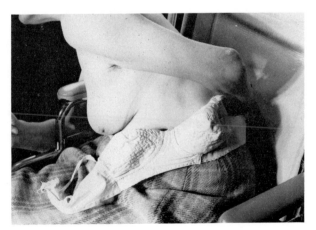

FIGURE 6-30

169

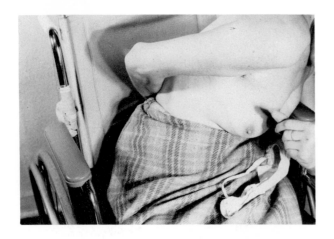 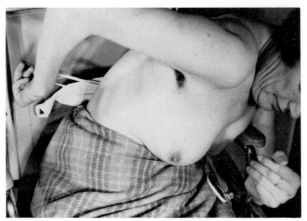

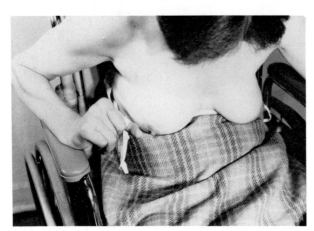

Method 2.   (Fig. 6-31) The brassiere is placed on the lap with the inside facing upwards and the shoulder straps towards the patient. The patient hooks the straps into thumbs or fingers, and flings the brassiere over her head, releasing one strap only when the brassiere is down her back and level with the wheelchair pushing handles. She reaches under her shoulder to retrieve the straps and pulls the brassiere down her back by bouncing her trunk forward in the chair and using a sawing motion with her hands. Some patients are unable to bounce forwards while their hands are in use. These patients must let go of the straps and pull themselves forward. The brassiere, if well placed, then slides down the back.

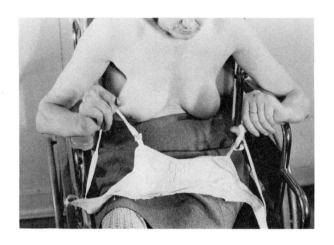
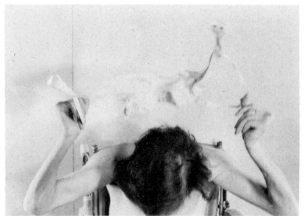
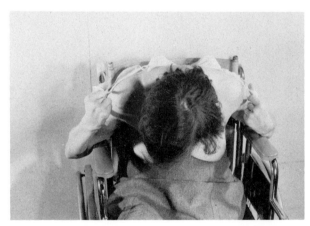
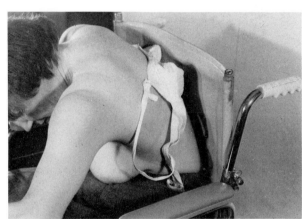
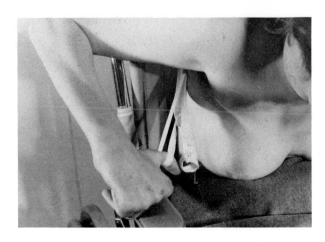
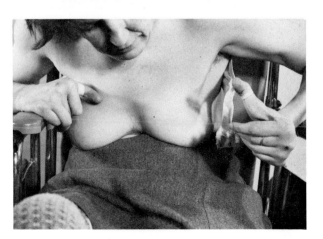

FIGURE 6-31

Method 3. (Fig. 6-32) The patient places the brassiere on her lap with the top towards her and the inside up, and slides her wrists down through the straps. She now hooks her thumbs under the brassiere and pushes it over her head. If she lacks range or power she may require a dressing stick to accomplish this. Without releasing the straps she works the brassiere down her back.

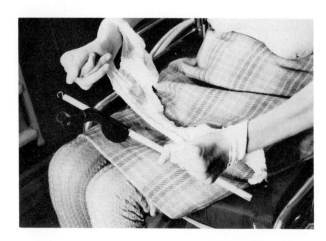

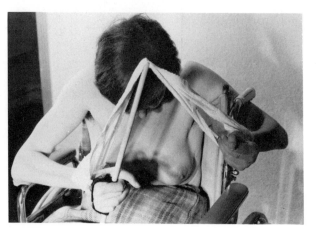

FIGURE 6-32

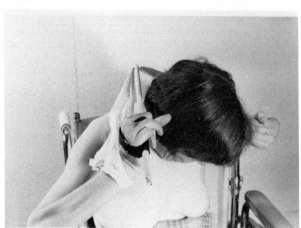

FASTENING

Method 1. (Fig. 6-33) The thumbs are inserted into the thumb loops and the ends are brought together for fastening. If the thumbs are rigid the hooks and eyes can be placed on the base of the backs of the thumbs so they can be easily opposed.

Method 2. (Fig. 6-34) If only one hand can be effectively used, the thumb may be hooked into one thumb loop while the other longer loop is hooked over the armrest. The free hand is placed under the fastening to bring it forward into position for fastening.

172

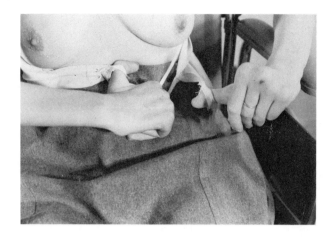
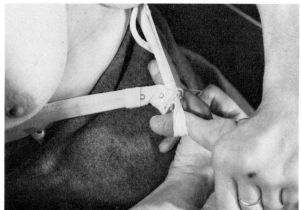

FIGURE 6-33

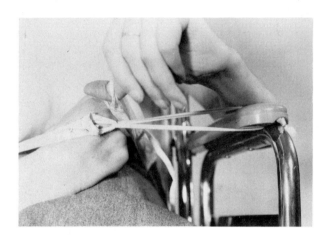

FIGURE 6-34

Method 3. (Fig. 6-35) The end of the velcro strap is threaded through the D-ring using the heels of both hands or a thumb hooked through a loop placed an inch or so back from the tip of the strap. The tip is then pulled using the heels of the hands until the loop is through the D-ring. The lower band of the brassiere is placed in position with the other thumb and the strap is pulled by the loop until the opening is closed before allowing the velcro strap to touch the opposing hook velcro. Once the bottom band is secure the top hook is easy to fasten since there is no strain on it. This may be accomplished using thumb loops under hooks and eyes or a short velcro D-ring fastening.

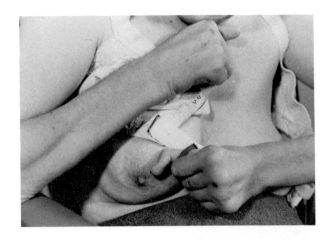 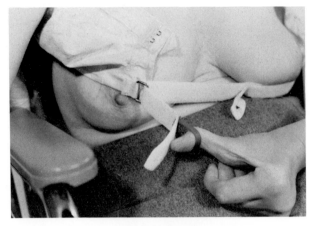

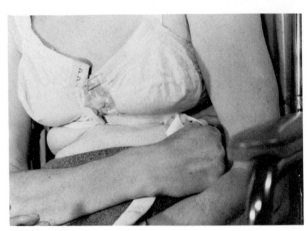 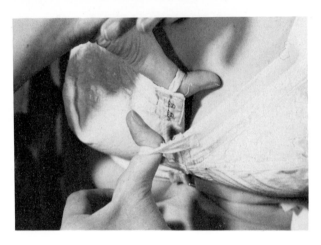

FIGURE 6-35

TURNING A BACK-HOOKED BRASSIERE AND PLACING STRAPS

After the hooks are fastened, the brassiere is turned around into position by pulling and pushing on the shoulder straps (Fig. 6-36). If possible, it should be turned so that the hooks pull into the eyes, i.e., to the left. When the brassiere is straight, one strap is hooked onto the opposite thumb web and either the elbow or the hand inserted through the strap. The other arm is inserted also and both straps are pushed up onto the shoulders. A dressing stick is occasionally required to enable a woman who does not have sufficient strength, who has restricted movement, or who is obese.

174

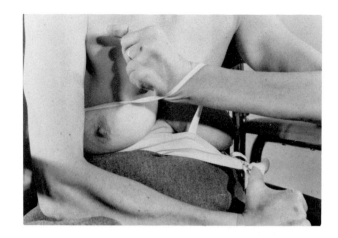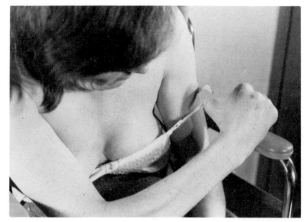

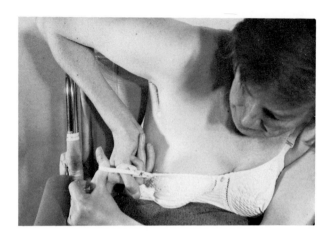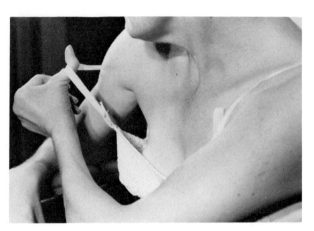

FIGURE 6-36

REMOVING

The brassiere strap is removed from the shoulder by hooking a thumb into it and pushing out and down (Fig. 6-37). The shoulder is extended when the strap reaches the elbow, slipping the forearm and hand out of the strap. Some patients, when the strap is nearly at the elbow, flex the elbow and remove the hand from the strap. The strap slides off the arm when the elbow is extended and the shoulder flexed. Then the other strap is removed. A brassiere with back hooks is turned by the straps so that the opening is at the front, ready to be unfastened.

UNDERPANTS AND PANTS

Jockey shorts may be used for male patients, because they do not wrinkle or bunch in the crotch as boxer shorts do. They provide good support, which assists in keeping the urine collection apparatus in position. For ease in placement and removal, open loops may be sewn at the waistband, one on either side forward of the side seams. Sometimes an additional loop at the back will be necessary. Obese patients may be able to wear boxer shorts only.

175

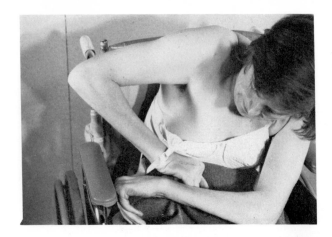
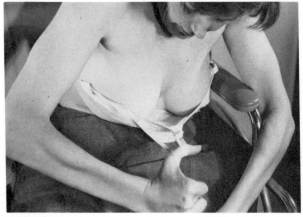

FIGURE 6-37

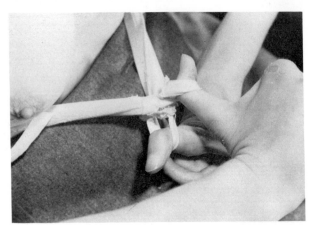

A loose knit cotton type of pantie is recommended for women. The afore-mentioned loops may be added if necessary. It is bad practice not to wear underpants as the softer material protects the patient from pressure areas and abrasions and absorbs perspiration. If there is difficulty in pulling the pantie on, a slippery material may be used instead, although this will not absorb perspiration well.

Outer pants should be on the large side, both for ease in putting on and for comfort when sitting. They should be made of a material that will enable the patient to slide easily, for instance a cotton-terylene mix. For comfort and cosmesis dress pants may be tailored to fit a seated person. Women will find a front fastening zipper easier to manage than a side zipper. A back zipper is contraindicated because it will be most difficult to zip up and may cause a pressure area.

PUTTING ON

Method 1. (Fig. 6-38) The low-lesion patient may put his pants on while in the chair. To gain stability he may first slide forward in his chair. He begins the technique either crossing one leg over the other knee or holding a leg up with his wrist. He slides his foot into the pant leg and pulls the waist over his knee. He puts

176

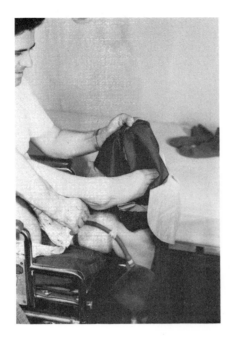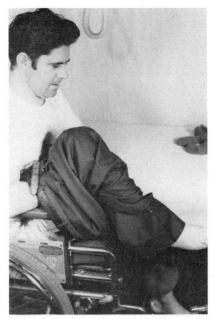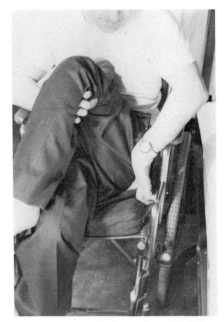

FIGURE 6-38

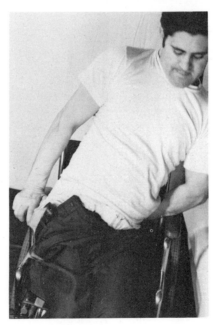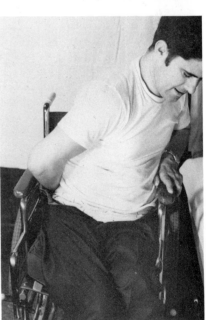

his foot on the footrest and repeats the procedure with the other leg. He tucks his pants as far under his buttocks as possible, lifting his legs alternately to do so. He now holds his pants at the side, using tenodesis or an extended wrist inside and under the waistband, and places his forearm on the armrest. As he does a quick pushup with the other arm, the armrest becomes a fulcrum, assisting his pull on the pants and also levering his buttocks up to enable the waistband to be pulled up.

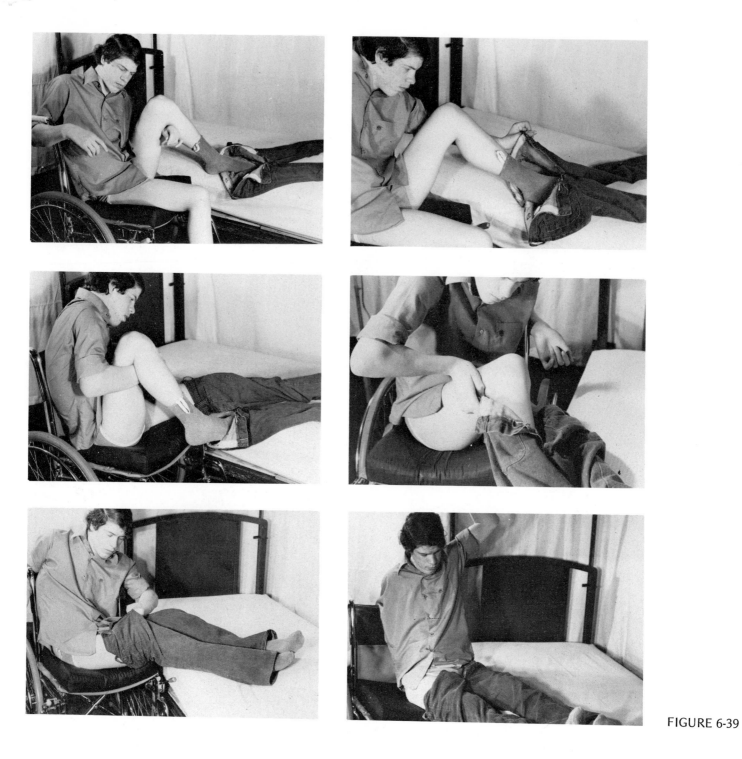

FIGURE 6-39

Method 2. (Fig. 6-39) In this method the patient sits in the chair with the chair in transfer position by the bed. He places his pants on the bed with the waist open in position to receive a foot when he lifts it onto the bed. He now holds the pants so that they do not move while his foot slips into the pant leg. The foot may require more than the force of gravity to slide it into the pant leg; in this case leaning forward may cause the knee to straighten or a push on the knee, internally or externally rotating the hip, will direct the foot down the correct pant leg. If necessary the leg and pant leg may be lifted together and then the pants held again while the leg slides further down the pant leg. The pant waist is pushed to below the knee so that the other leg can also be slipped into the pant leg. The pants are pulled up as far as possible before the patient transfers to the bed. He completes pulling his pants over his hips on the bed.

Method 3. (Fig. 6-40) The patient sits on the bed and flicks his pants out so that they lie straight in front of him. He inserts a wrist under his calf from the inside so that when he picks his leg up, it is externally rotated with the toe pointing toward the top of his pants. He works the pant leg opening over his foot with his free arm and then places his foot on the bed. While he holds the top of the pants, he allows the weight of the leg to force his foot down through the pant leg. The other leg is inserted in the same way. The pants are pulled up as far as possible by friction of the hands on the material and by a wrist pulling against the crotch. When the pants are pulled up to the buttocks, he leans back on alternate elbows to roll from side to side using the free arm to pull the pants over the hips.

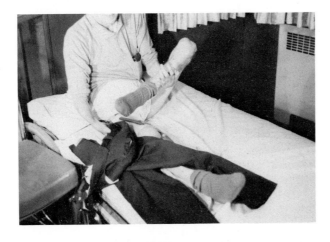
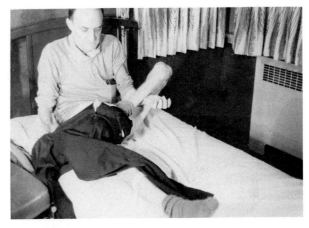
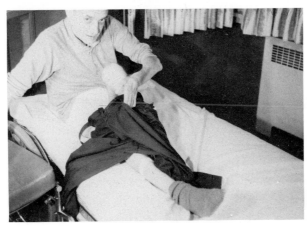
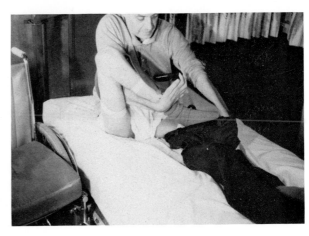

FIGURE 6-40

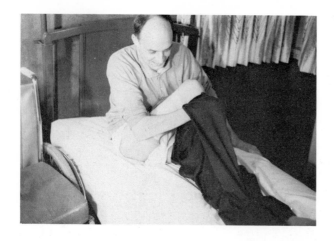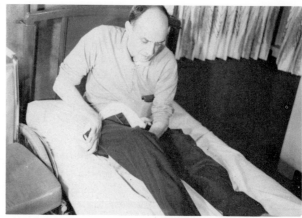

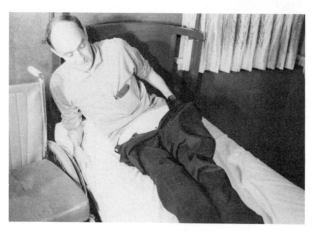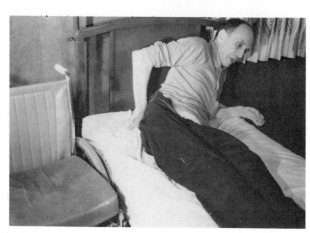

Method 4. (Fig. 6-41) The patient lies on his side on the bed, leaning on an elbow. He reaches down with his free arm to pull his upper leg towards himself and rests the knee on the extended wrist of the lower arm. The free arm is used to pull the pants over the foot and work the material up until the foot is free and the waistband is at the knee. Either the upper or the bottom leg may be inserted into the pants first. The top of the pants is opened so that the other leg can be directed towards the opening and the pants are pulled onto the leg. The pants are pulled up as far as possible by holding the material between the heels of the hands or by using an extended wrist under the waistband and one at the crotch. Then the patient rolls from side to side to pull his pants up.

180

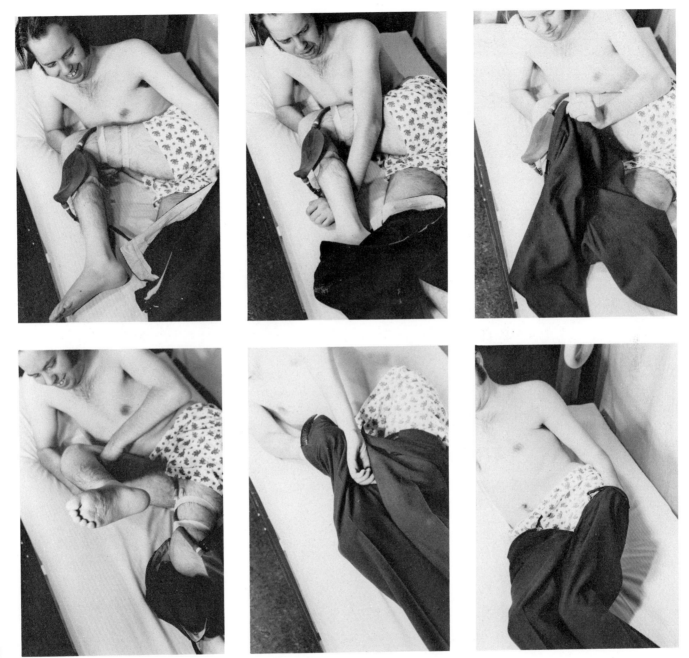

FIGURE 6-41

Method 5. (Fig. 6-42) The patient leans forward with one elbow resting on the bed. He inserts a wrist under his calf and levers his foot off the bed. The other arm pulls the pants over the foot until the waistband is clear of the heel. Still resting on one elbow he uses friction of his two hands in opposition to pull the pant leg up and over his foot. He gathers his pant leg down around his knee to allow the waistband to be scooped around his other foot.

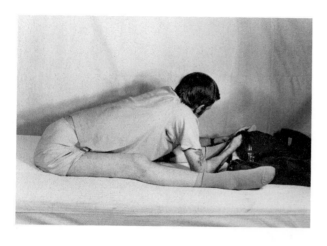
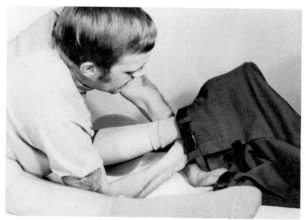

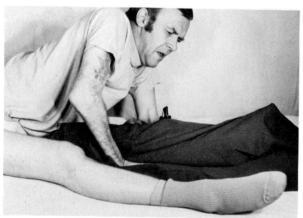
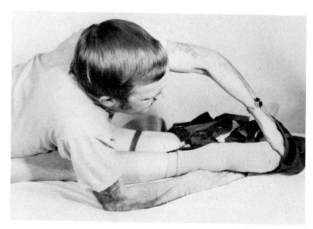

FIGURE 6-42

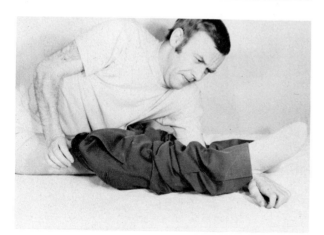

Method 6. (Fig. 6-43) The patient sits up on the bed and hooks his knee with an extended wrist. When he drops back onto the bed his leg is raised towards his chest, enabling him to slip the pants over his foot with the free arm. He works the pants up the leg using hands and teeth. He sits up again and repeats the procedure

with the other leg. The patient may put the pant leg on in the lying position or he may sit up and allow the weight of the leg to help straighten itself and slide into the pant leg. He lies down to roll from side to side to work his pants over his hips.

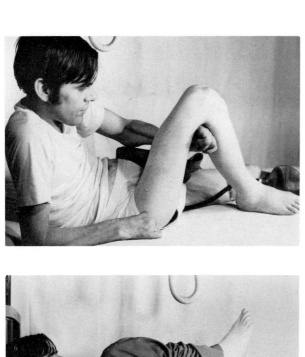
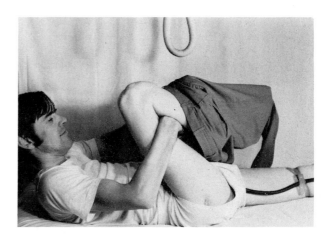
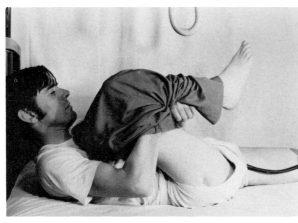
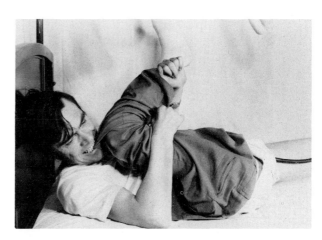
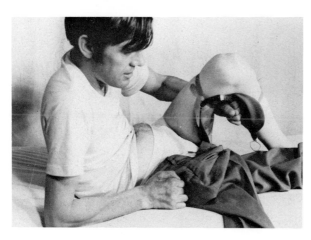
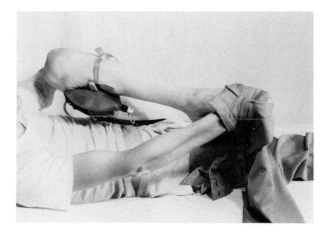

FIGURE 6-43

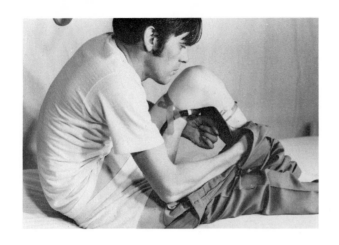
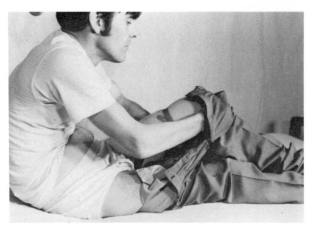

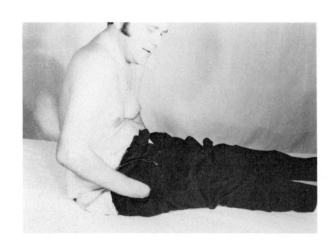
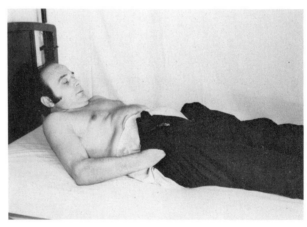

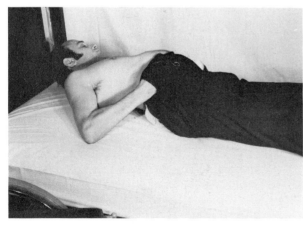
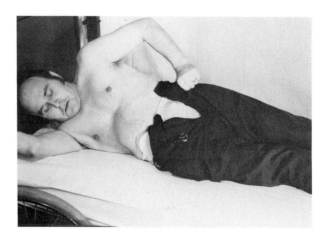

FIGURE 6-44

Method 7.   (Fig. 6-44) After the patient has his pants pulled over his legs, if he puts his hands in his pants pockets and drops back onto the elbows this will pull the pants up so that when he rolls he can pull the pants clear of his hips easily. Reciprocal pulling with the hands in the pockets and the elbows on the bed after the pants are pulled up will align them for fastening.

Method 8.   (Fig. 6-45) The patient lies on his side and works his trunk into flexion. If he has flexor spasm this position will encourage his legs to flex so that they are within easy reach. If he does not have flexor spasm he must work his trunk into sufficient flexion so that he can place a wrist around the back of a leg to pull him into a jackknifed position. Using both hands, he threads his lower foot into the pant leg; then he straightens his leg by pushing on the knee or thigh while keeping the waist of the pants in position with the other hand. The other knee is pulled up and the other pant leg is slipped on. The pants are worked up as far as possible before the patient rolls from side to side to pull them over his hips.

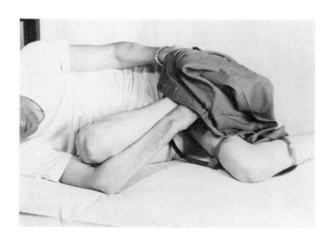
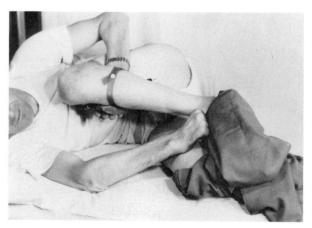
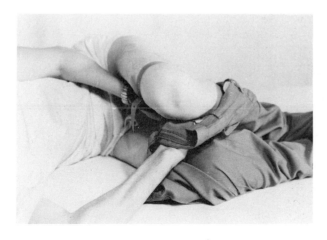
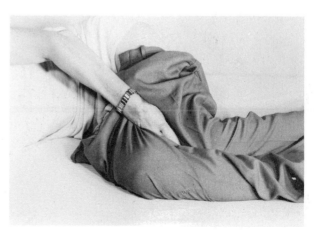

FIGURE 6-45

185

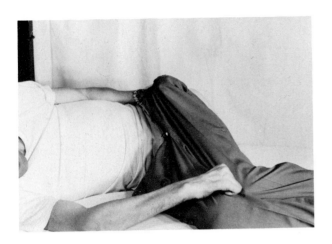
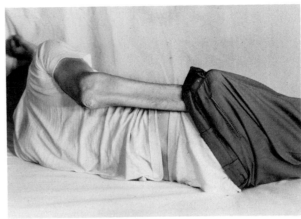

Method 9. (Fig. 6-46) The patient sits against the head of the bed and flings his pants out so that they lie straight in front of him. He uses an extended wrist to pick up a knee and pulls it close to his chest so that the foot can be threaded easily into

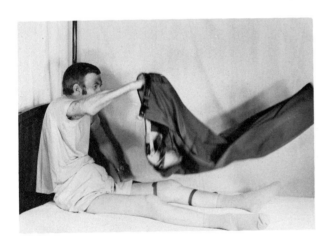
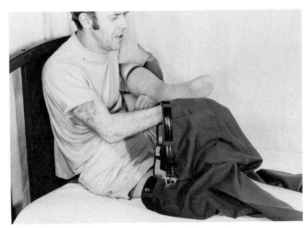

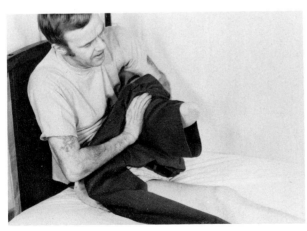
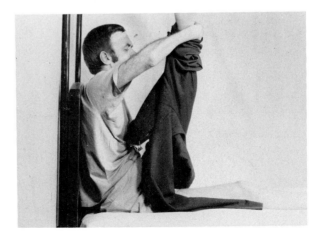

FIGURE 6-46

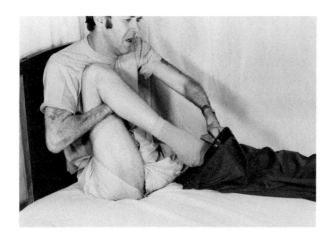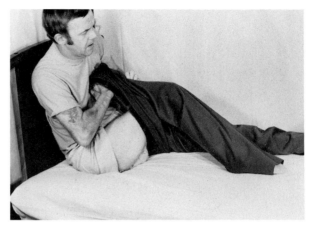

the pant leg. The pant leg is worked up using friction of the hands until the foot is free. If the patient is sufficiently flaccid he can straighten his leg so that it is vertical, allowing the pants to fall into position. The other leg is now pulled up and inserted into the waistband. The pant leg may be pulled up the leg in the same manner as before or the leg may be allowed to slip down into the pant leg by gravity while the pants are held in position at the waistband. The patient now moves down the bed so that he can roll from side to side to enable him to pull the pants over his hips.

Method. 10. (Fig. 6-47) A patient with extensor spasm may make use of this spasm by sitting against the head of the bed and holding his pants inside the waistband or with his hands in his pockets. He pulls on the pants with extended wrists while initiating his extensor spasm. This will slide him down the bed and into his pants.

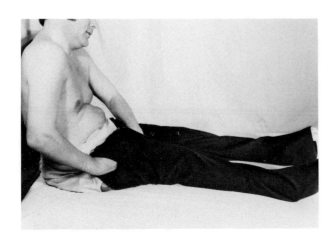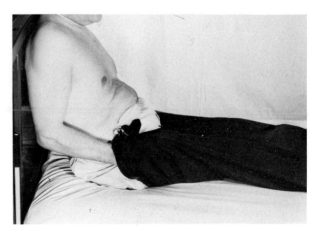

FIGURE 6-47

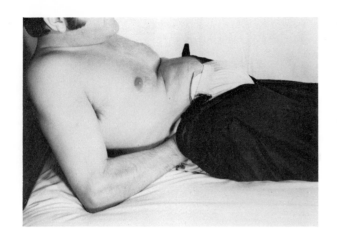
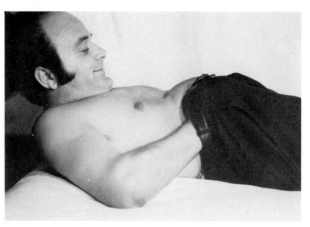
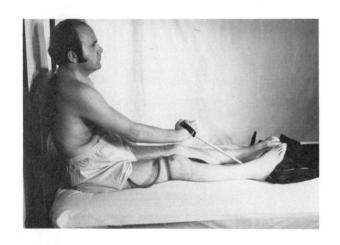
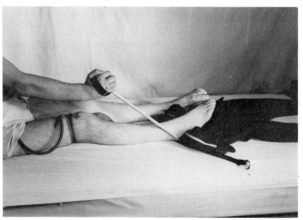
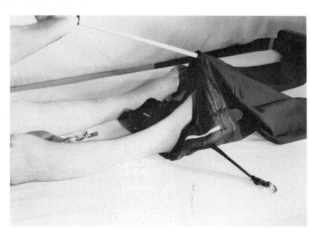
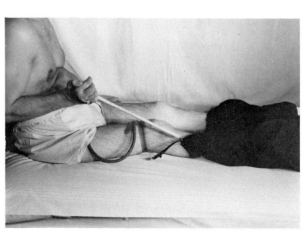

FIGURE 6-48

188

Method 11. A patient who must lean against the head of the bed or the raised head gatch for balance may be unable to pull his feet within reach and, therefore, must use a dressing stick (Fig. 6-48). A patient with flexor- or extensor-type spasm or a patient with tight hamstrings may find that his heels dig into the mattress on any attempt to lean forward. This patient will need a dressing stick as a substitute for forward flexion. A dressing stick may be required in the early stages of training in any situation in which the patient cannot reach to slip his pants over his feet.

REMOVING

Method 1. (Fig. 6-49) The patient sits in his chair and unfastens his pants. He places one hand inside his pants at the back and leans away from this side. While he leans over the arm of the chair he synchronizes a pushup and a scoop of the hand under the freed buttock. He repeats this action on the other side. With practice the pants can be freed of the buttocks in two moves. The patient lifts one leg at a time to push the pant legs off.

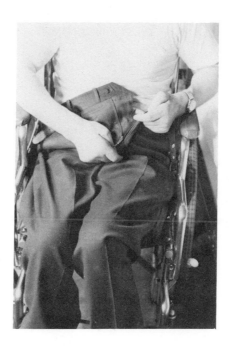 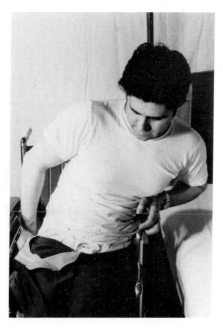

FIGURE 6-49

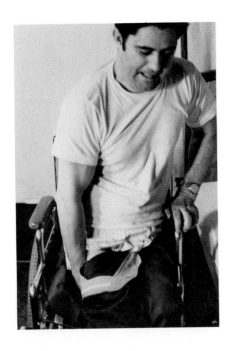
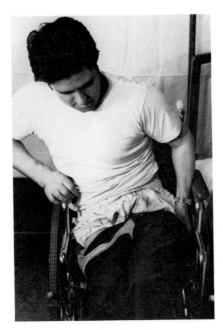
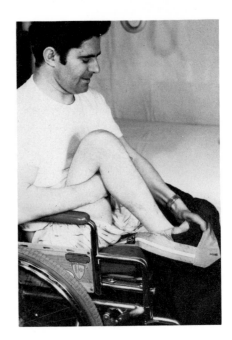

Method 2.   (Fig. 6-50) The patient sits on the bed and unfastens his pants. He hooks his thumbs over the waistband of his pants, locks his elbows, and does a pushup. He flexes his trunk and head forward so that his buttocks move back and out of his pants.

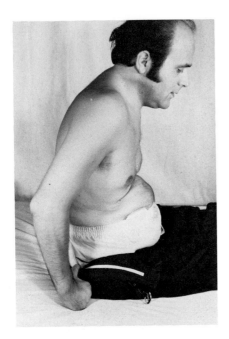
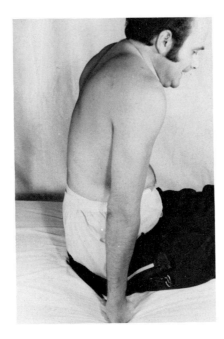
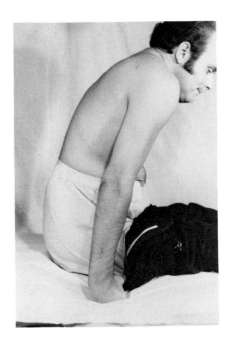

FIGURE 6-50

190

Method 3. (Fig. 6-51) The patient sits on the bed and hooks one arm into an overhead strap while the other hand catches the waistband at the back of the pants. He jerks up and pushes the pants under his buttock simultaneously. He switches arms to release the other side.

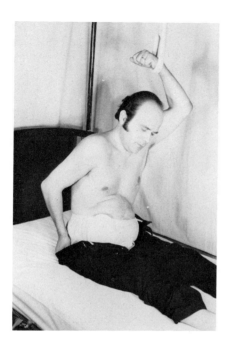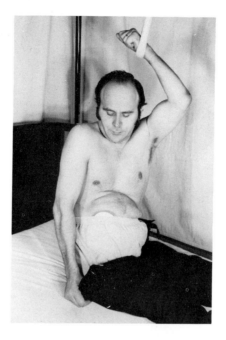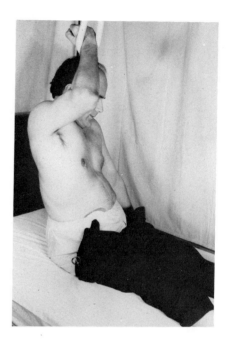

FIGURE 6-51

Method 4. (Fig. 6-52) The patient sits on the bed and unfastens his pants. He leans back supported on one elbow while the other hand pushes the pants down over the freed buttock. He leans to alternate sides repeating the process until the pants are below his hips. He sits up to push the pants below his knees. Holding the pants down with one hand he pulls up a knee to lift a leg out of the pants. The process is repeated for the other side.

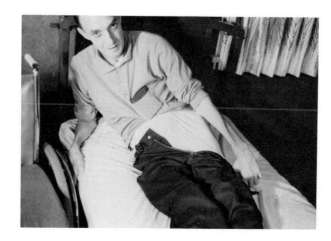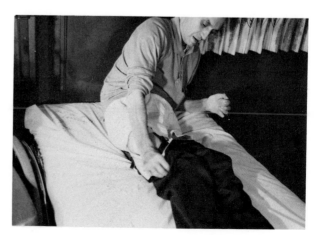

FIGURE 6-52

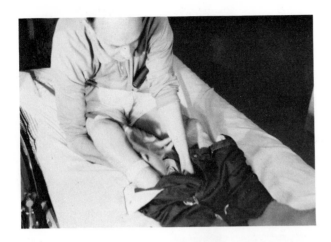

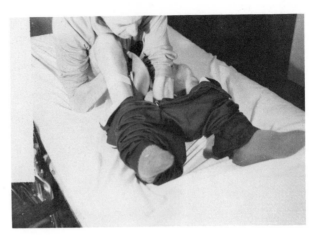

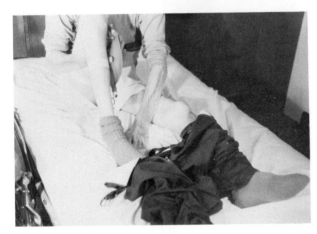

Method 5. (Fig. 6-53) The patient hooks his wrists under his knees and pulls them up as he falls back onto the bed. He now hooks both knees with one arm while he pushes the pants down over his knees. He places a wrist under each knee and kicks them off by pulling alternately with his arms.

Method 6. (Fig. 6-54) The patient works his pants clear of his buttocks

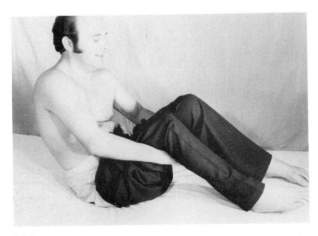

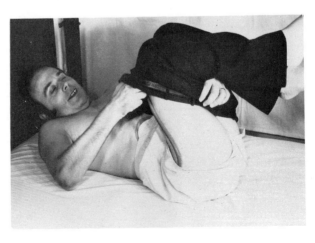

FIGURE 6-53

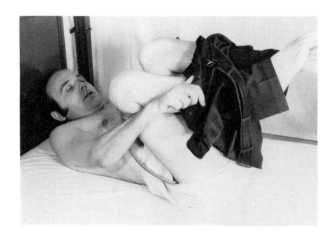
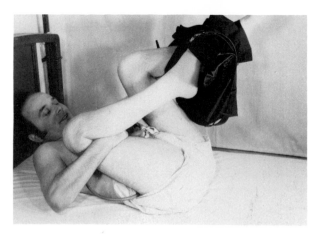

using one of the previous methods. He sits up and leans forward on one elbow and uses friction of both hands to work his pants down. He may lean on first one elbow and then on the other to push the pant legs down. When the pants are at his ankles he inserts a wrist under the calf while still leaning on his elbow and extends his wrist and flexes his elbow to lever his foot off the bed. The free arm pushes the pants away under the heel.

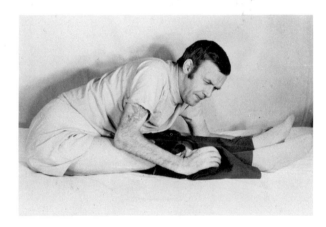

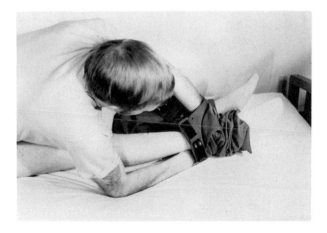
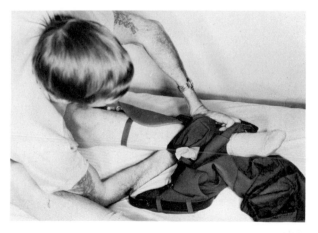

FIGURE 6-54

Method 7. (Fig. 6-55) The patient sits on the bed and leans back on alternate elbows to push the pants down past his hips. He remains in this position and hooks a wrist under a knee to pull it up. He pushes the pants down over his knee and then hooks a wrist under his bared knee. He pulls and slackens on the knee alternately to kick his leg partially out of the pants. He repeats the process with alternate legs until the pants are worked off.

Method 8. (Fig. 6-56) The patient lies on the bed and, rolling from side to

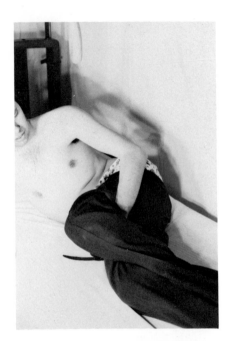
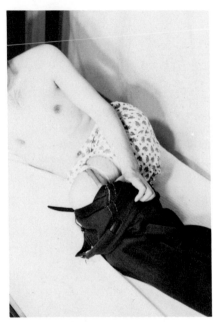
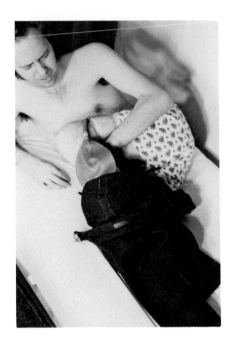

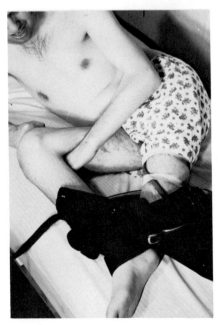
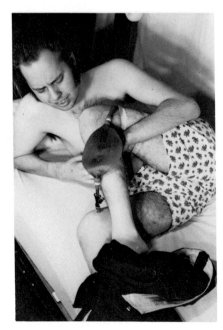

FIGURE 6-55

194

side, pushes his pants down past his hips. He works his trunk into a flexed position so that he can hook a wrist behind his leg to pull it up to his chest. He uses one arm to maintain the position of the leg while the free arm pushes the pants down past his knee. He now hooks the bared knee with an extended wrist and pulls it up as far as possible so that he can push the pant leg off his foot with his free arm.

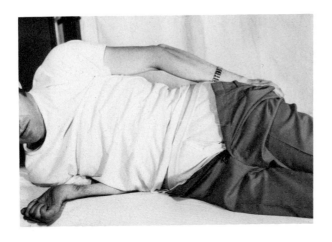
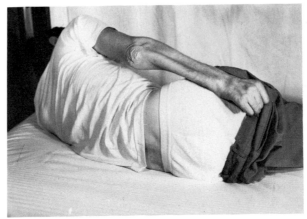
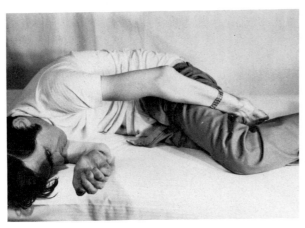
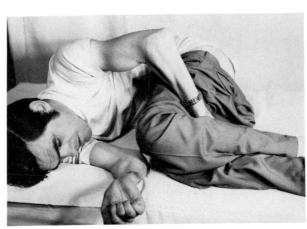
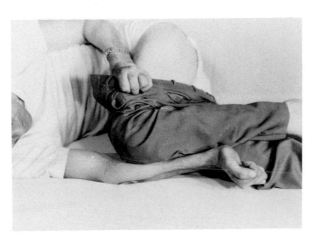
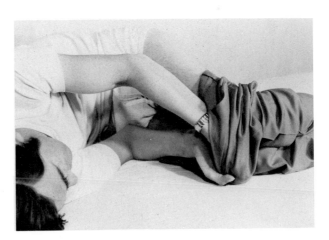

FIGURE 6-56

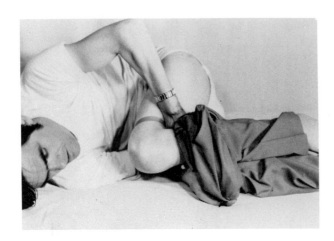
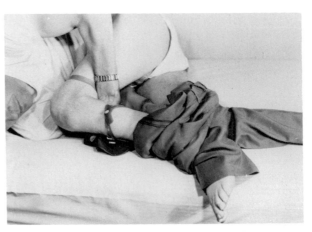

Method 9. (Fig. 6-57) The patient works his pants down over his hips using one of the previous methods and then sits close to the head of the bed and places his hand under a knee. He rocks back, picks up his knee, and leans against the head of

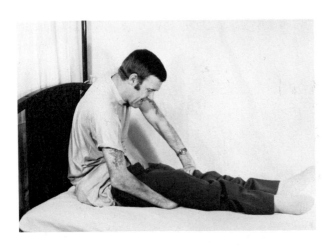
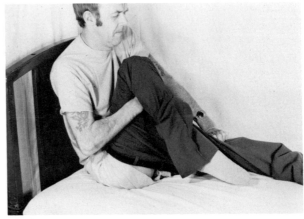

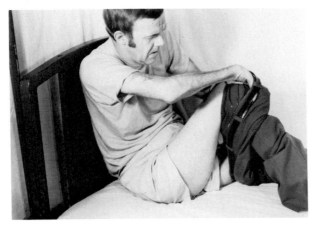
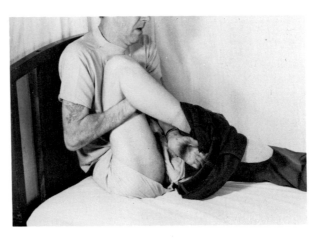

FIGURE 6-57

the bed. This frees both hands so that one arm can hold the knee while the other works the pants off the leg.

Method 10. The patient lies on the bed to work his pants down over his hips using one of the previous methods. He now moves up to the head of the bed and leans against it so that both hands will be free (Fig. 6-58A). By moving up the bed he will drag the pants part way down his legs. If the patient is unable to lift his knee so that he can reach his feet, he will require a dressing stick to push his pants over his feet (Fig. 6-58B). Some patients may use this method reclining against a raised head gatch.

A
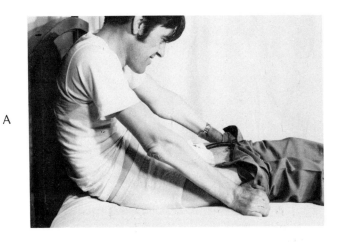
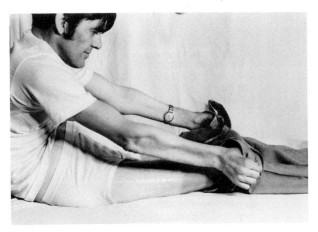

B
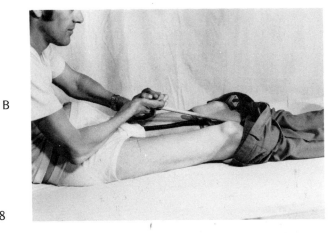
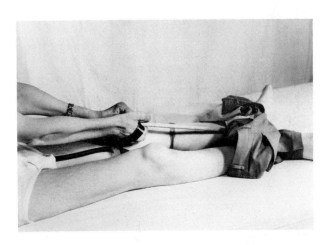

FIGURE 6-58

FASTENING PANTS

Waistband

An elastic waistband saves the necessity of fastening the pants, provided that it is not too difficult to pull the pants up. If elastic is not satisfactory, a hook fastening is easier to manage than either a press stud or a button.

Adaptations. For ease in fastening, a loop just large enough to insert a thumb is sewn to the extreme edge of the hook side of the waistband (Fig. 6-59A). A similar loop is sewn to the inside of the waistband underneath the eye (Fig. 6-59B).

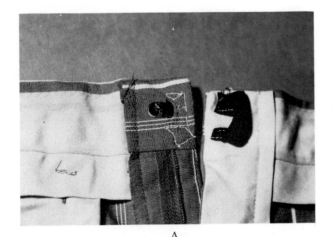

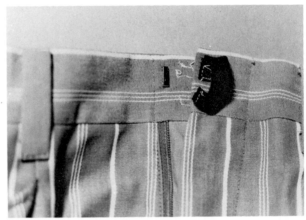

FIGURE 6-59

A   B

A D-ring maybe sewn on the hook side of the waistband and 4 inches of hook velcro is sewn to the eye side on the waistband (Fig. 6-60A). Four inches of the opposing velcro is sewn to the hook velcro at the fly so that it will fasten when folded back. A thumb loop is sewn to the free end (Fig. 6-60B) or a thumb hole is cut near the tip. The velcro can be backed with leather to give the cosmetic effect of a dress belt when fastened.

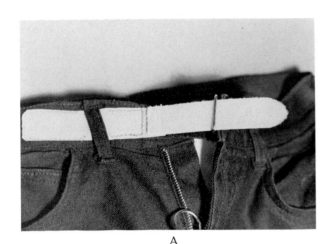

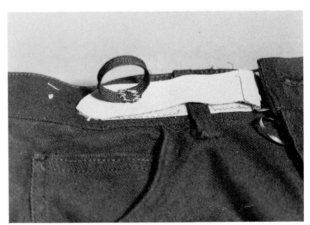

FIGURE 6-60

A   B

Procedures. A patient may hook the fastening of his pants by depressing the eye side into the abdomen with the heel of one hand. The other hand pushes the hook side over and down into position. The hand on the eye side is released to allow the abdomen to expand and snap the hook into the eye. A conventional hook-type fastener may be fastened using the belt loops of the pants. A thumb is inserted into the loops on either side of the fly and brought together until the hook is in position. If necessary the hook may be spread for easier fastening. The leather-faced velcro is threaded through the D-ring and then pulled back using the thumb loop. If this is difficult a hook may be pushed through the D-ring to catch the loop and pull it through.

Zippers

Fly zippers may require a loop fastened to the tab. The loop must be large enough to accommodate a thumb. It can be made of shoelaces, split rings, key chain, leather thong—in fact, any material strong enough to withstand laundering and a strong pull but at the same time able to meet cosmetic demands. To pull up the zipper, one hand holds the material at the base of the zipper while the thumb of the other hand, inserted in the loop, pulls the tab up. Usually the patient leans back if he is sitting in a chair (Fig. 6-61), thus eliminating the folds in the front of his pants and reducing his girth.

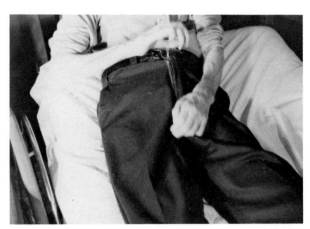

FIGURE 6-61

Pant Leg Zippers

Pant leg zippers are sewn to the inner seam of each pant leg unless there is adductor spasm or tightness; then they would be sewn into the outside seam to prevent possible pressure sores. The zippers are used for any of three reasons. First, they facilitate checking and emptying the urinal apparatus. In addition, they facilitate dressing. Also it may be practical to use standing splints or braces to improve circulation and as a prophylactic for G.U. malfunction; if so, the zippers simplify applying and removing braces.

Zippers should reach within 4 or 5 inches of the crotch. The zippers should be heavy duty and sewn so that they do not catch in the material. Dress pants should have a hidden zipper for cosmesis. The zippers must have a loop of strong and unobstrusive material fastened to the tab. A small zipper opening in the pants will suffice if emptying the urinal bag is the only concern.

Managing the zipper.   The following method is for the patient who is able to flex forward at the hips so that his chest rests on his knees and who then can return to the upright position. When leaning down, the patient places one thumb in the cuff of the pants by the zipper or, in lieu of a cuff, in an unobtrusive thumb loop. He places the other thumb or a finger in the zipper loop and pulls it up to the knee. In order to check the urinal apparatus, he will have to open the zipper completely. To do this he sits upright and holds the material taut at the knee with the palm of one hand while pulling the zipper up with the other hand. In order to close the zipper the patient holds the material at the top of the zipper with one hand and pushes the zipper down past the knee. Holding onto the back of the chair with one wrist, he leans forward and completes closing the zipper.

If the patient is unable to return to the sitting position after leaning forward, he can manage by raising his leg and placing his foot on a raised object such as the leg strap on the chair, the toilet bowl, or a footstool. This will place the zipper tab within reach.

If the patient must hold onto the back of the chair with one wrist to maintain his balance, the bottom of the pants must be held down in some manner. For instance, an elastic under the instep as in ski pants or an eye attached to the shoe and a corresponding hook on the pant cuff.

SHOES, SOCKS, AND STOCKINGS

Shoes should fit well to prevent foot deformities. Inside seams should be smooth to avoid pressure areas. An oxford-type shoe with a wide opening and front-lacing is suitable. The shoe should be large enough to permit the heel to be inserted without the use of a shoehorn. Slip on shoes must fit well so that the shoe will slide onto the foot easily but will not drop off accidentally. Cosmesis demands a work and a dress shoe, but women should avoid a high-heeled dress shoe because of the difficulty of positioning the feet on the footrests. Fastening by zipper lacing is very satisfactory. Five or six hole zippers in black or brown are obtainable and are easily placed in the shoe by following the manufacturer's instructions. If the shoe has fewer holes, the zipper must be stabilized at the closed end either by sewing it to the shoe with strong thread or by threading the lace through two holes made in the shoe at the appropriate point.

It is often necessary to stabilize the tongue of the shoe on one side. This can be done by making two holes in the tongue under the two top eyelets in the shoe and threading the lace through them. A thumb loop is fastened to the tab on the zipper. Elastic shoe laces may be used instead of zipper laces if the shoes can be slipped onto the feet and the shoes are secure. Some patients need a thumb loop at the back of the shoe to assist in donning the shoe (Fig. 6-62). This should be large enough for the thumb and of the same coloured leather as the shoe. It should be sewn neatly to the outside without bulky stitching on the inside.

A shoehorn may be required if the back of the shoe folds down when pushing the foot into the shoe. In this case it is usually too difficult to hold a shoehorn and push the foot into the shoe at the same time. A special homemade shoehorn will help. Instructions follow. Two shoehorns may be placed one on the other and rivetted together at the top with a washer between them to separate them sufficiently (Fig. 6-63A). A length of cord may be fixed to the top so that the shoehorns may be easily pulled out after the shoe is on (Fig. 6-63B). A clip-on shoehorn can also be made by bending the top of a metal shoehorn back to clip over the back of the shoe (Fig. 6-64). A cord with a loop at the other end may be fixed at the bend for easy release. In either design of shoehorn, it is attached to the shoe before the shoe is positioned to receive the foot.

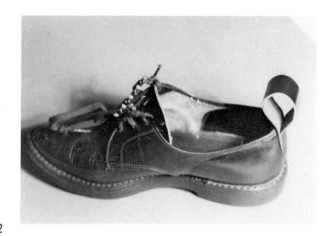

FIGURE 6-62

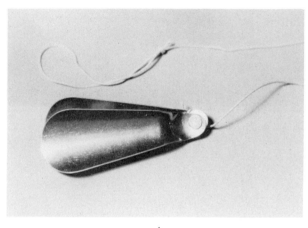

FIGURE 6-63

A

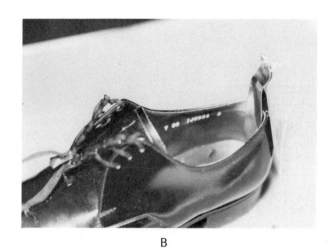

B

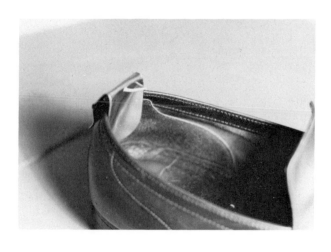

FIGURE 6-64

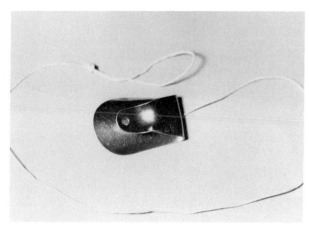

Socks should be of a loose knit without tight tops. If there is elastic in the tops, some of it can be removed provided that the top elastic is left intact (otherwise the sock will unravel). Thumb loops may be required inside the top of the sock. Loops should be sewn so that they are open and protruding above the top of the sock; they should match the socks in colour as closely as possible. A loop on either side of the sock is usually adequate.

Many types of stockings are manufactured with a patent semielastic top to hold them up, a factor which is very satisfactory provided the tops are not tight. Pantyhose will not be practical if a catheter is used and they make it difficult to handle clothing during toiletting.

BASIC POSITIONS

Various positions can be used by an individual patient; however, the aim is maximum stability so that, if possible, two hands are free to work and clear the heel from a surface. Socks are easiest to put on if two hands are used, but putting on shoes and taking off shoes and socks may often be accomplished with one hand only. Where possible the position should enable counterpressure to be applied. The methods of handling socks and shoes is described at the end of this description of positions. It is always necessary to work out the optimum position first and then the handling method.

Position 1. (Fig. 6-65) A patient who has a good hip joint and good balance will slide forward in his chair for stability and then pick up his leg. He stabilizes it and applies counterpressure with one arm while working with the other.

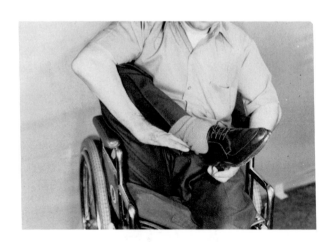

FIGURE 6-65

Position 2. (Fig. 6-66) If the patient sits in the chair with one ankle crossed over his knee he is in a very stable position which, in addition, secures the foot so that his two hands may be free to work. If the ankle is inclined to slip off the knee, an arm may be used to hold it but the hand can still be left free to assist in dressing.

Position 3. (Fig. 6-67) The patient sits in the chair in the transfer position and places one leg on the bed. He crosses the other leg over so that the foot is within reach. This position is extremely stable and will probably enable him to use both hands.

202

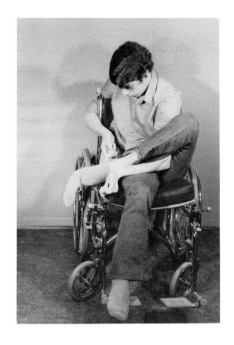

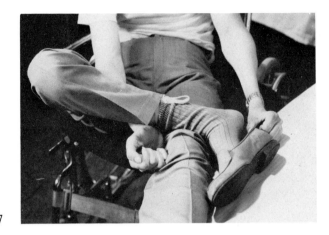

FIGURE 6-66   FIGURE 6-67

Position 4. (Fig. 6-68) The patient sits in his chair with one knee crossed over the other. This position leaves the heel free and counterpressure applied by the other knee. Since the position usually leaves only one hand free it is usually used for removing socks and shoes.

Position 5. (Fig. 6-69) The patient sits in his chair with one arm hooked around the pushing handle for stability. He lifts his leg with the other arm hooked under his knee so that he can lower his foot into his shoe.

Position 6. (Fig. 6-70) The patient, sitting in the chair, faces the bed about a foot away. He applies his brakes and lifts one leg to rest against the edge of the mattress. This position allows him to keep his leg flexed, so freeing both hands while his foot remains within reach. If he wishes to apply pressure, any flexion of his arms will cause him to lean forward so pushing against his knee with his chest.

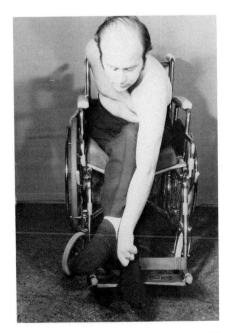

FIGURE 6-68

203

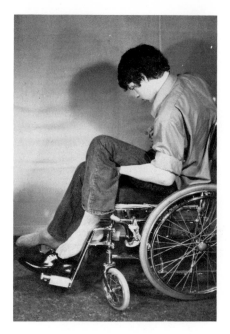

FIGURE 6-69

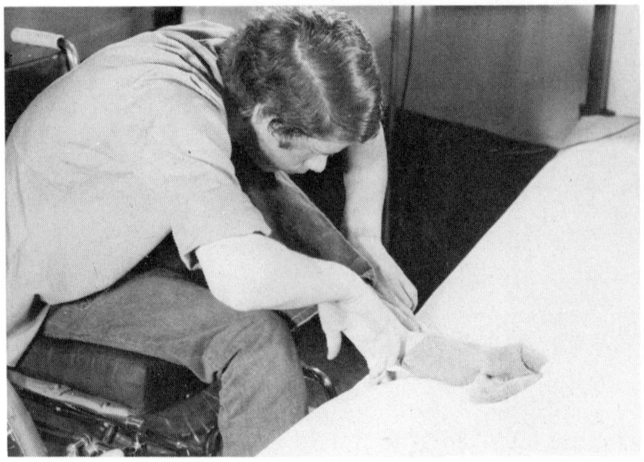

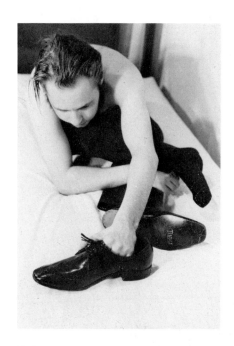

FIGURE 6-71

Position 7. (Fig. 6-71) The patient sits on the bed with one calf crossed over the other leg. This raises the foot from the bed and leaves both hands free to work. Extra stability may be gained by leaning on one elbow.

Position 8. (Fig. 6-72) The patient sits on the bed with his elbow on the bed and lifts his heel using wrist extensors and elbow flexors. This position leaves only one hand free. The leg cannot flex when pressure is applied to the sole of the foot because his chest and shoulder prevent it.

Position 9. (Fig. 6-73) The patient sits in the chair with the chair in transfer position and places one foot on the bed. He pulls the leg up and into outward rotation with a wrist under his knee. This position places the foot on its side leaving the heel free. If necessary for extra stability he may hook the arm near the bed around the chair back upright, pull the knee up with the other hand, and transfer the knee to the wrist of the arm holding onto the chair back.

Position 10. (Fig. 6-74) The patient sits in the chair in the transfer position with both legs on the bed. This position is very stable and permits the use of both hands.

Position 11. (Fig. 6-75) The patient lies on the bed with one knee pulled up to his chest. He holds it in external rotation with his arm inside the knee and over the lower leg. This position leaves both hands free and his heel within reach.

Position 12. (Fig. 6-76) The patient lies on the bed with his knee pulled up to his chest with his forearm, thus leaving one hand free to work.

Position 13. (Fig. 6-77) The patient sits against the head of the bed and pulls his knee up with his leg in external rotation. He holds it in position with an elbow in front of his knee, leaving two hands free to work.

204

FIGURE 6-70

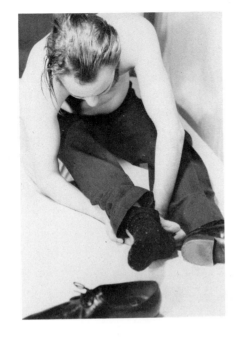

FIGURE 6-72

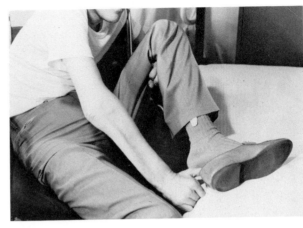

FIGURE 6-73

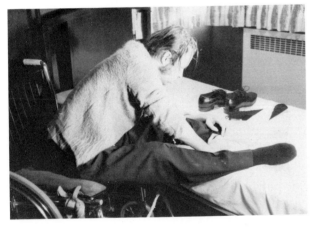

FIGURE 6-74

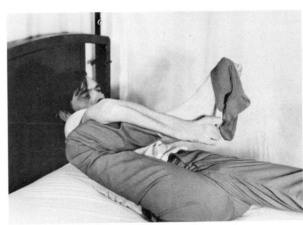

FIGURE 6-75

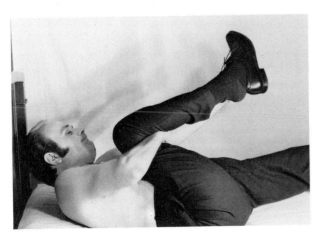

FIGURE 6-76

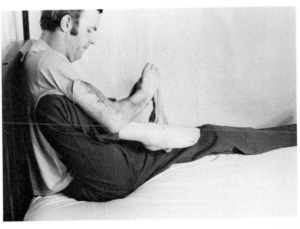

FIGURE 6-77

Position 14. (Fig. 6-78) The patient sits against the head of the bed and rests his foreleg in an appropriately placed sling. This position leaves both arms free to work.

Position 15. (Fig. 6-79) The patient sits against the head of the bed and uses a dressing stick to reach his feet. This position is used if the heels dig into the bed on forward flexion of the trunk or if the patient is unable to reach his feet.

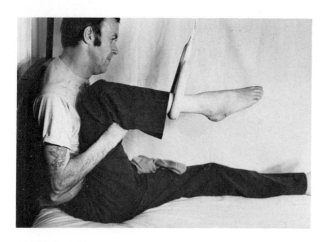

FIGURE 6-78

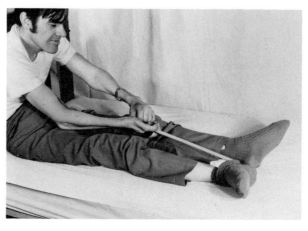

FIGURE 6-79

SOCKS AND STOCKINGS

Methods of Handling—On

Method 1. (Fig. 6-80) The top of the sock is stretched open using the thumbs and, if necessary, the teeth. The sock is slipped over the toes with a hand on each side of the foot so that the toes line up with the opening. As the sock is moved up the foot, the patient internally rotates his hands to maintain the thumb position as a hook in the sock. He slides his thumb to the back of the sock to clear the heel. Friction of the hands may be used to smooth the sock into position.

Method 2. (Fig. 6-81) The fingers or thumbs are inserted in the sock loops and the socks are stretched out so that the opening lines up to accommodate the toes. The socks are pulled up and twisted so that the loop is pulled under the heel. The hands must be turned so that the mechanical pull on the thumb or finger is maintained. If one hand must be used to maintain the position of the foot or to lift the heel from a surface, the loops may be pulled alternately. The hands are turned so that the pull against the thumb occurs when the thumb is in extreme extension so that it will hold without any muscle action (a pull on the back of the thumb will merely flex it and allow the loop to slip off but a pull against the inside of the thumb will cause it to maintain its extended position). Talcum powder sprinkled inside the sock or on the foot will facilitate sliding the sock onto the foot.

206

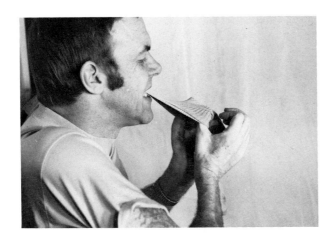
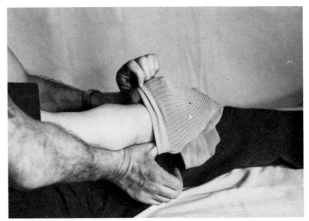
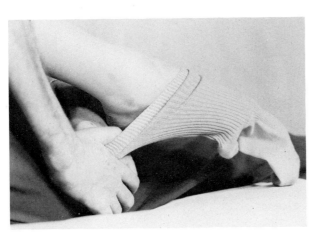
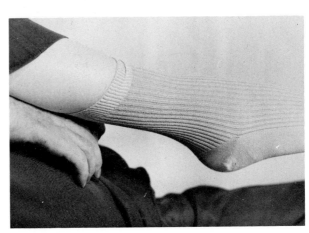

FIGURE 6-80

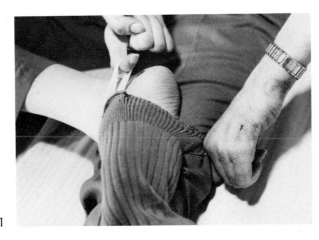
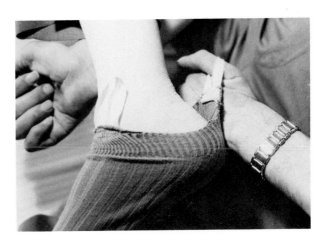

FIGURE 6-81

207

Method 3. (Fig. 6-82) A dressing stick might be required to pull on the sock loops. This may be particularly useful if a patient's heels dig down into the mattress when he reaches for his feet. Since usually only one hand is free to use a dressing stick there is more difficulty starting the sock on the foot. The sock may be manoeuvered onto the big toe, which will hold one side of the sock while the other side is stretched over the little toe.

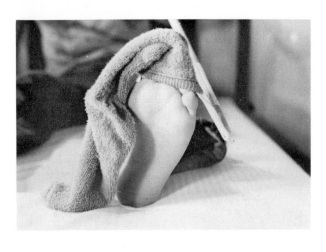
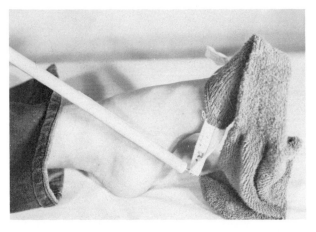
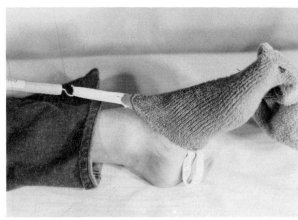
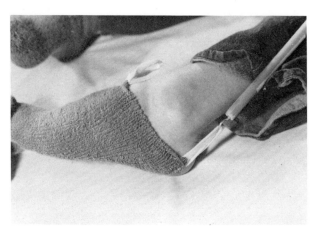

FIGURE 6-82

Putting Stockings On

The patient assumes her normal position for donning socks. She slips the stocking onto one hand and holds the other side, stretching it with her thumb (Fig. 6-83). She slides the stocking onto her foot keeping her hand inside the stocking for as long as possible. She works the stocking up by alternately pulling on the top and stroking the stocking. Loops at the top of the stocking will probably cause it to ladder. Garters may be permanently attached to the tops at side or front with a pulling loop but again will ladder all but the sturdiest hose.

208

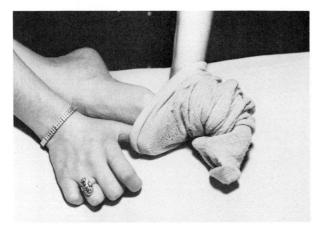
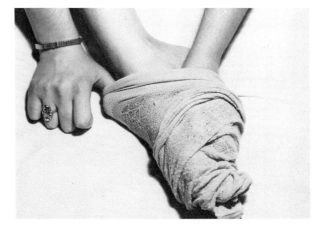
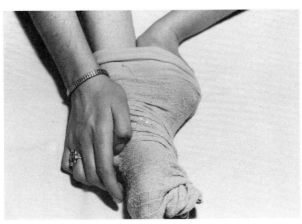
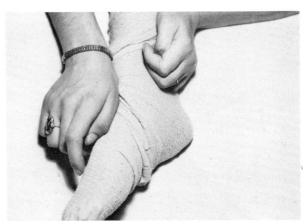

FIGURE 6-83

Removing Socks and Stockings

Socks are easy to push off provided that the heel can be lifted slightly. The thumb or fingers form a natural hook when pushing under the sock top or in a loop (Fig. 6-84). A dressing stick may be required if the heels dig down hard or if the feet are not within reach. The dressing stick may be notched so that the base of the V catches the sock top.

SHOES

Methods of Handling—On

Method 1.   (Fig. 6-85) The patient uses tenodesis to pick up the shoe under the instep and pushes it onto his foot using the side of his hand or thumb against the heel.

Method 2.   (Fig. 6-86) The patient picks up the shoe by placing a hand inside it and slips the shoe over his toes. He now catches the shoe under the instep

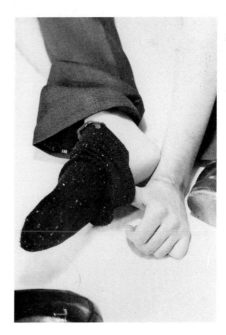

FIGURE 6-84

209

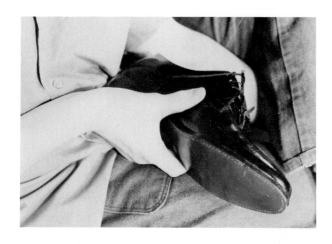
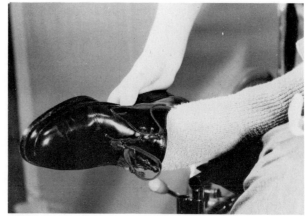

FIGURE 6-85

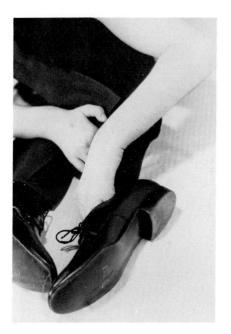
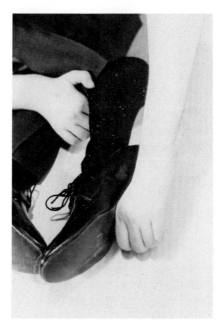
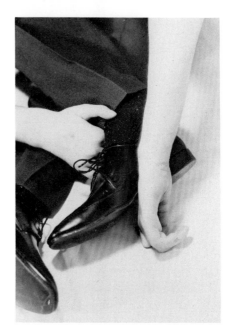

FIGURE 6-86

against the heel. He pulls the shoe on by using the side of his hand. Counterpressure is applied by the other arm against the knee or by the force of gravity.

Method 3. (Fig. 6-87) The patient sits in the wheelchair and, if necessary, stabilizes himself with one arm over the back of the chair. He moves his foot over, leaving room for the shoe to be placed on the footrest. He lifts his leg with a wrist under the knee so that the toe points into the open shoe and lowers the leg so that the forefoot slides in. He now extends his wrist against the calf pushing the foot and the shoe forward until the heel catches on the front edge of the footrest. If gravity does not slide the foot into the shoe, pressure on the knee will do so. Wheeling the chair against a wall will also push the shoe onto the foot.

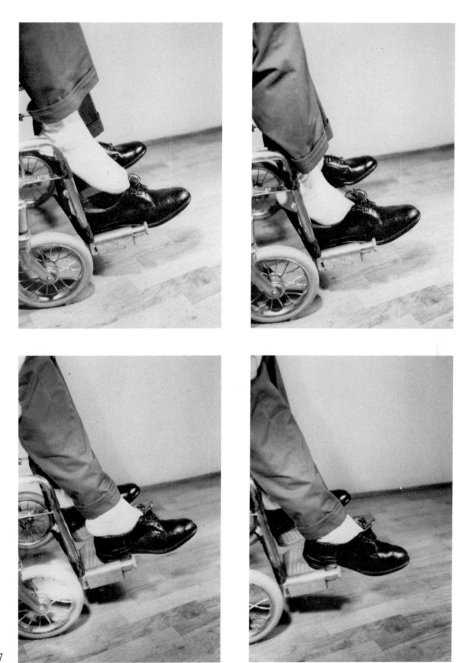

FIGURE 6-87

Methods of Handling—Off

Method 1.   The patient holds his leg in position with one arm. He uses the heel of his other hand against the heel of the shoe to push it off (Fig. 6-88).

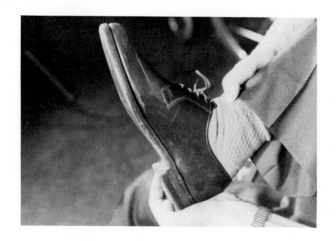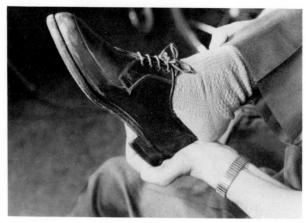

FIGURE 6-88

Method 2. The patient places his foot within reach, and pushes the heel of the shoe off with his thumb or dressing stick (Fig. 6-89).

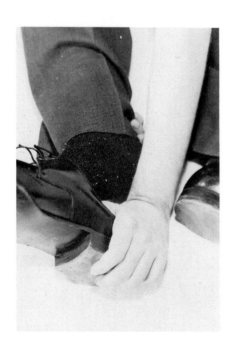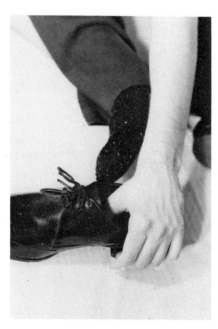

FIGURE 6-89

Method 3. (Fig. 6-90) The patient lifts his leg and, by extending his wrist behind his calf, he pushes his lower leg forward allowing his foot to drop in front of the footrest. He now lifts his knee, gently catching the heel of the shoe on the front of the footrest. His shoe will slide off as he replaces his foot on the footrest.

Method 4. The patient lifts his leg under the knee and shakes his leg, causing the shoe to slide from his foot onto the footrest. Retrieving it will be easier from the footrest than from the floor.

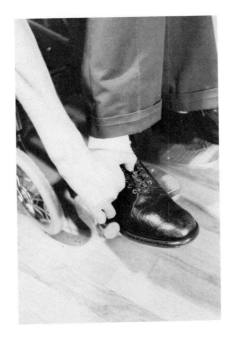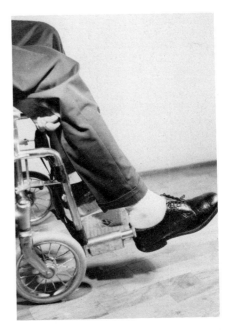

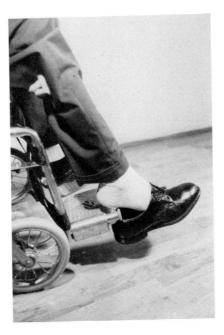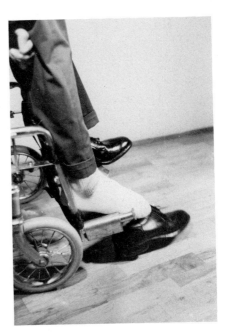

FIGURE 6-90

DRESSES AND SKIRTS

If dresses have fastenings they should be at the side or the front. When the dress is fitted the patient should be seated since length and skirt fullness may require adjustment in this position. Most patients prefer not to sit on a skirt owing to the difficulty of tucking it under and untucking it. For this reason full skirts or skirts with

213

fullness at the back may be selected so that the skirt can be bunched behind and still appear smart in front. Some women prefer to have a split in the skirt at the back so that they do not sit on the skirt. This may be useful if the woman is transferring frequently to the toilet or if occasional incontinence is a problem. Methods of putting on dresses are very similar to methods of putting on skirts or sweaters, and once she has mastered these she should require no further instruction. Skirts are put on over the head and are fastened in the same manner as a pant waistband.

COATS

Jacket-length coats are more convenient to put on and wear. Roomy armholes in a slippery and light material are advantages. Zippers that must be joined at the bottom are difficult to manage, if necessary, buttons or velcro should be substituted. Ponchos are easy to put on and require no fastening. A rain poncho is excellent protection for a patient seated in a chair.

TIES

Clip-on ties are the easiest to manage for most patients. However, ties may be permanently knotted and the slip knot adjusted to put it on over the head. An open loop may be required at the inside of the small end of the tie to enable the patient to hold while pulling the tie knot up.

WATCHES

Watches should be self-winding or electric. If the watch is not self-winding, a large winding stem can be turned by friction with the heel of a thumb. The strap must be an expansion type or a velcro D-ring fastening substituted for the buckle. When putting it on, the watch is worked over the hand using the thumb or fingers of the opposite hand. It is easiest to work the watch well down one side of the hand, so that it will stay in position when the hand is pressed onto some stable object, such as a thigh, while the strap is pushed over the other side of the hand. The thumb may be used to push the watch off, sliding the thumb from one side of the strap to the other. Friction on the pant leg or arm of the chair may be used in conjunction with this.

7

Bowel and Bladder Management

"Bowel training" is the program designed to reactivate the patient's regular bowel habits. "Bowel management" follows bowel training and explains the methods and equipment used to teach the patient to manage his own bowel regimen.

BOWEL TRAINING

TIMING

The patient must be toiletted at the same time each day. If, after a reasonable length of time, the bowel movement shows a pattern of being more successful on alternate days or every third day, the regimen should be changed to accommodate this pattern. Some patients find it desirable to evacuate their bowels in the evening. This may be due to practical reasons—pressure of time in the morning before work, previous habits—or because bowel initiation is easier in the evenings. If the patient is dependent on family or orderly for assistance in his bowel evacuations, it may be more convenient during the evenings. Later, during the training, the patient may experience certain signs that indicate the bowel contents are starting to descend. These signs may be goose pimples, headache, sweating, muscular twitching, abdominal fullness, indigestion, or strong spasms.

TECHNIQUES

The patient must be able to tolerate sitting for at least half an hour before bowel training is started. Little is gained by starting earlier. The physician may choose to prescribe a mild laxative the evening before in order to ensure that the stools are of normal consistency. He may also prescribe a suppository to be inserted high in the rectum half an hour to an hour before the toiletting.
The patient transfers or is transferred onto a raised toilet seat or commode, and his feet are placed on a footstool to compensate for the additional height. A backrest adds to the security and comfort of the patient. Side bars may be neces-

sary to give the patient complete security. Care must be taken when placing the patient on the toilet. It is especially important that the buttocks are not parted to cause tension on the skin of the natal cleft. On the other hand, the buttocks must not be compressed, thus inhibiting reflexes of evacuation. The patient must be comfortable if a bowel movement is to be achieved. The patient may initiate evacuation by pressing down on the abdomen, by holding a deep breath, by allowing the trunk to forward flex, or by raising the knees. Kneading the abdomen by hand or forearm along the level of the colon from right to left may assist.

The assistant's hand is gloved and a finger is well lubricated with vaseline. A gentle massage with the finger on the skin around the anus will often be sufficient to relax the external anal sphincter. A finger may be inserted to further relax the sphincter if external massage is insufficient. The stool will then be expelled if it is of a soft consistency and is in the lower rectum. If the stool is too firm, it may have to be removed manually to prevent impaction. Plenty of lubricant must be used and extreme care taken to avoid damage to tissues. Two fingers may have to be used to break up the stool and gently work it out. If the stool is too firm the laxative doses may be adjusted by the physician and possibly mineral oil added. The fluid intake may be increased and the diet adjusted to include more bulk and roughage to prevent recurrence.

After evacuation the initial cleansing is done gently with toilet tissue. A protective pad or paper is placed on both wheelchair cushion and bed before the patient transfers. A pubic wash is done on the bed using pHisoHex or, if this is too drying, the prescription may be changed to Cetavlon. The skin is now checked for abrasions or obvious pressure before drying and powdering.

BOWEL MANAGEMENT

When bowel regulation has been achieved and the initiation of evacuation methods has been established, the patient is ready to begin looking after his own bowel management. By this time the patient should have learned to transfer himself to commode or toilet seat and to control his own laxative or diet regulation. Bowel movement may be initiated with no aids, by the regulation of diet or prescribed laxatives, or by kneading his abdomen and flexing his trunk forward. He may require suppositories or digital stimulation. As the management methods are developed, any equipment necessary to enable the patient to be independent, must be provided.

SUPPOSITORIES

Patients with some finger function may be taught to hold the suppository and insert it adequately. Many patients will require a suppository inserter (Fig. 7-1). This flanged suppository inserter has been in use for over 14 years and has proved to be both safe and efficient. The flange controls the depth of insertion and the soft rubber tube is shaped and lubricated to prevent any damage to delicate tissues. The handle may be adapted so that it can be held firmly and at the correct angle. An additional handle may be made, which can be attached to a standard suppository inserter and adjusted to establish the optimum angle for any patient who cannot manage the conventional angle. The appliance is inserted until the flange makes contact with

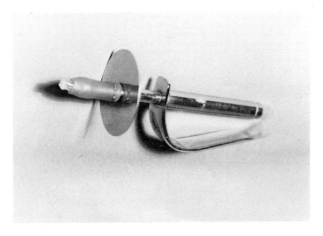

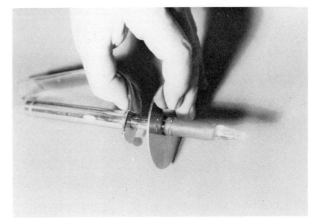

A

B

FIGURE 7-1. *A,* Suppository inserter; *B,* Compression ejects suppository; *C,* Additional handle if adjustment is required.

C

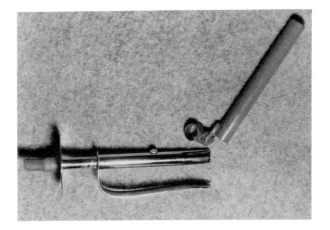

the buttocks. Further pressure compresses the spring and moves the plunger down to eject the suppository (Fig. 7-2).

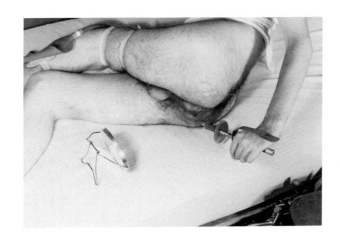

FIGURE 7-2

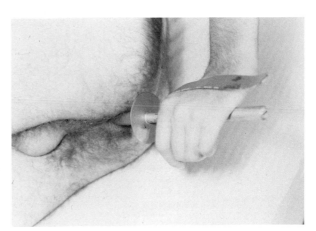

217

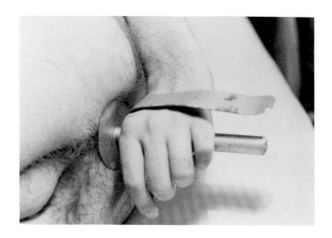 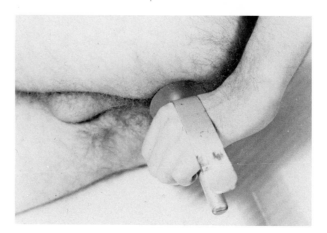

A wrist-driven flexor-hinge or tenodesis-type splint is not recommended as the wrist must be flexed in order to reach the anus. The flexor-hinge splint will close only when the wrist is extended.

Positions for Insertion

Position 1. The patient lies on his bed with the dominant arm uppermost, the upper leg fully flexed at the hip and knee, and a mirror with a broad base pre-positioned on the bed. This position tends to turn the patient slightly onto his abdomen and makes it easier for him to reach.

Position 2. The patient lies on his side on the bed with both knees flexed. This position parts the buttocks more than other positions but makes the anus harder to reach because he is lying on his side.

Position 3. The patient places his chair by the bed in side transfer position. He remains in the chair or commode chair, but rests his upper body in side lying on the bed, leaving his feet on the footrests or placing them on the bed. This position reduces the number of transfers required.

Position 4. He may insert the suppository while in position on the commode chair or toilet, using a position as described in Positions for Insertion and Digital Stimulation.

Positions for Insertion or Digital Stimulation

The patient positions himself on the toilet. He stabilizes himself with one arm, enabling him to reach his anus with the other using one of the following methods:

Position 1. (Fig. 7-3) A table is placed by the side of the toilet. The height is adjusted so that the patient's elbow rests comfortably on the top. The patient leans over this elbow, so raising his buttock from the toilet seat on the opposite side. This permits digital stimulation without reaching under the toilet seat.

Position 2. (Fig. 7-4) The patient flexes his trunk so that he can reach from the front through an open front toilet seat. Depending upon the build and the ability of the patient, he may rest one forearm across his thighs or he may rest his trunk upon his thighs. To use this method, he must be able to regain his upright position.

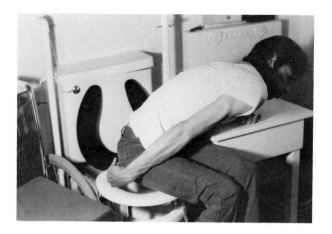

FIGURE 7-3

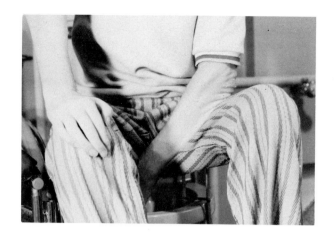

FIGURE 7-4

Position 3. The patient hooks one forearm over a side bar at elbow height (Fig. 7-5A) or places his wrist in an overhead strap placed above his shoulder (Fig. 7-5B). He leans away from the bar or strap to reach under the side of the raised toilet seat.

Position 4. (Fig. 7-6) The patient places one wrist in an overhead strap and leans forward to reach through the front of an open front toilet seat. The overhead strap enables the patient to pull himself to an upright position.

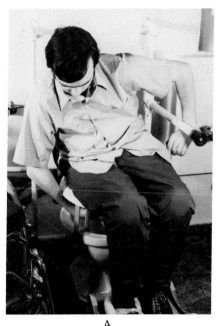

A

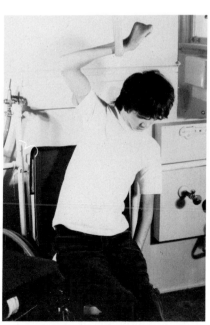

B

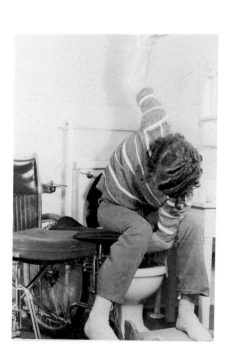

FIGURE 7-5

FIGURE 7-6

EQUIPMENT FOR DIGITAL STIMULATION

Disposable gloves are donned and the finger to be used is lubricated. The patient may be able to use a gloved finger for digital stimulation but, where this is not possible, splints and aids may be used.

A length of ⅜-inch I.V. tubing (Fig. 7-7A) is looped around the base of the middle forefinger and is drawn over the palm to a wrist strap. The tension should be adequate to pull the finger forward so that it is held straight and away from the other fingers (Fig. 7-7B). Where there is difficulty in holding the other fingers back, a bar may be attached to the tubing behind the middle finger. The bar runs in front of the remaining fingers (Fig. 7-7C). The bar must be washable and adequately formed or padded to prevent pressure areas.

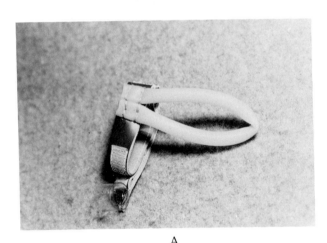

A

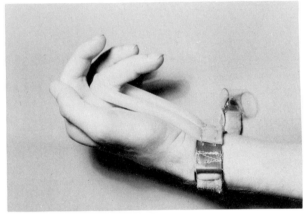

B

FIGURE 7-7

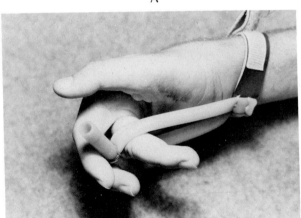

C

A plastic dorsal wrist splint may be fitted to hold the wrist in flexion. A metal bar extends from the dorsum of the shell to beyond the proximal interphalangeal joint of the middle finger. A ring is attached to the end of this bar to fit around the finger. For ease of application, the ring may be constructed so that it swivels where it joins the bar (Fig. 7-8A). This holds the wrist in full flexion and the finger is flexed at the PIP joint and extended at the metacarpophalangeal and distal interphalangeal joints (Fig. 7-8B). This is a functional position for reaching the anus.

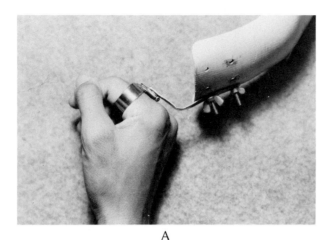 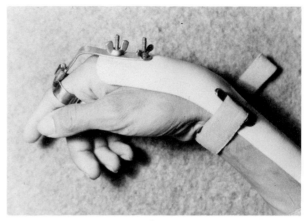

| A | B |

FIGURE 7-8. Digital stimulation splint. This model has an adjustable finger piece for trying optimum positions. Note wing nuts.

A smooth plastic stimulator may be attached to a rocker bar with the fulcrum under the toilet seat and the adapted handle protruding beyond the seat (Fig. 7-9). The stimulator may be covered with a disposable rubber-finger cot. This method is not recommended unless the patient is a careful person who will use a mirror or who has sparing of sensation around the anus. A rear-view mirror may be permanently attached to the toilet seat or a commode chair in a convenient position where it will not interfere with transfers.

FIGURE 7-9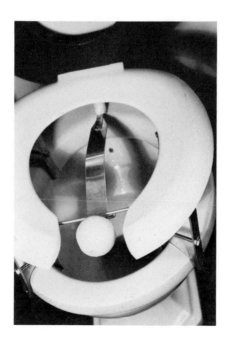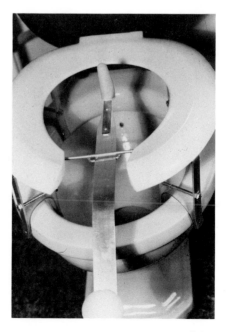

CLEANSING

The positions adopted for digital stimulation, mentioned previously, will also stabilize the patient for the first steps in cleansing.

Using Toilet Tissue

The patient who has some ability to grasp may find that he needs more tissue to provide a firm grip. A large amount of toilet tissue may be wound around one hand. Wiping is done with the paper on the dorsum or radial side of the hand.

A toilet-tissue holder may be constructed (Fig. 7-10A). The handle must be adapted to attach to the patient's hand firmly enough to provide good control. The shaft is curved as required and the length is adjusted to the patient's needs. The holder at the tip may be made of two or three horizontal coils of wire. Coat hanger wire is suitable for experimentation and easily obtained, but stainless steel wire should be used in the permanent appliance. The two ends of the wire should finish at the handle so that there are no unprotected ends. Toilet tissue is inserted into the centre of the coils and arranged so that it folds over the wires (Fig. 7-10B).

The patient transfers onto his chair and then to bed, so that he can wash to ensure cleanliness.

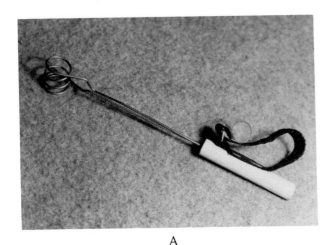

A

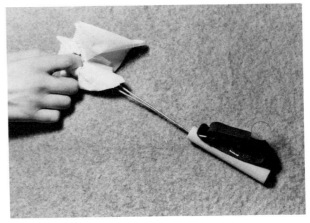

B

FIGURE 7-10

Pubic Wash

Before transferring to the bed, the patient places a basin of water and his washing equipment in a convenient position by the bed. He is careful to test the temperature of the water before placing the basin on his knees or lapboard to transport it. He then spreads a plastic or flannelette sheet or an absorbent pad on the bed. After transferring to the bed, the patient will roll onto his side and flex the upper leg. The patient reaches over his buttock to wash the posterior area thoroughly with a washing cloth or mitt. The anterior area may be washed conveniently when lying supine or sitting up. Since the patient is unable to wring out the wash mitt, he must

222

verify that the pad or plastic is well placed to protect the bedding. He dries the area and applies powder, using powder directly from the container or using an adapted powder puff (Fig. 7-11). The puff may be made of artificial sheepskin sewn to a metal or plastic handle, which may be curved and adapted for an adequate grip.

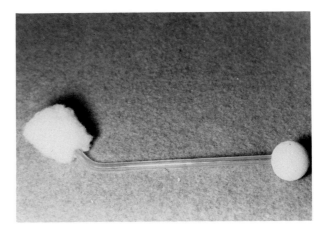

FIGURE 7-11

BLADDER MANAGEMENT

Male and female patients may with training achieve automatic bladder function; this is the optimum method of management. This type of management may be impractical for a woman who is unable to transfer independently to the toilet; therefore, the prognosis of eventual transfer abilities should be made before attempting to discontinue use of the catheter. If a woman must be toiletted by others it may make care of the patient an unnecessary burden or it may curtail work or social life for the patient. All factors must be taken into consideration before attempting to achieve an automatic bladder.

A satisfactory and safe method of external urine collection for quadriplegic women has not been developed. At the moment these women are limited to the choice of an automatic bladder with toilet transfers or to the use of a catheter. Partly owing to this limited choice, more women than men are motivated to achieve an automatic bladder.

A man may achieve an automatic bladder without the necessity of achieving independent toilet transfers. He may use a urinal or, if he knows that he will not be able to reach a toilet at the requisite time, he may apply a urine-collecting apparatus for the occasion.

The urine-collecting apparatus may be used by the man who is unable to achieve an automatic bladder. This consists of a condom which is cemented to the penis and attached to a tube by tape or a plastic plug. Alternatively a commercially available Texas catheter may be used; this consists of a condom already attached to a short length of tubing. The tubing leads to the collecting bag. A modified emptying apparatus is usually necessary.

Some patients have an ileostomy for medical reasons. Some patients learn to apply the urine-collecting system provided that the bud is conveniently placed and the patient is sufficiently dextrous.

223

When the method of urine collection has been established it becomes desirable for the patient to perform the task of assembly and attachment himself. This equipment should be assembled and the smaller items kept on a tray so that they are accessible. Quadriplegic patients with adequate grip will manage the application using no aids. The flexor-hinge hand splint is a most useful aid for many others who could not otherwise accomplish application of the drainage system. Many patients, who initially rejected the use of a hand splint, find its use so vital for this task they perceive its use in other situations as well and accept it.

If a patient cannot apply a condom by unrolling it with his thumb or fingers, the condom may be modified. A large number of condoms may be prepared for the patient at one time by unrolling them over a length of dowelling. A double length of thread can be laid down on either side before the condom is rerolled for use. The ends of the thread are tied in a loop so that they can be used as thumbloops (Fig. 7-12). The condom will unroll easily by pulling on the threads once the condom is started on the penis and making contact with the cement.

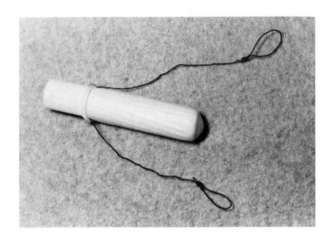
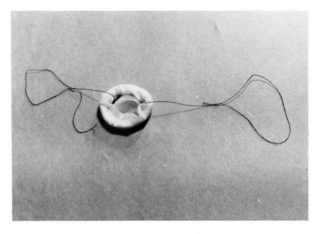

FIGURE 7-12

Insertion of Condom into Tubing

The tubing is made of a pure gum surgical tube 3/8 x 3/16 inches. The plug (Fig. 7-13) is made of 1/2-inch (outside diameter) and 1/4-inch (inside diameter) acrylic plastic tubing cut into 1-inch lengths. It is turned down on a lathe to 3/8 of an inch (outside diameter) except for 1/8 of an inch left at one end as a collar.

The following are methods used to insert the plug through the condom into the tubing and sink the plug. In all cases the condom must be punctured before application. An orange stick is generally used for this purpose.

Method 1. (Fig. 7-14) The patient uses tenodesis to hold the tubing and leans the condom against the end. The plastic plug is manoeuvered into position against the condom and tube, using the heel of the hand and the table surface to tip it. Once the plug has been started into the tube the hands can be repositioned to enable more force to be applied to sink the plug home.

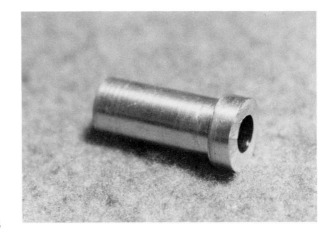

FIGURE 7-13

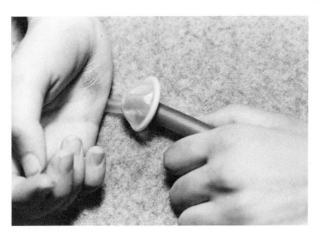

FIGURE 7-14

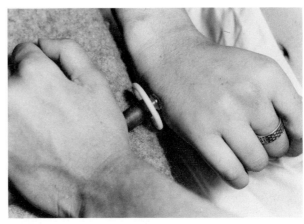

Method 2. (Fig. 7-15) The patient rests the condom over the end of the tube, using tenodesis to hold it in position, and starts the plug into the tube, holding the plug with a flexor-hinge splint. Once it is started he changes position so that he can drive it home. This may be done by holding the tube down with the side of his hand and using the thumb of the splinted hand to push the plug all the way down to the collar.

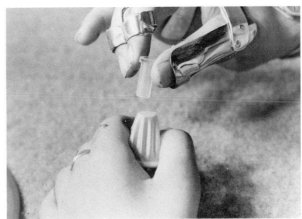

FIGURE 7-15

225

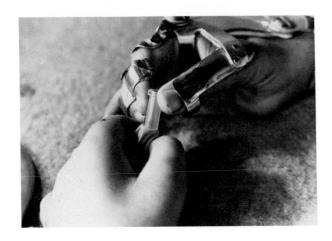 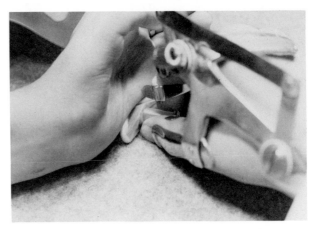

Method 3. (Fig. 7-16) The patient uses two flexor-hinge splints to attach the condom to the tube in a normal fashion. He may complete pushing the plug into the tubing with one rigid thumb tip.

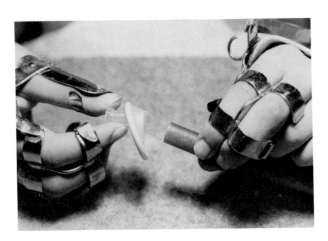 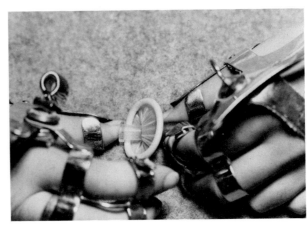

FIGURE 7-16

Method 4. (Fig. 7-17) A simple clamp may be made of two pieces of wood, lined with foam and hinged at the end with leather. This requires little pressure to hold the tubing firmly while the plug is inserted.

Method 5. (Fig. 7-18) A wooden pencil is held between the teeth and the sharpened end is inserted into the flanged end of the plastic plug. This holds the plug firmly while enabling the patient to see what he is doing. He holds the urinal tubing either between the heels of his hands or, using his splint, manoeuvres the condom until it rests over the tubing. The condom is placed so that it will unroll towards him. Using the pencil in his teeth, he inserts the plastic plug into the tubing through the condom. He checks to ensure that the condom is punctured.

Method 6. (Fig. 7-19) A jig may be made to hold the plug securely for both assembly and disassembly of condom and tube. A length of two-by-two is sanded smooth, and a groove is cut down one side to fit the depth and diameter of the collar of the plug. A thin sheet of metal or plastic has a slot cut into it to fit the body of the

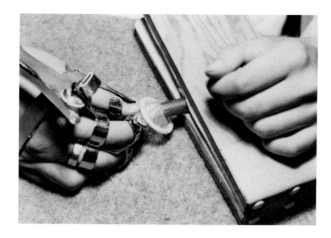
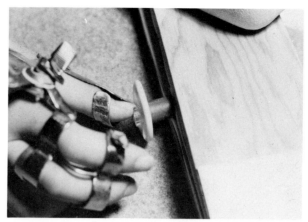

FIGURE 7-17

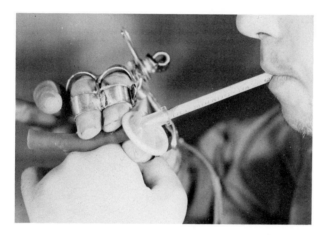
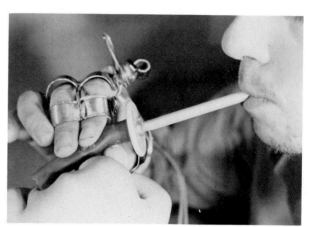

FIGURE 7-18

plug. The slot is aligned over the groove and fastened down so that the plug can be dropped in and held in place by the collar. If a clamp is used to hold the tube, the plug height should be regulated to align with the tube. A hole may be drilled through the two-by-two using the hollow plug in place as a guide, so that the condom can be punctured through it following assembly.

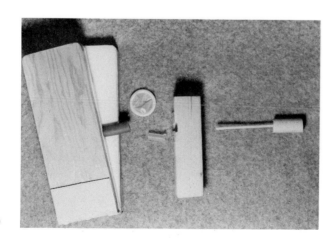
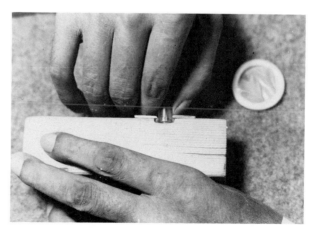

FIGURE 7-19

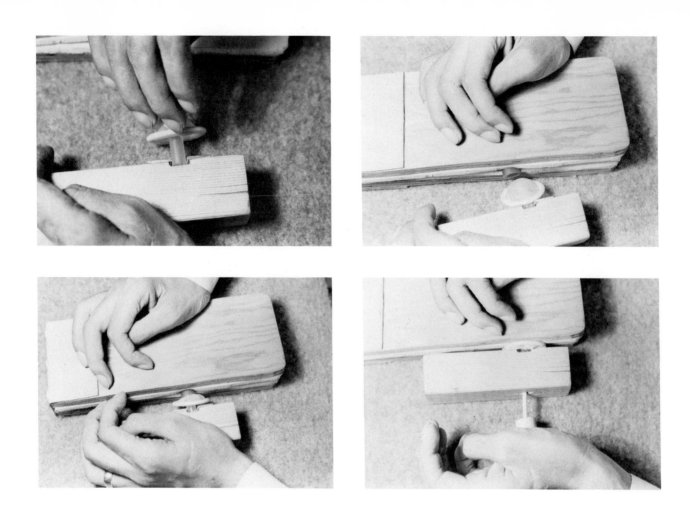

Method 7.   (Fig. 7-20) If a plastic plug is not available the condom may be attached to the tubing with 1/2-inch adhesive tape. The condom is first pulled down over the tubing and taped. It is then pulled back over this tape and is taped again. This method requires considerable dexterity.

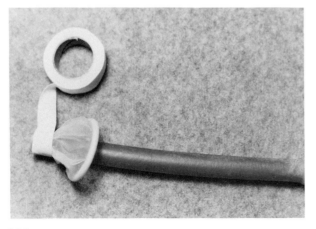 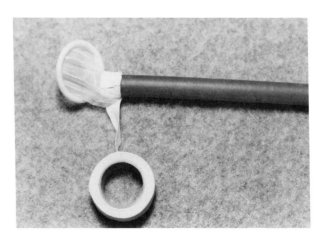

FIGURE 7-20

228

Method 8. (Fig. 7-21) A condom may be attached by using two rubber bands cut off the tubing. One band is slipped about an inch down over the tubing. The condom is pulled down over the tubing and the other ring is slipped over condom and tubing about 3/4 of an inch down. The condom is now pulled back and the first ring is lifted over the second. This is the same principle as the tape method. It is unlikely that a quadriplegic patient will be able to manage this method himself.

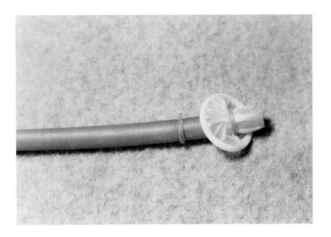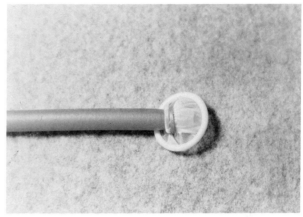

FIGURE 7-21

Securing Tubing and Urinal Bag

The urinal tubing extends approximately 6 inches to be slipped over a 3-inch plastic connector tube (Fig. 7-22). The connector is used to observe flow of urine and also to reconnect to the night drainage system if it is used. Once the system has been established, some patients prefer not to use a connector as it creates additional assembly problems. The connectors are made of 3/8 of an inch (outside diameter) and 1/4 of an inch (inside diameter) acrylic plastic tubing. These are tapered at either end on a sander. The urinal bag has a tube permanently attached and adjusted in length for the individual patient. The patient attaches this to the plastic connector (Fig. 7-23).

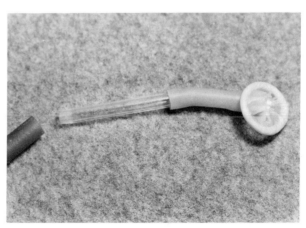

FIGURE 7-22

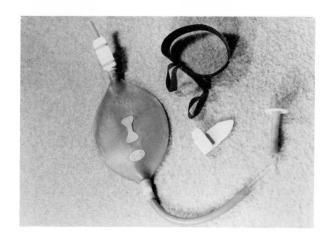

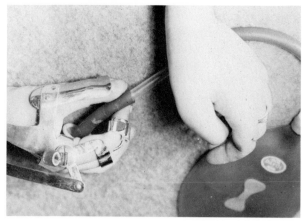

FIGURE 7-23

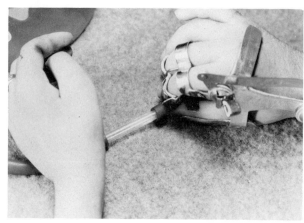

The conventional rubber leg strap is removed, and a plastic clip is placed in the rubber slot (Fig. 7-24). A strip of 1-1/2 inch elastic with loops at either end and a velcro fastening forms a garter (Fig. 7-25A). This is wrapped around the lower leg just below the knee and the plastic clip is slipped behind it (Fig. 7-25B). The clip is made of a thermoplastic material such as plexiglass or sansplint. A jig will simplify

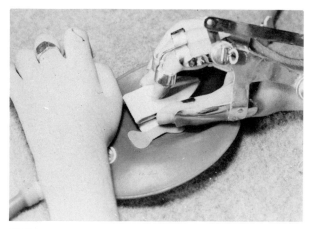

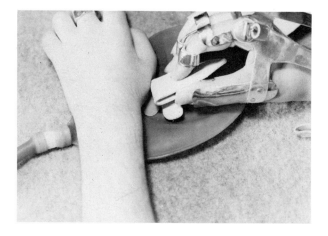

FIGURE 7-24

manufacture of these. The clip is designed to fit into the slot on the urinal bag and, therefore, must be made for a left or right leg so that the bag does not slip off the clip.

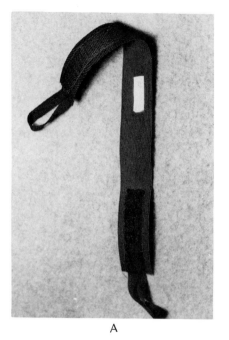 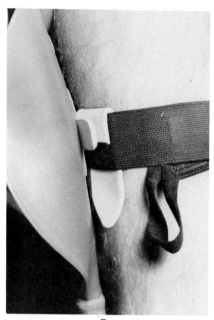

FIGURE 7-25

A   B

The same pattern of plastic clip may be bent to form a left or a right clip (Fig. 7-26). The small projection is placed pointing to the left and bent back for a left clip and facing right and bent back for a right clip. A three-piece jig may be made to be used to make the clips accurately and quickly. The heated material is held over the number one jig which is on a solid base. The number two jig is pressed down over the material forming the first bend. Number three jig is pushed over both jigs and the plastic projection to form the final bend (Fig. 7-27).

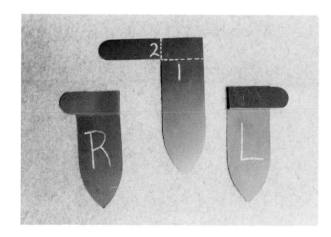 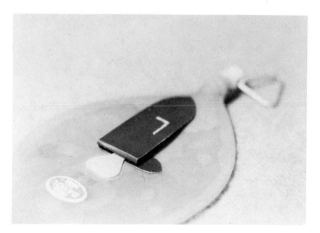

FIGURE 7-26

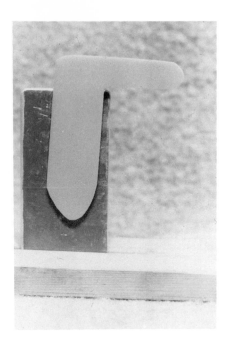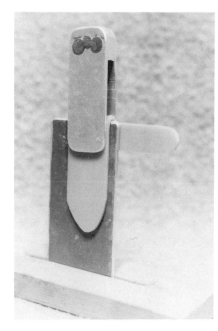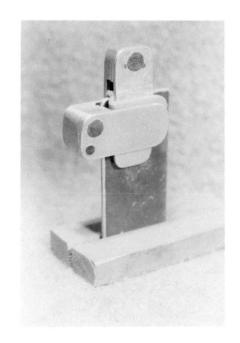

FIGURE 7-27

Usually a garter of the same style is used to position the tubing above the knee (Fig. 7-28). Sufficient tubing must be allowed so that the condom will not be pulled off when the patient changes leg position.

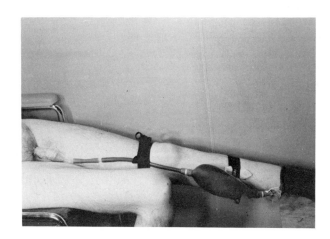

FIGURE 7-28

A short length of urinal tubing is attached to the urinal bag outlet with the cutoff clamp in place (Fig. 7-29). A modified lever-type-tubing cutoff is placed on this short tubing. A ring is cut off the tubing and slipped over the end of tubing to maintain the clamp in position. The cutoff is modified by rivetting a plastic loop to the lever and fastening a base plate beneath the cutoff so that if can be held firmly while the cutoff is operated.

232

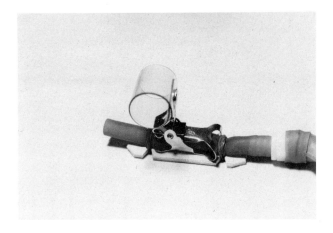

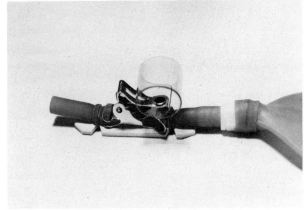

FIGURE 7-29

A, Clamp closed

B, Clamp open.

A cutoff clamp can be made of solid stock, hinging the lever so that the tubing is shut off with a roller-cam action (Fig. 7-30). Nonferrous wire is used to modify the cutoff plugs on the end of the urinal bag (Fig. 7-31). This is short and easy to camouflage and provides leverage to twist the plug.

APPLICATION OF URINE-COLLECTING SYSTEM

The patient assembles all his equipment and places it within easy reach. Some patients will prefer to sit up in bed so they can lean against pillows placed against the back of the bed. Other patients may find it more convenient to sit in the wheelchair with feet either on the footrests or on the bed. A patient may slide his buttocks forward on the chair seat to improve his balance and free both arms.

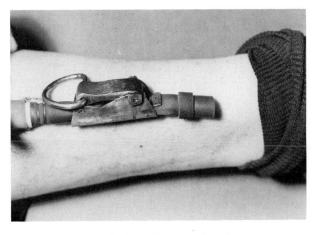

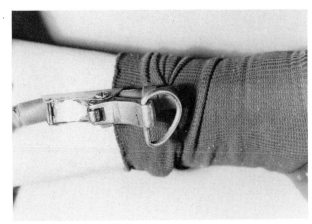

FIGURE 7-30

A, Cut-off clamp closed

B, Cut-off clamp open.

233

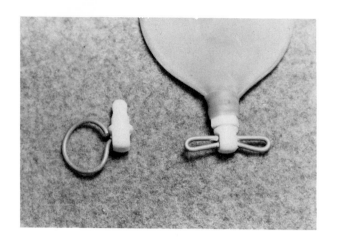

FIGURE 7-31

The patient applies benzoin simple to the shaft of the penis using a swab stick or gauze (Fig. 7-32). The screw top of the benzoin bottle may require adaption and occasional cleaning if the threads become sticky. A benzoin allergy patch test must be done prior to use. While the benzoin is drying the patient squeezes skin cement into a small receptacle. He uses his finger tips or a swab to apply the cement to the shaft of the penis (Fig. 7-33). Cement may be bought in a tin can with a brush fastened to the inside of the screw top lid. This is a very convenient utensil for brushing on the cement. If pubic hair interferes with cementing or application, the hair should be clipped.

When the cement is tacky the patient unrolls the condom for about an inch to ensure that the plastic plug does not touch the head of the penis (Fig. 7-34A). He puts the condom over the head of the penis until the roll makes contact with the cement. Once the condom has made contact with the cement, it can be rolled on easily (Fig. 7-34B).

The prepared condom is used in the same manner but, instead of unrolling it in the normal way, the two thread loops are pulled simultaneously to roll the condom on (Fig. 7-35). The condom is pressed in position all around to ensure good contact.

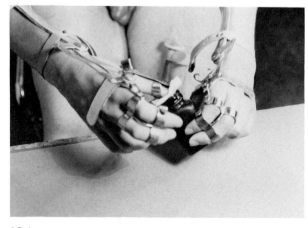

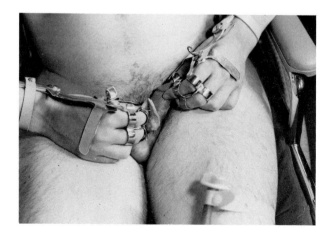

FIGURE 7-32

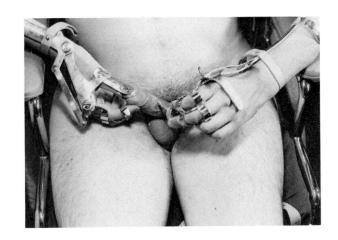

FIGURE 7-33

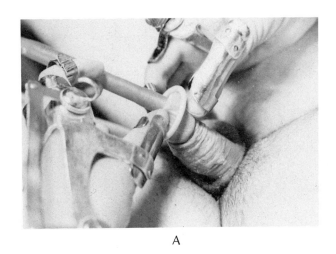

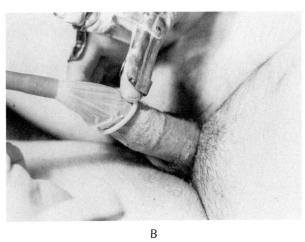

FIGURE 7-34

A

B

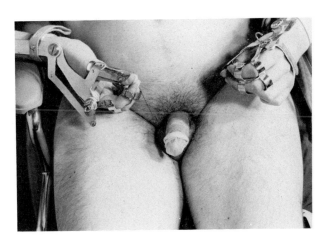

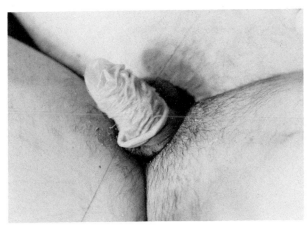

FIGURE 7-35

235

The patient pushes the blunt point of a pair of bandage scissors under the collar of the condom and cuts the collar by using the thumbs of both hands to close the scissors (Fig. 7-36). This prevents constriction of the penis. The scissors are pointed towards the patient's abdomen to ensure that he will not snip his skin. Some patients will remove the entire collar to eliminate any possible pressure area.

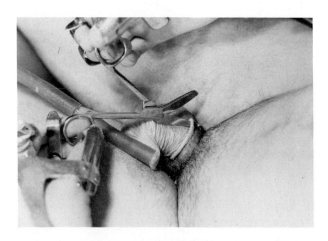
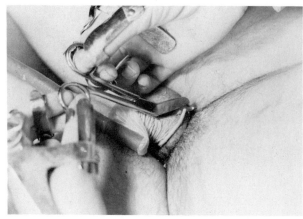

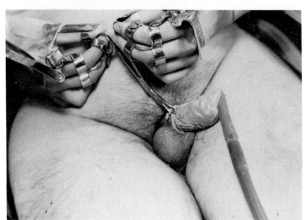

FIGURE 7-36

DRAINING THE URINAL

If the quadriplegic patient cannot attain complete independence he should be taught at least to empty his own urinal bag. Independence in this aspect of management is of great psychological benefit and enables him to remain unattended for a greater length of time.

Method 1. (Fig. 7-37) The patient positions himself by the toilet and reaches down to unzip his pant leg or, if he does not use a zipper, he pulls the pant leg up. He lifts the bag by pulling the clip out of the garter and rests the bag across his knee. He holds it down with one hand so that he can insert a thumb into the plastic loop and pull it open. He closes the clip by pressing down with the heel of his hand

236

or with his thumb. The firm base on the clip prevents the tubing from tipping or buckling during closure.

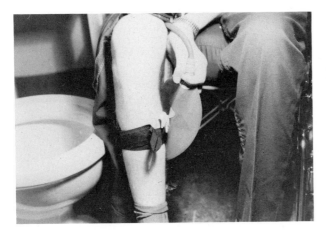 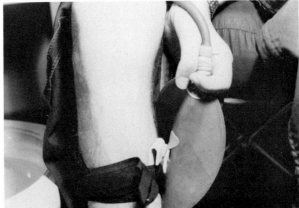

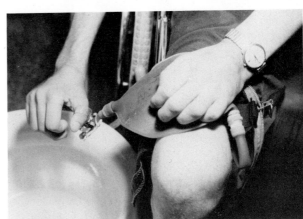

FIGURE 7-37

Method 2. (Fig. 7-38) The patient lifts his leg onto the toilet seat and reaches down to unfasten the drainage clamp. He may unclip the bag from the garter if he must rest the bag on the edge of the toilet seat in order to open the clamp. This position is stable and also prevents him from leaning so far forward that he may not be able to sit up again.

NIGHT DRAINAGE

The patient places an absorbent pad under the connector when he is in bed. He disconnects the urinal bag tube and attaches the connector to a long I.V. tube that leads down to a receptacle such as a gallon plastic bleach bottle, which is left on the floor under the bed. A patient must be encouraged to change position every two hours even if he must use an alarm clock to rouse himself at first. He usually starts the night on one side, then turns to supine, and then to the other side. Each

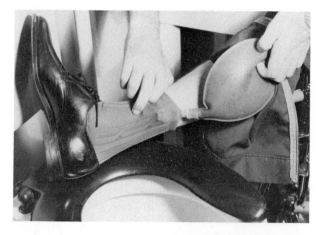
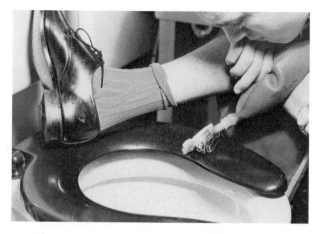
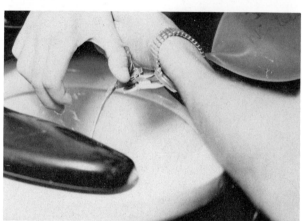
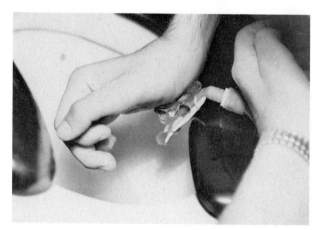

FIGURE 7-38

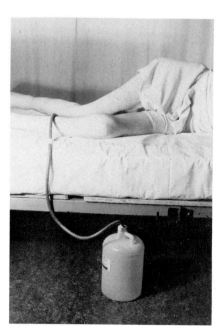

FIGURE 7-39

time he turns he must make certain that the urinal tube crosses his leg below the knee so that drainage is ensured (Fig. 7-39).

Sometimes a patient should lie prone because of pressure areas or because a dependent patient requires turning less frequently in this position. When a male patient is prone, he may require elevation with pillows, leaving a space between genital area and bed (Fig. 7-40) so that he does not lie on drainage tubing or penis and so that involuntary erections will present no problem. The patient's night connection may lead to a disposable plastic bag that hangs from a detachable hook on the bed (Fig. 7-41). This position is used mainly by the dependent patient because of the difficulty of placing pillows.

REMOVING AND DISCONNECTING THE URINE-COLLECTION SYSTEM

The clip of the urine-collection bag is slipped out of the lower garter and the garter above the knee is removed. The bag is placed on the bed or on a convenient

238

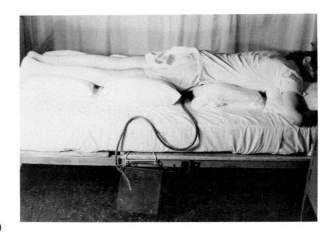

FIGURE 7-40

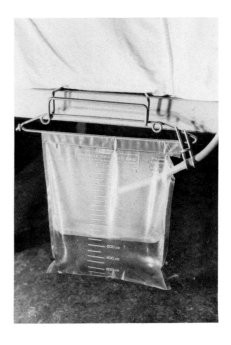

FIGURE 7-41

surface below the level of the condom to ensure continued drainage. The condom is peeled off, using hand friction, and the whole assembly is dropped into a receptacle. Skin cement should be removed completely once a week, using a cement solvent or ether. Cement solvent will scald the skin if used too generously or if left on too long. The area should be thoroughly washed and powdered before reapplying the clean urine-drainage system.

All plastic connectors should be moved from side to side to work them out of the tubing. Pulling will merely clamp the tubing tighter. The assembly apparatus may also be used for taking apart. The tubing connected to the top or bottom of the urinal bag is removed only periodically for thorough cleaning. Only quadriplegic patients with good finger function will be able to perform this task.

CARE OF URINAL APPARATUS

The urine-collecting apparatus is completely disconnected. Connectors are checked for sediment. The bag and tubing is rinsed well in cold water before soaking it in green soap or 20 per cent Dettol for 30 minutes. The equipment is suspended to dry.

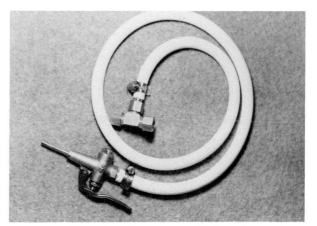

FIGURE 7-42

239

Two bags may be used, one every other day to permit proper cleansing and disinfecting. A flexible hose may be "T'd" into the cold water line of the toilet or sink. A nozzle with a long nose to insert into the urinal tubing is clamped to the hose (Fig. 7-42). This nozzle should have a lever-type release, operated by depressing it. This nozzle will require shop modification to lengthen the nose. This system is valuable, as the water pressure washes the urinal apparatus with little trouble to the patient.

MENSTRUAL MANAGEMENT

Management of the menstrual period may be a major problem for some women, especially those with a heavy flow, who need to change sanitary napkins or tampons frequently or have limited time or access to bathroom facilities during work or recreation time.

TAMPONS

Tampons are used by preference by many because of cleanliness and safety. A female quadriplegic patient with fair grasp may be able to insert and extract a tampon, positioning herself either on the toilet or on the front edge of her chair. Tampon inserters similar in mechanical principle to suppository inserters may be practical with certain patients but this apparatus has not been satisfactorily developed yet. Another possible adaptation is the addition of a longer cord with a loop tied at the end to facilitate extraction. Some women who are learning bladder control may find that tampons create too much pressure on the bladder; they should use pads until the pattern is well established. The dependent patient may be managed most satisfactorily by using tampons, eliminating hazards of pressure from pads.

SANITARY PADS OR LARGE DRESSINGS

Sanitary pads can now be obtained with a strip on the back which will cling to underpants and keep the pad in place. A pad may be placed in the crotch of the underpants before pulling them up. This will normally be accomplished in whatever position the patient uses for putting on her pants. The front of the crotch of a pair of stretchy underpants may be cut from leg opening to leg opening and a velcro closure and loop sewn in. When the patient is seated on the toilet she can undo the crotch flap to replace her pad.

Many women cannot tolerate sitting on a normal sanitary pad owing to a combination of the bulk of material, dampness, and their particular skin tolerance and build. Large dressings may be used by some women because they are less bulky and can be placed to cover a larger area, so distributing pressure and reducing risk of soiling.

CONTROL THROUGH MEDICAL MEANS

The physician may prescribe birth control pills to be taken on a daily basis in an attempt to eliminate the menstrual period entirely. Menstrual periods may be such a problem to some women that they and their physician may consider surgery.

240

8

Holding and Manipulating

MANIPULATING

The quadriplegic patient lacking only the intrinsic muscles of the hand should not needs aids or splints. He will lack some dexterity and strength that could hinder him in some vocational and avocational pursuits but should not interfere with his self-care.

A patient who lacks finger flexion may pick up, hold, and manipulate to a varying extent using tenodesis, i.e. the normal finger flexion caused by extension of the wrist (Fig. 8-1). The fingers must have contracted a little to make their grip functional. Care must be taken not to overstretch fingers for this reason, but range must be maintained in the thumb web space and the distal joint of the thumb. A patient may require padded handles (Fig. 8-2) to use his tenodesis effectively if his fingers are not sufficiently contracted or if his grip is weak. Padding should be made of lightweight, nonslip material and be either washable or removable. Plastizote, ground to shape, is an excellent padding material. Another is foam-backed leather with velcro or press-stud fastenings to allow cutlery to be removed for washing.

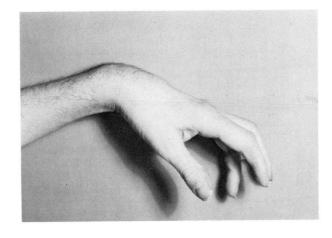
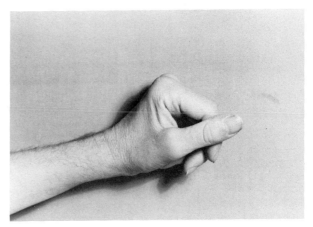

FIGURE 8-1

He may hold and use a thin-handled tool by weaving the handle into the fingers, i.e. over the first, under the second, over the third, and under the fourth, or vice versa (Fig. 8-3). He may tighten the grip by using tenodesis.

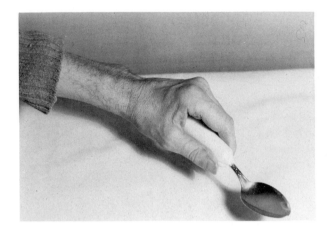

FIGURE 8-2

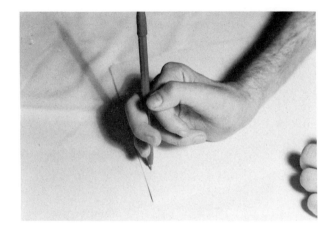

FIGURE 8-3

Many objects may be held between the heels of the hands. Legible writing is possible and may be useful if a small amount of writing such as a signature is required (Fig. 8-4). This method does, however, preclude using a telephone and holding the paper down simultaneously.

The patient may push or pull by placing his hand and arm into such a position that a digit can be put into its extreme of joint range, so using ligaments rather than muscles (Fig. 8-5).

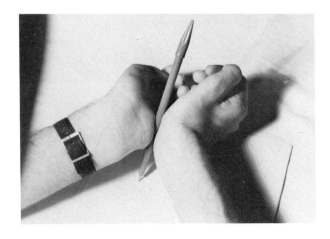

FIGURE 8-4

242

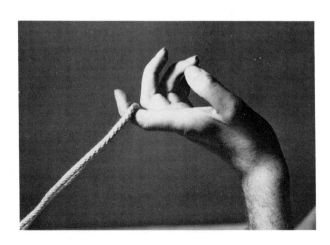

FIGURE 8-5

Type 1. A wrist-driven flexor-hinge splint may be prescribed. This is a plastic or metal splint that causes the first two fingers to meet the thumb when the wrist is extended (Fig. 8-6A). The splint must be carefully fitted both to prevent pressure areas and to ensure that the thumb and fingers meet correctly. The wrist extensors must be strong enough to take some resistance plus gravity. The patient must be capable of maintaining his hand in a pronated position while holding his wrist in extension. It is preferable to fit the leading hand even though it may be a little weaker.

If the patient requires the second splint it may be constructed so that it opens wide, whereas the first splint is made so that the wrist is only slightly extended when the fingers and thumb meet. This enables the patient to grip a greater variety of objects. A spring pencil holder attached near the MP joint of the splint provides a stable point for many tools as well as a pen or pencil and is a valuable addition (Fig. 8-6B).

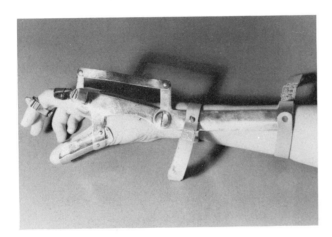
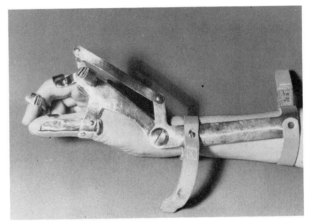
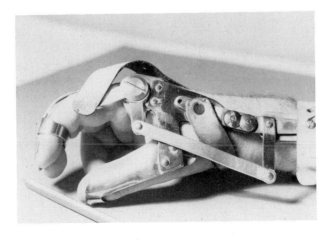
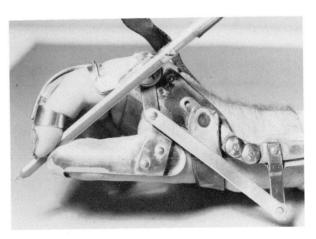

FIGURE 8-6

B, Drive bar below

243

Training a quadriplegic in the use of his splint is very similar to amputee training. This includes counselling the patient in the advantages and disadvantages of the splint, in gradually working up wearing time, in checking for pressure points, and in gradually increasing strength, dexterity, and endurance. Some activities performed with flexor-hinge splints include hobbies such as mosaic work, carpentry, and sewing. Work activities may include writing, operating typewriters, telephones, calculators, etc. Everyday activities may include cooking, eating, and housework.

Type 2. A patient may use a splint with a pocket in it to fit common tools such as a spoon, tooth brush, or pencil (Fig. 8-7). This splint may be made with velcro and a D-ring, putting the pocket on the palmar side of the hand, the narrower end of the pocket at the ulnar border. The strap is fastened around the hand proximal to the metacarpophalangeal joints. This splint is both easy to put on and to secure.

The velcro D-ring pocket splint is made from approximately 8 inches of 1-inch-wide pile velcro, with 4 inches of hook velcro sewn to the end facing in the same direction. To form the pocket, a 3-inch length of pile velcro is sewn facing the pile velcro strap 1½-inches from the end of the pile velcro. The pocket is usually tapered, wide to grip tools at one end and narrow to grip a pencil at the end where the hook velcro is sewn. Modifications may be made—a sewn base to the pocket or a 2-inch width of velcro sewn to the 1-inch strap to fit cooking utensils, etc. A square 1-inch D-ring is sewn to the free end of the pile velcro. The hook velcro is threaded through it, and an open loop of plastic is rapid-rivetted to the back of the free end of the hook velcro (Fig. 8-8). The plastic loop may be made of .040 gauge polished polyethylene chloride sheeting, 1-inch wide by 3 inches long.

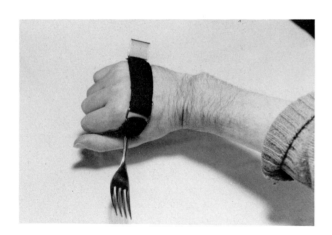

FIGURE 8-7

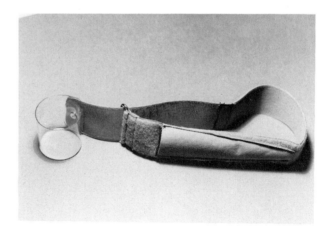

FIGURE 8-8

Type 3. Loop handles of plastic, leather and elastic, velcro and D-ring metal, etc. may be permanently fixed to the tool. The loop should be placed proximal to the metacarpophalangeal joints, firmly enough to prevent the tool from sliding around the hand (Fig. 8-9). The rigid loop handle with an open end will be practical and easier to put on than a handle with a complete loop, particularly for those with very wasted hands or those with large metacarpophalangeal joints. Velcro and D-ring fastenings are practical for the majority. Tools must be fixed to the loops so that they are in the optimum positions. This should be ascertained by temporary taping before the loop is permanently fixed.

Type 4. A firm grip that will not release can be provided using a glove with the fingertips fastened to a strap. The fingers are then drawn down and the strap is fastened around the wrist (Fig. 8-10). If the strap is fastened with velcro it may be undone independently but most quadriplegic patients who require this aid will be unable to put the glove on alone.

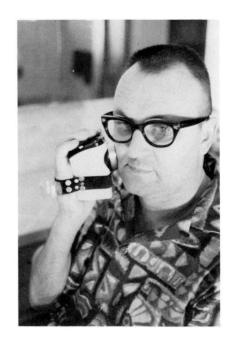

FIGURE 8-9

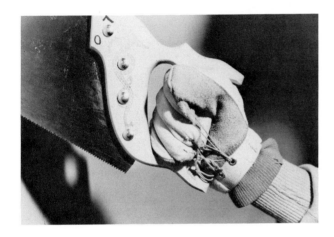

FIGURE 8-10

Type 5. A patient may stabilize objects in clamps (Fig. 8-11) or vises (Fig. 8-12). When a scissor action tool such as a side cutter, pliers, or a leather punch is frequently used, a clamp may be permanently brazed under the lower lever arm so that it may be fastened to the working surface and one lever only operated (Fig. 8-13).

FIGURE 8-11. Leather-hinged wooden clamp rubber lined for optimum grip.

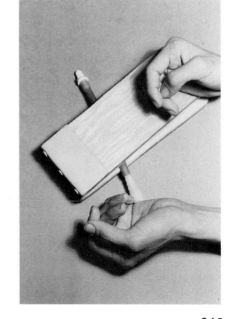

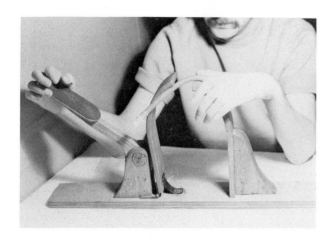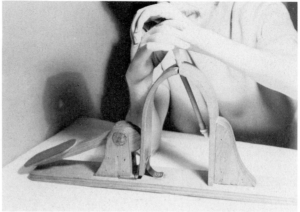

FIGURE 8-12. Leather worker's vise leaves both hands free.

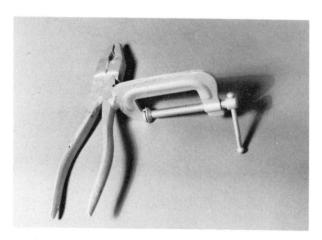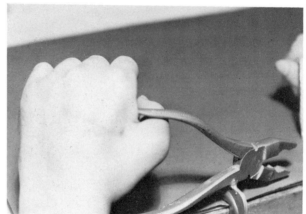

FIGURE 8-13

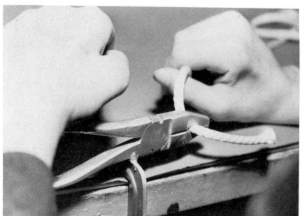

Type 6.   Pliers may be adapted for use with a wrist-driven flexor-hinge splint. A ring is brazed to the lower lever of the plier to fit around the thumb and elastic is fitted over the fingers and fastened to the top lever (Fig. 8-14). The pliers may be used to handle small objects with an accuracy that may not be possible with the fingers.

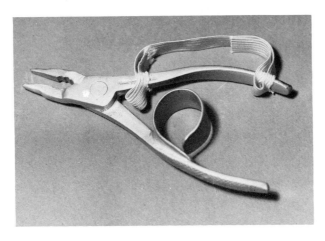

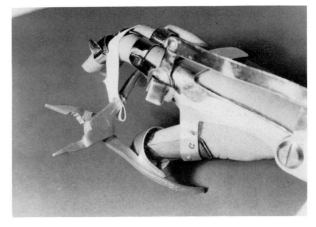

FIGURE 8-14

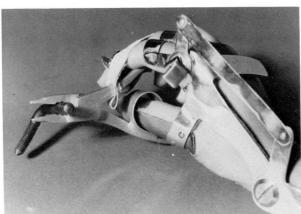

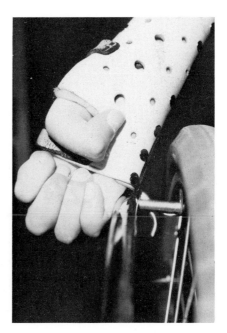

Type 7.   Fibreglass or plastic splints may be made that immobilize the wrist and are fitted with metal sockets for holding the tools most commonly used by the patient, i.e. projections for propelling the wheelchair, typing sticks, and pen (Fig. 8-15). This is used for patients with flail wrists but with elbow flexion and shoulder control.

FIGURE 8-15

Type 8. The commercially available ball-bearing feeder may be prescribed for a patient with a high lesion but very little spasticity (Fig. 8-16). This feeder usually requires a supinator attachment. The feeder requires careful adjustment and training in its use (see Adjusting a Ball-Bearing or Rocker Feeder). The arm trough may be replaced by moulded plastic or fibreglass so that pressure areas are avoided and the arm is stabilized in the trough.

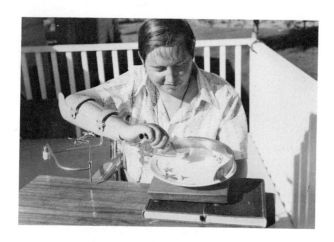

FIGURE 8-16

Type 9. More commonly used is the rocker feeder suitable for quadriplegic patients who have some degree of spasticity (Fig. 8-17). This may be clamped to the table or to the wheelchair arm. Usually a supinator attachment is necessary. The rocker feeder has a universal joint under the trough which may be more or less mechanically restricted in movement, depending on the degree of control of the patient. A rocker feeder may have a horizontal arm to permit some horizontal motion, the length again depending on the amount of control possible. This arm fits vertically into a tube on the clamp or wheelchair arm and then is bent at right angles.

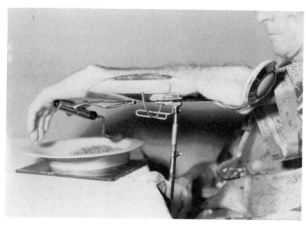
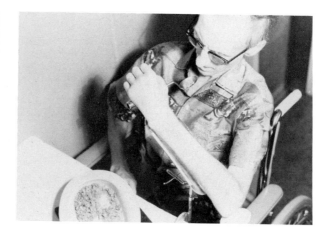

FIGURE 8-17

An adjustable stop may be fitted to the vertical part of the arm. The height of the apparatus, length of the arm, and point of balance of the rocker require adjusting to the individual patient. (Details on adjustment procedures will be found under Adjusting a Ball-Bearing or Rocker Feeder.) The metal trough in this feeder may also be replaced with a moulded fibreglass or plastic trough.

Type 10. Overhead slings may be prescribed (Fig. 8-18). The sling support bar should be easily detachable from the chair to enable transportation. The height of the bar can be varied to increase or decrease the pendulum action. The bar is raised for the patient with more control and vice versa. The suspension unit can be spring or webbing, again, the spring for the patient who can control it but who can benefit from the feeling of liveliness and from the increased reach. The suspension can clip directly to an elbow sling and must be adjustable to the most useful height. This height is often decided by the spoon-to-mouth test.

Two slings may be used, one for the elbow and one for the forearm (Fig. 8-19). These have adjustable webbing straps that clip to either end of a horizontal metal strip above the two slings. The strip has holes drilled in it at 2-inch intervals. The strap or spring from the overhead bar is clipped to one of the holes in the metal strip, thus creating a fulcrum and allowing the metal strip to pivot. The position of the fulcrum is adjusted so that the forearm can be held horizontally when relaxed. Further adjustments for optimum function can be made from this point. A patient who must use slings will usually require a splint to support his wrist. A slot may be incorporated to accept frequently used tools.

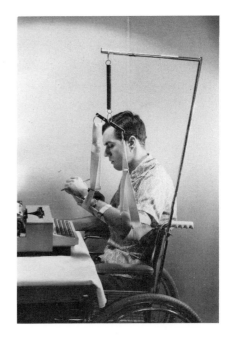

FIGURE 8-18

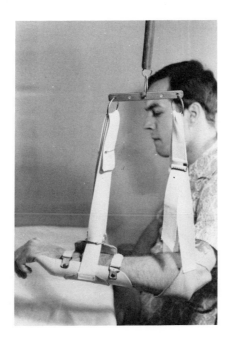

FIGURE 8-19

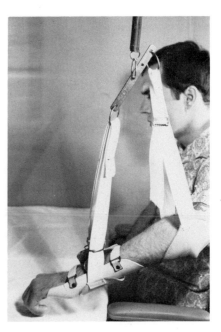

Type 11. When a patient cannot operate a splint with his own muscle power, external power may be selected. This power may be electrical or CO_2 muscle power (Fig. 8-20) and may be activated by mechanical pull of a valve or switch, by myoelectric-operated solenoid switches, or by contact-operated micro switches. The type of switch and the movement required to operate it must be selected so that the device can be operated in a near natural manner, unrestrictive to other functional movements. The device must not take an excessive amount of time to put on and must be acceptable and useful to the patient. Many patients using external power will need to have the apparatus put on for them.

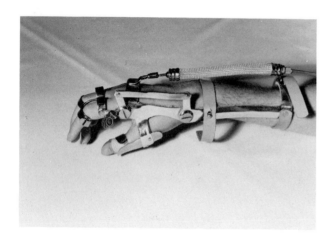 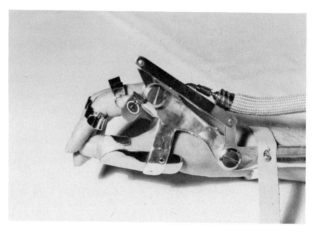

FIGURE 8-20

Type 12. A patient may use a mouth- or head-controlled stick for page turning, controlling an electric wheelchair, painting, writing, typing, etc. (Fig. 8-21). If a patient uses a mouthstick a great deal of the time, he may require a plate fitted over his teeth by a dentist in order to protect his teeth and maintain a good bite. The patient should be able to rest a mouthstick in a holder, so that it can be retrieved easily.

Type 13. Apparatus may be mounted in a stable and convenient position and operated by head movement. Such apparatus may be an electric razor, toothbrush, comb, or electric switches (Fig. 8-22).

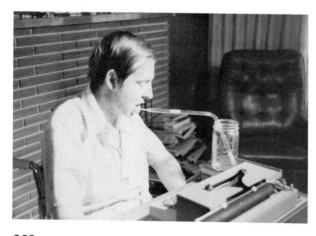 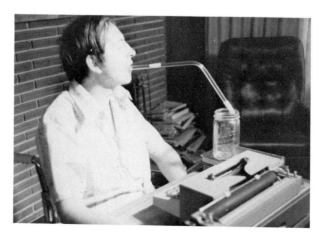

FIGURE 8-21

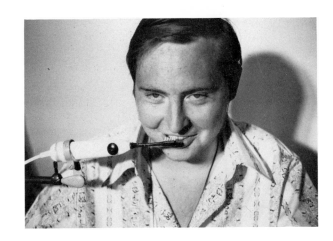

FIGURE 8-22

Type 14.   Such specialized electronic equipment as POSSUM or PILOT may be presecribed for environmental control, typewriter operation, etc. for a patient who cannot manage in any other fashion. This equipment may be operated with either minimal movement or by controlling inspiration and expiration of air (Fig. 8-23).

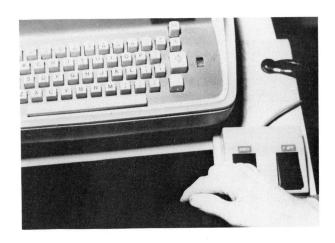

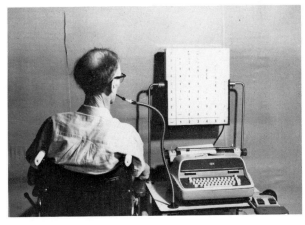

FIGURE 8-23

HOLDING METHODS APPLIED TO SPECIFIC TOOLS

TOILETTE

As stated previously, the patient's own care for his personal needs is of psychological importance to him. His daily toilette is one of these aspects.

Tooth Care

Toothpaste.   Toothpaste is stored within reach with the cap screwed down just enough to hold. It is picked up by tenodesis or between the heels of both hands. The cap is removed by using the teeth and tongue, and the amount of toothpaste desired is sucked from the tube. The cap is replaced with a minimal twist given by both head and hands. The toothpaste can be squeezed onto the toothbrush bristles by using the heels of the hands, by using a flexor-hinge splint to squeeze the paste out, or by using the teeth while holding the bottom of the tube in the mouth.

Toothbrush. The toothbrush may be picked up by using tenodesis, the palms of both hands, a padded handle, a loop on the handle, a flexor-hinge splint, or a pocket splint (Fig. 8-24). An electric toothbrush is managed in the same manner. It should be possible to swivel the toothbrush so that the inside and outside of the teeth can be cleaned. The toothbrush should point towards the back of the mouth so that a turn of the head will allow the teeth on both sides of the mouth to be cleaned. The toothbrush handle may be bent or the holder angled to allow all the teeth to be reached.

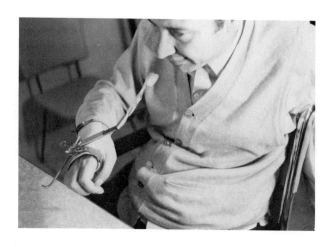

FIGURE 8-24

With an ordinary toothbrush, a combination of hand and head movement is used for brushing. Up-and-down brushing is difficult and side-to-side brushing is substituted. To save swivelling the toothbrush twice, the outside of one side and the inside of another is cleaned, then the toothbrush is swivelled using the tongue and teeth. Teeth may be further cleaned by eating raw carrot, etc., if tooth brushing is inadequate. Frequent visits to the dentist will help to preserve the teeth, the equivalent of the quadriplegic patient's third hand.

Dentures. Dentures can be ejected with the tongue into the cupped hands or into a container of denture cleaner. The dentures may be cleaned by using a nail brush fastened to the sink with suction cups. They may be held by tenodesis or between the heels of the hand to replace. The arms may be stabilized by resting the elbows on a solid surface.

Care of the Hair

Short hair is easiest to manage for both men and women. Bobby pins, rollers, etc., are not practical, and visits to a hairdresser or help at home must be available for longer or more complicated hair styles. Because the patient may have a problem with excessive sweating his hair may have to be shampooed frequently.

Brush. A military-style brush may be adapted by fastening a length of elastic to either side of the brush with screws and washers. The elastic must fit snugly over the hand. D-ring and velcro can be substituted for elastic. A brush with a handle may have an elastic loop, a D-ring and velcro, or a padded handle (Fig. 8-25). For mechanical advantage the hand should be placed close to or over the back of the brush rather than on the handle where the leverage will work against the patient. If the patient is unable to reach parts of his head, he should rest an elbow on a table or dresser and flex his neck and upper trunk until his hand reaches his head. This is a method of obtaining increased shoulder flexion. A flexor-hinge splint may be used to hold the handle of a hairbrush.

Comb. A rat-tailed comb may be held in a wrist-driven flexor-hinge splint, in a pocket splint, a rigid splint, a wall-mounted bracket, or by using a padded handle (Fig. 8-26). The rat-tailed comb may be twisted, bent, or lengthened to allow all parts of the head to be reached.

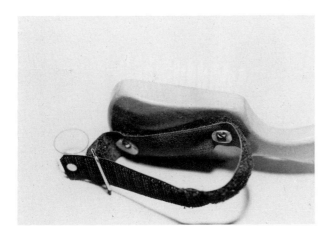

FIGURE 8-25

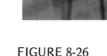

FIGURE 8-26

Shaving

Electric Razor. A strong tenodesis can be used to hold an electric razor; vibration will cause the razor to slide out of a weak grip. A flexor-hinge splint may be used to hold most makes of razor, weight being the limiting factor. During training a long elastic may be taped to the razor and hung round the neck as a safety measure. A plastic handle may be bent to fit the hand and fastened to the razor with epoxy cement. The handle must be positioned so that the beard can be completely shaved.

Velcro and D-ring, as in a pocket splint, may be taped to the razor (Fig. 8-27A) to establish the correct angle before permanently rivetting the velcro D-ring to a detachable leather razor jacket (Fig. 8-27B).

The razor may be attached to a bar which may be slipped into a slot in a rigid cock-up splint (Fig. 8-28A). The angle of the razor should be adjusted so that all the face can be shaved. The razor may be fixed to a swing away bar projecting from the

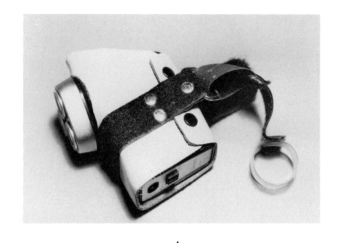

FIGURE 8-27

A

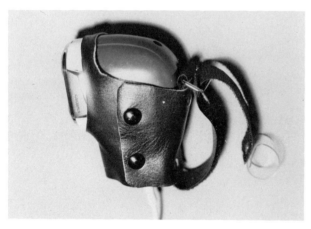
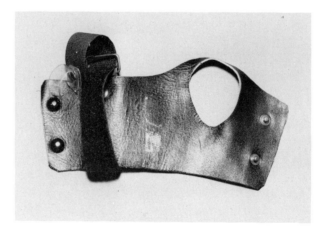

B

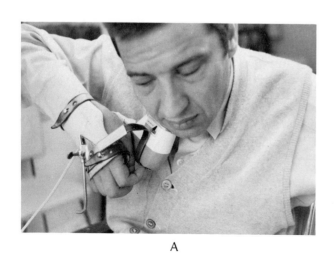

A

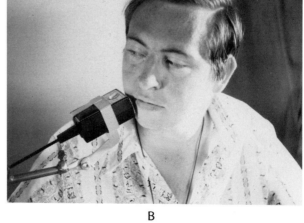

B

FIGURE 8-28

254

wall (Fig. 8-28B). The patient can move his chair around so that he can reach both sides of his face. The plug on the electric cord may be enlarged for easier handling by jamming an empty spool (such as an adhesive tape spool) permanently over the plug. A metal spool should be insulated for safety. It may be easier to adapt the plug than to adapt the razor switch which is often small or inset. The use of cordless razors may be an advantage, but weight, shape, and cost must be taken into consideration.

Safety Razors. The person who cannot be counselled to use an electric razor must have a safety razor adapted. The razor may be held in a flexor-hinge splint, or by padding the handle. Since there are so many makes of safety razor with as many different methods of inserting and extracting blades this problem must be worked out individually.

FOOD MANAGEMENT

Spoons and Forks

Some patients manage an unadapted spoon but many spoons must have two bends of about 120° giving a step effect. One bend should be by the bowl and the other about 2 inches up the handle, thus the rest of the handle and the bowl will be approximately parallel (Fig. 8-29A). The spoon can now be used in a deep bowl and the fingers will be kept out of the way (Fig. 8-29B).

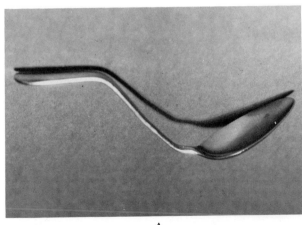
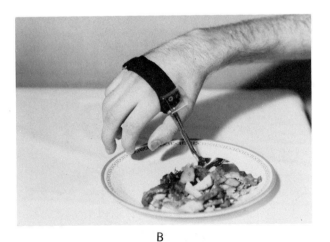

FIGURE 8-29

A   B

A spoon may require not only a double bend but also a twist so that the spoon tip will point towards the mouth. Patients with inadequate range may require a lengthened handle (Fig. 8-30A). A length of stainless steel or plastic is fixed to a spoon and then bent back to form a loop which is fitted proximal to the metacarpophalangeal joints (Fig. 8-30B). This spoon handle is easy to apply.

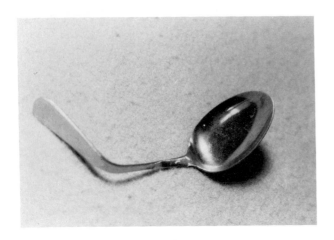
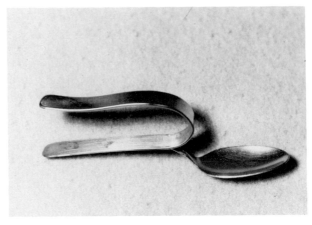

A

B

FIGURE 8-30

Spoons or forks may be held by threading the handle through the fingers or by the use of a pocket splint, a padded handle, or a flexor-hinge splint. A rigid cock-up splint may have a slot on the palm to receive the modified handle. This spoon may be a swivel-handled spoon with stops and two bends in order to keep the bowl level (Fig. 8-31 and 8-32).

Adjusting a Ball-Bearing or Rocker Feeder

The patient is seated in his normal position in the wheelchair. The trough, elbow, and hand piece are adjusted for length and comfort and a tentative point of balance is found (Fig. 8-33A). The final point of balance is dependent on the height and position of the trough. The height of the feeder is adjusted so that when the elbow is down it clears the table or chair arm. The hand should be about level with the nose (Fig. 8-33B).

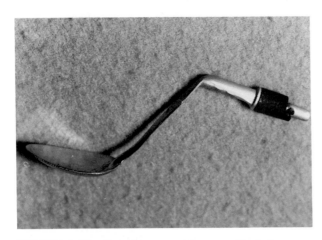
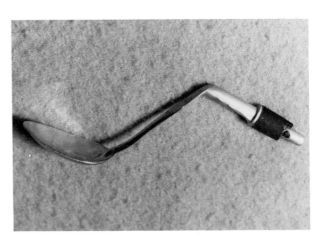

FIGURE 8-31. Swivel spoon with stops. Black sleeve fits into metal slot on the splint under the palm of the hand.

256

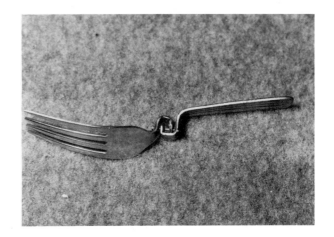

FIGURE 8-32. Simply constructed swivel fork made by cutting and bending the fork handle, drilling a hole through the bent ends, and inserting a cotter pin as an axle.

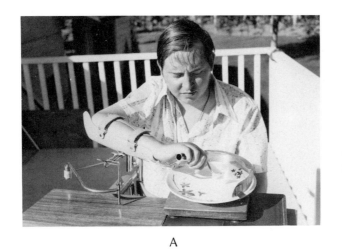

A

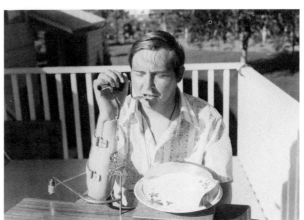

B

FIGURE 8-33

C

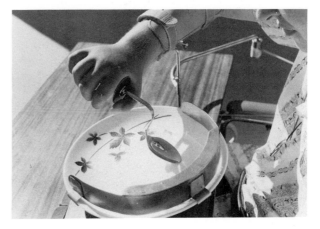

The double angles of the spoon should be as shallow as possible so that the hand does not have to be raised high but should be long enough so that the lever arm is sufficient to maintain the spoon bowl in a horizontal plane. Much depends on the efficiency of the swivel which must not bind. Once the length of the drop in the spoon is established, the spoon-to-mouth test will be used to establish final positioning. If either the up or down movement should be difficult, the balance may be adjusted to compensate.

The rocker feeder may have two points permanently marked on the vertical adjustment; one for eating which often requires considerably more height than other activities, i.e. typing.

The table or plate height is adjusted so that the spoon reaches the plate Sometimes the plate must be raised on a block so that the elbow can clear the table (Fig. 8-33C). The plate may require a plate guard, or a Mannoy plate made by Melaware may be used. A nonslip pad may be required to stabilize the plate. A turntable may also be required to compensate for limited movement if the patient is unable to reach parts of the plate. Finally the stop on the swivel spoon is fixed so that the spoon remains stable while picking up food but is able to swivel freely as the spoon travels towards the mouth.

Plates

Plates may be fitted with plate guards or a Mannoy plate may be used if the patient has difficulty pushing the food onto fork or spoon. A nonslip pad will stabilize the plate. Soup bowls may be more functional than a dinner plate for some patients because the rounded shape fits the spoon bowl and enables more food to be picked up.

Water may be spooned when working out mechanics so that the levels can be easily seen and little mess made. Spooning dried foods is useful for working out plate-level mechanics. During eating training a patient should be given privacy until he becomes proficient. Type of food chosen for training is important. Foods which tend to stick to the spoon such as purees or stews are preferable to dry food or thin soups.

Knives

Cutting can be a difficult and lengthy procedure for some quadriplegic patients. In these cases it is preferable to have meat cut beforehand so that the patient can eat a hot meal. The patient may hold a sharp knife between the heels of both hands and use direct pressure rather than a sawing action. Greater pressure and some rocking action can be achieved by using the knife tip although the area cut is less.

A rigid metal or plastic handle may be attached to the knife near the blade and bent back over the dorsum of the hand (Fig. 8-34). The other end is not attached to the knife handle but left open for easy insertion of the hand. The knife blade may require some bending for better function. The knife must be firmly held to enable the patient to apply adequate pressure. The knife may be held conventionally so that the blade points toward midline or, if more pressure is required, the knife may be reversed so that supinators which are generally stronger may be used effectively (Fig. 8-35).

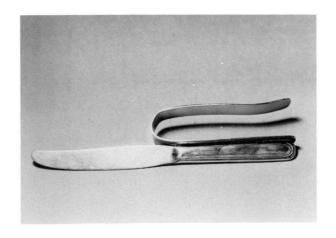

FIGURE 8-34

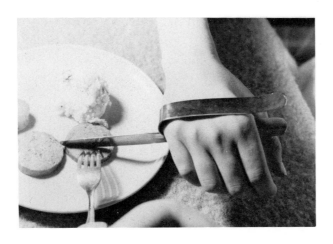

FIGURE 8-35

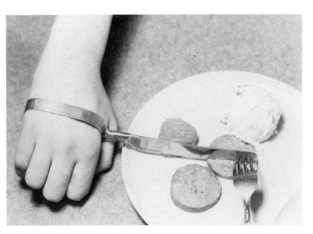

Water glasses and Cups

Many quadriplegic patients have finger flexors adequately contracted to use tenodesis for holding a cold glass. The glass is pushed into the hand with the other hand (Fig. 8-36). A wrist-driven flexor-hinge hand splint may be used to pick up a small glass provided the drive bar is above the hand. A plastic straw may be used for hot or cold liquids.

Mugs and some cups may be managed by pushing the thumb into the handle and with the wrist extended the lower part of the mug rests against the dorsum of the flexed fingers. Care must be taken that hot cups do not cause burns on anaesthetic fingers. The heels of both hands may be pressed against the opposite sides of the glass and the glass raised to the mouth. Resting the elbows·on the table while raising the glass adds to stability.

Quadriplegic patients have been known to pick up a glass in their teeth and drink, but this method is not recommended because of the possibility of breaking teeth or glass.

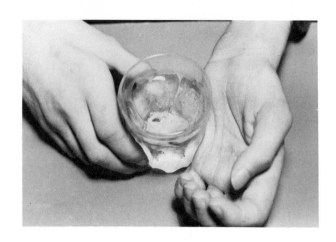 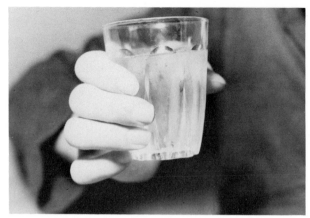

FIGURE 8-36

WRITING

The table surface must be at a comfortable height and the chair must be wheeled well under it so that the elbows can rest on the table. A ballpoint pen can be heated and bent down if the point touches the paper at too acute an angle. A felt-tipped or nylon-tipped pen may be used if a patient cannot exert adequate pressure.

Tenodesis may be adequate to hold a pen in the normal manner. The eraser end of the pencil rests in the thumb web and the other end under the terminal phalanx of any of the first three fingers. The elbow is usually raised to compensate for the extended wrist, and the hand is not completely pronated.

The pencil may be held by threading it through the fingers, i.e. over the first, under the second, over the third, or vice-versa. This is not usually a very firm hold but may be useful for writing a small amount, i.e. a signature. A pen may be held between the heels of both hands pressed together. This precludes the use of a telephone or holding down a paper at the same time. In addition it is hard to see around the hands to watch the pen tip, therefore the pen tip must usually be tipped towards the writer. This method is useful mainly for writing a signature when equipment is not at hand.

If writing is shaky, the patient should be counselled to write faster. Practise and writing exercises are usually helpful. Shakiness may not be reduced but will not be as obvious in the writing.

If a patient is found to require a writing splint, assessment of the optimum hand angles, pen angles, and methods of holding the fingers and pen may be worked out using adhesive tape. It should be remembered that the pencil or pen will be held more firmly with tape, but there will be a good indication of which fingers or thumb should be incorporated in a splint.

A pocket splint may be useful for writing, particularly when control of pronation and supination is good. The pencil is pushed through the pocket so that the point projects about an inch below the ulnar border of the hand. The pencil must be held firmly in the pocket.

A flexor-hinge splint is very useful for writing, particularly with the addition of a hook or spring loop to hold the eraser end of the pencil near the metacar-

260

pophalangeal joint (Fig. 8-37). The position is determined by temporarily taping the pencil in position for writing, then marking the correct placement for the spring clip.

A writing splint made of plastic or metal to hold the pencil between the thumb pad and finger may be constructed (Fig. 8-38). All the interphalangeal joints may need to be stabilized in this splint, thus creating a solid triangle, the finger forming one side, the thumb another, and the thumb web the third.

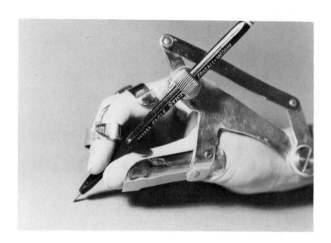

FIGURE 8-37

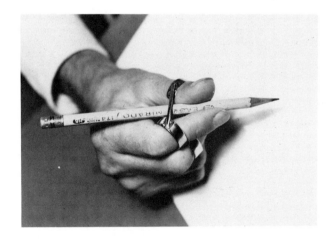

FIGURE 8-38

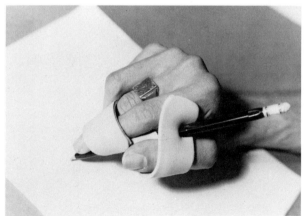

A great variety of plastic or metal splints may be constructed so that hand and pen are held comfortably (Fig. 8-39). If the writing aid is to be permanent it must be made so that it will last, be easy to put on, and be unobtrusive.

If a quadriplegic patient requires aids such as ball-bearing feeders, rocker feeders, overhead slings, or a mouthstick, he will find it more practical to type.

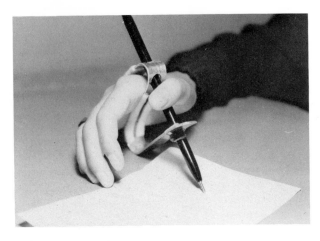 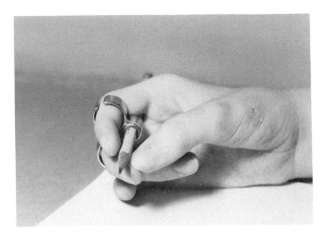

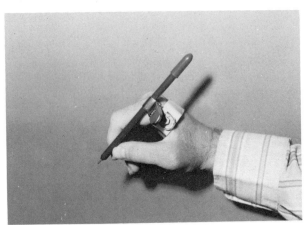 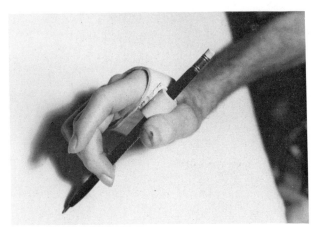

FIGURE 8-39

TYPING

The typewriter should be placed at a comfortable height and distance to reduce fatigue. One finger of each hand may be used if the fingers are in a suitable position and the other fingers do not hit the keys inadvertently. Methods used by the patient for holding his pencil can be used with the pencil reversed so that the eraser hits the keys.

A plastic finger cot may be made with a typing stick projecting from the tip (Fig. 8-40). Arm slings or ball-bearing feeders may be used with a detachable typing stick firmly fitted to the handpiece. Typing sticks should be rubber tipped so that they do not slip on the keys or damage them. They must be fixed at an angle and length to allow the patient to see the keys as he hits them. The typing stick should be short to reduce the length of the lever arm. Typing sticks may be constructed from pencils with erasers at the tip or, if the sticks require a curve, metal rod such as welding rod may be used with detachable slip-on erasers plugged to fit over the tips.

A mouthstick may be used (Fig. 8-41) but care must be taken that the teeth are not damaged by excessive use with poor fitting. A dental plate incorporating the mouthstick may be fitted over the teeth by a dentist to prevent this damage. The mouthstick should be made just long enough so that the patient can look with comfort at the keys he is touching. The head should be held in a comfortable position.

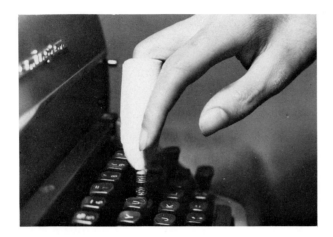

FIGURE 8-40

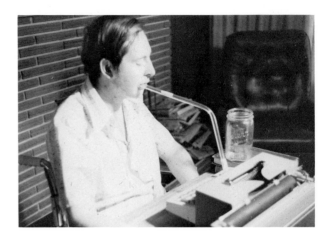

FIGURE 8-41

A POSSUM or PILOT system may be used to operate a typewriter by a patient with minimal or no movement.

If a manual typewriter is impracticable an electric typewriter may be used. Care should be taken when selecting a typewriter to see that margin setting and carriage return buttons are within reach and that the paper can be inserted independently. The paper may be rolled into an electric typewriter using the carriage return button, once the paper is placed in position. The typewriter may be adapted to take a continuous roll of paper to eliminate frequency of loading.

Similar methods to the above may be used to operate many business machines.

TELEPHONING

Dialing

The receiver may be placed on a convenient surface while dialing. Dialing is facilitated by using immovable telephones, telephones placed on a nonslip surface, telephones with deep dial holes and a light return spring.

A rigid finger may be used for dialing. When a high number is dialed the right hand must be pronated and the shoulder internally rotated. As the number is rotated around the dial the shoulder is externally rotated and the hand supinated so that the finger remains in the same position relative to the dial. This is reversed for the left hand.

A pencil reversed in a pocket splint may be used with or without a flexor-hinge splint worn simultaneously to hold the receiver. Dialing may be accomplished using a reversed pencil in the pencil holder of a flexor-hinge splint. Pushbutton dialing or a speaker phone may be substituted for a conventional phone.

Picking up the Receiver

Picking up the receiver is easier if the receiver is a light-weight type (the modern plastic receiver). The receiver may be pushed off the rest onto the table while the number is dialed or, less commonly, may be held in position while dialing. The receiver may be picked up using tenodesis, the heels of both hands, or a flexor-hinge splint, or it may be held permanently in position on a stand.

A simple economical stand may be made for the patient who cannot hold a receiver. A lamp stand with a flexible arm may be used with broom handle clips fastened to the top to hold the receiver (Fig. 8-42). The flexibility makes it easy to position the receiver for the individual.

Because the receiver is permanently off the telephone rest, another means must be used to depress the contact buttons. A wooden base is made for the telephone with a 3-inch-square projection in line with the buttons. A corner brace is used to fasten a length of solid stock ½-inch by ½-inch, and a hole is drilled in it, level with the contact button. Another length of stock is drilled so that one contact button is held down when the two pieces are attached at right angles (Fig. 8-43A), using a bolt as an axle. Washers are used as spacers to eliminate friction. An elastic is hooked around two screw eyes, positioned so that when the movable lever is vertical (Fig. 8-43B), the elastic moves behind the fulcrum. A stop is necessary at the base to prevent the arm from moving past the vertical.

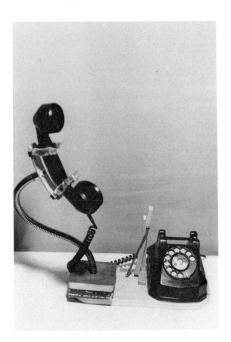

FIGURE 8-42

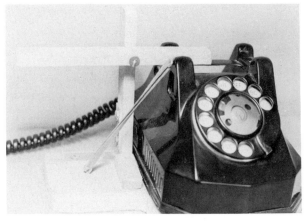

A

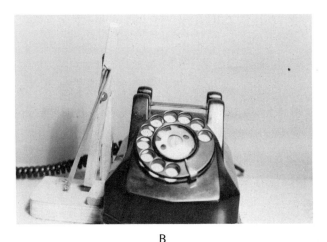

B

FIGURE 8-43

Holding the Receiver

After placing the receiver in position it may be held as it was picked up. It may be held by shoulder shrug as in holding a violin. Many types of receiver rests or speaker telephones are available, but solving telephone problems will depend to some extent on the types available in different localities.

CUTTING WITH SCISSORS

The method presented here (Fig. 8-44A) may be useful for the quadriplegic patient, not only for hobby purposes but also for trimming pubic hair and cutting the ring of the condom. Pressure down onto the table closes the scissors while gravity will open them (Fig. 8-44B). The scissors must be chosen carefully so that they will open easily and still cut without requiring any twisting force.

Electric scissors may be adapted by using an elastic band around the scissors strong enough to depress and hold the switch. A thumb loop tied around the elastic band enables it to be pulled onto or off the switch (Fig. 8-45).

FIGURE 8-44

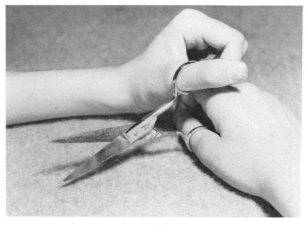

A

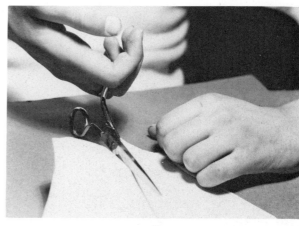

B

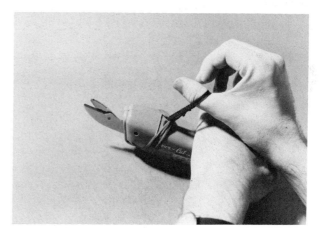

FIGURE 8-45

SMOKING

A table lighter may be used, or a pocket lighter may be stabilized by fitting it into a wooden base (Fig. 8-46). Grip may be aided by slipping elastic bands around

265

the lighter or gluing sandpaper to it. The lighter should not require continuous pressure to maintain a flame.

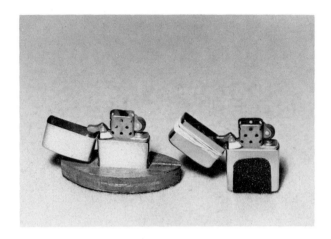

FIGURE 8-46

Cigarette holders are recommended to prevent burns on anaesthetic hands or hands that cannot easily drop a cigarette which is burning them. The cigarette holder must be tested for easy insertion of the cigarette. A cigarette holder attached to the ashtray with a length of flexible tubing to the mouthpiece may be utilized safely by the dependent patient, but people who can manage conventional holders generally prefer to use them.

An ejector type may be held between the teeth while the body of the holder is pushed in using the sides of both hands in order to eject the butt. The cigarette holder may be picked up using the teeth or by hand using tenodesis. The holder may be placed in the pencil holder of the flexor-hinge splint provided the angle does not allow the fingers to be burnt, or it may be held in the normal manner in a flexor-hinge splint. The normal adduction of the fingers or when the fingers are flexed by tenodesis is often adequate for the cigarette holder to be held between the fingers. The holder may also be held between the heels of the hands.

If a patient prefers not to use a conventional cigarette holder, he may use a ring which fits around the cigarette and attaches with an extension to finger rings (Fig. 8-47) or a handle to be held by tenodesis. For some patients a stand must be made for the cigarette holder with an ashtray placed under the cigarette. The patient reaches the holder by using head and neck movements and need not use his hands.

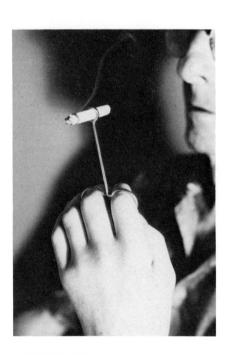

FIGURE 8-47

9

Car Transfers and Driver Training

CAR TRANSFERS

EQUIPMENT

A bridge board is the basic piece of equipment needed in car transfers. They may be of different types.

A rectangular bridge board, 10 inches by 30 inches, may be made of ¼-inch tempered hardboard, bevelled at the ends and with all edges rounded (Fig. 9-1). The only finish required is polish, which may be either a good floor polish and/or talcum powder.

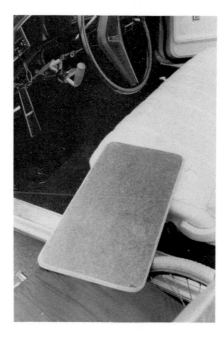

FIGURE 9-1

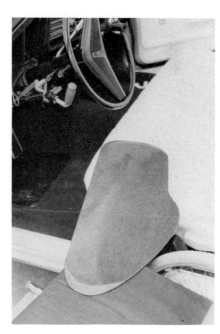

FIGURE 9-2

A tempered hardboard bridge board is rounded at the ends to make it easy to slide under the buttocks and shaped for the individual's car (Fig. 9-2).

A rectangular bridge board may be made of ⅜-inch plywood cut to 10 inches by 30 inches with the edges bevelled and sanded. The top surface and the edges are padded with ¼-inch foam rubber and covered with nylon material (Fig. 9-3A). Nonslip matting may be applied to the undersurface at either end (Fig. 9-3B).

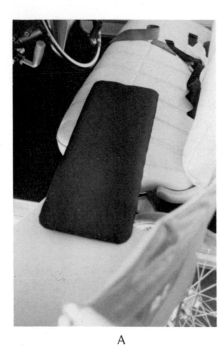

A

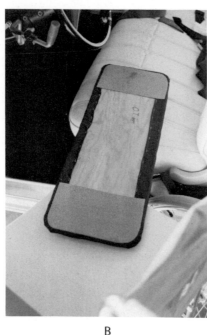

B

FIGURE 9-3

A bridge board, with a post and flange to fit into the front chair arm socket and with a cut out to accommodate the wheel of the chair, overlaps both chair cushion and car seat. It may be made of unpadded tempered hardboard or it may be made of ⅜-inch plywood with the edges chamferred; the board is padded with ¼-inch foam and nylon covered. This board should be only lightly padded or it will create a high ridge to slide over since it does not abut to the seats. The floor flange is fastened to the board with counter-sunk flat-head bolts (Fig. 9-4A). The part of the pipe that has not been machined down acts as a stop, which regulates the height of the bridge board. The machined part should be short enough so that it does not extend below the chair arm socket. The board, when in position, extends about 2 inches over the chair cushion and about 4 inches on to the car seat, depressing both slightly (Fig. 9-4B).

A palette-shaped bridge board is made of ½-inch plywood, the edges of which are chamferred and smoothed. A length of ¾-inch pipe is machined down to fit into the front chair arm socket and is threaded into a floor flange (Fig. 9-5). The position of the floor flange on the underside of the board is determined by placing the board between chair and car and placing the pipe in the chair arm socket. Another floor flange and pipe are placed as a leg to the floor of the car to provide stability. This board may be padded and covered.

268

FIGURE 9-4

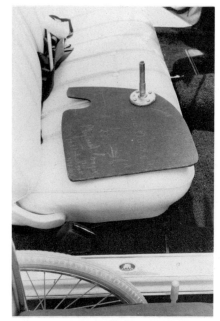

A

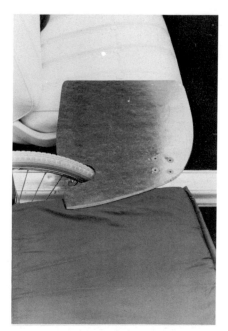

B

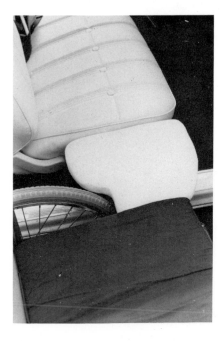

FIGURE 9-5

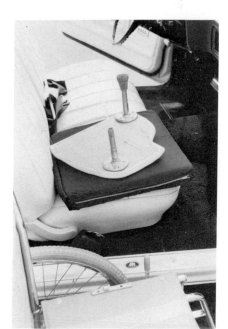

A very stable bridge board, similar to the previous board, including the projection fitting into the chair arm socket, has a leg by the front corner of the car seat, which extends from the bridge board to the car floor, and another leg projecting down from the back corner of the bridge board, resting on the doorsill.

The board can be padded and nylon covered, with an extra roll of padding at the rear to prevent the patient from sliding off the back of the board. This board does not project over either car seat or wheelchair cushion; it abuts on both. The board should extend from the front edge of the wheelchair seat to the front edge of the car seat (Fig. 9-6).

Different makes of cars may necessitate some modification of design (Fig. 9-7).

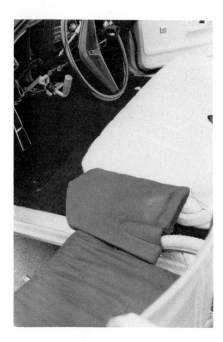
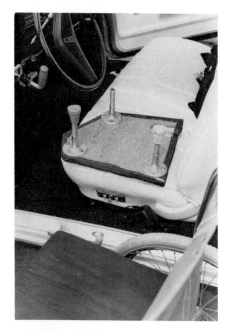

FIGURE 9-6

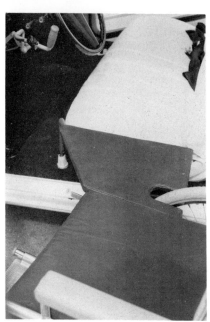
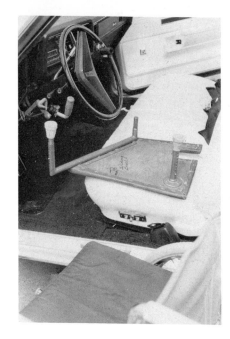

FIGURE 9-7

An overhead strap may be required. It may be permanently fixed to the ceiling of the car or detachable, with a hook which will fit into the guttering over the car door (Fig. 9-8).

Bridge boards and car seats may be sprayed with silicone or dusted with talc to facilitate sliding. The type of clothing worn and the type of seat covering must be taken into consideration. While the patient is first learning transfers, a synthetic and cotton-mix material for pants or a nylon material, which will move with the patient, can be effective to reduce friction. A hard nylon fabric is preferable for car seats, since vinyl tends to become sticky and plush-type material tends to cling.

CHAIR TO CAR

It is often easier to transfer on the driver's side so that the steering wheel may be utilized as an aid for pulling. Quadriplegic individuals use parking lots whenever feasible to eliminate variations in levels. However, if street parking must be used, it is safer to use the curbside door.

In all transfers the patient opens the car door and wheels his chair as close to the seat as possible, turning the front of his chair towards the car at about 30°. He applies the brakes and removes the wheelchair arm nearest the car.

Method 1. (Fig. 9-9) The patient who is able to do a pushup will probably use no sliding board. He places his feet in the car before transfer because he gains a mechanical advantage as he flexes his trunk forward, placing a significant amount of weight on his feet. To transfer, he places his hands well back, one on the chair and one on the car seat. Flexing his trunk forwards, he depresses and flexes his shoulders and twists his upper trunk away from the car to pivot onto the seat.

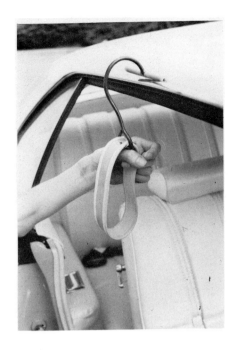

FIGURE 9-8

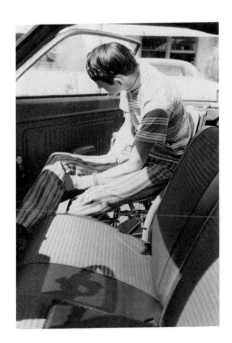

FIGURE 9-9

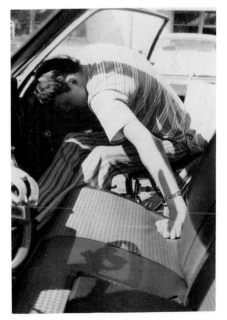

271

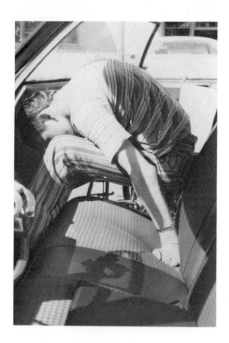
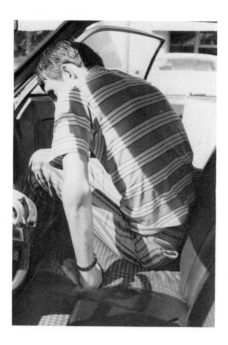

Method 2. (Fig. 9-10) The bridge board is placed in position first; then the patient turns away from the car and places both hands against the chair arm rest or on the cushion against the chair arm. He leans away from the car pushing himself backwards towards the car using his shoulder and elbow flexors. He repositions his hands, one on the dashboard or on the door and the other hand close to his buttock. He leans towards the chair and pushes his buttocks onto the car seat. He now lifts his legs into the car.

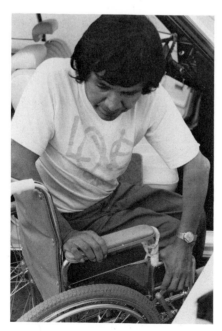
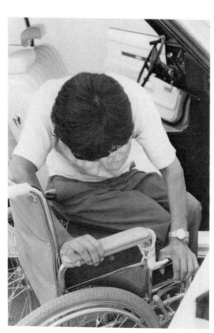
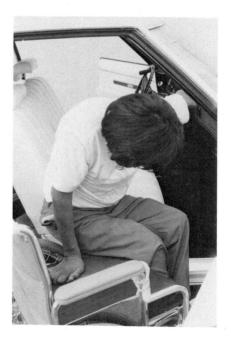

FIGURE 9-10

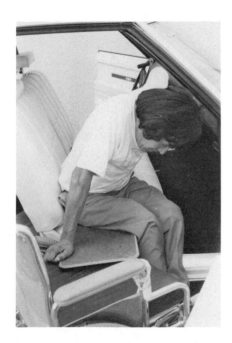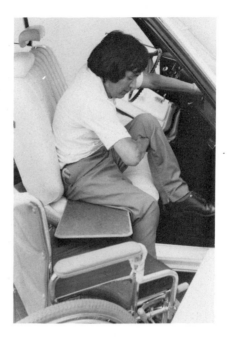

Method 3. (Fig. 9-11) The patient leans away from the car to insert the sliding board well underneath his buttocks with the other end resting on the car seat. He shifts forward in the chair and lifts both feet into the car. He must place his feet so that his knees will flex when he transfers, or he may find that he is blocked by a knee locked in extension. He leans on one elbow on the car seat and hooks the other wrist through the steering wheel. He pulls with both arms to slide onto the car seat. He pulls himself partially upright with the arm near the chair, using the steering wheel or the door frame; this enables him to lock his other elbow and stabilize his position.

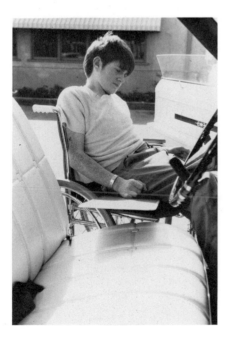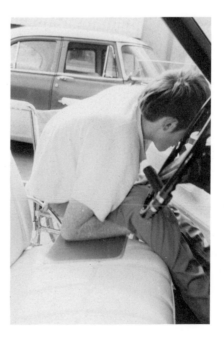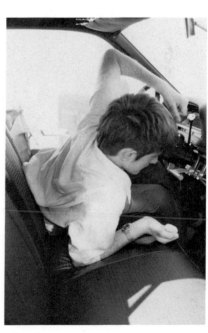

FIGURE 9-11

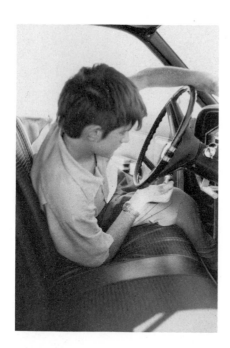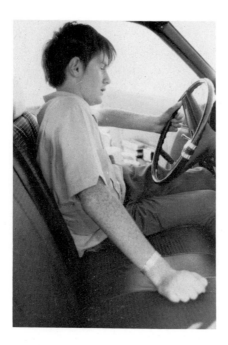

Method 4.   (Fig. 9-12) The patient leans away from the car to place the bridge board in position. He hooks his sling into the car roof gutter and places his forearm in it to maintain balance while he leans away from the car again. He places his thumb web against the front upright of the chair arm, pushing strongly with this arm while the arm in the sling is internally rotated to pull and swivel him into the car. He then lifts his legs into the car.

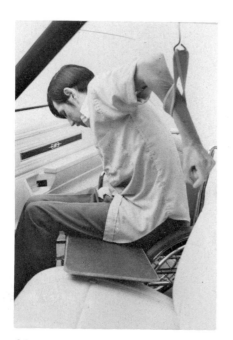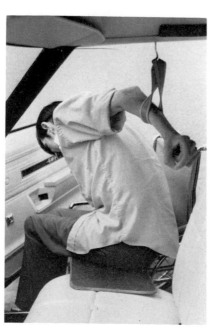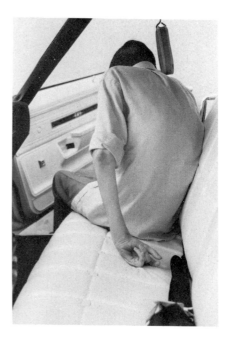

FIGURE 9-12

CAR TO CHAIR

Method 1. (Fig. 9-13) The patient who is able to do a pushup will probably use no sliding board after he has mastered this technique. His feet remain in the car while he places his hands, one on the car seat close to his buttocks and one on the chair seat as far away as possible. He flexes his trunk forward and pushes up with his arms while he turns his upper trunk towards the car to pivot onto the chair seat.

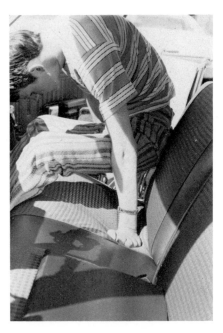 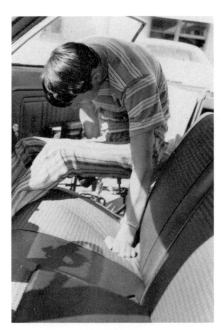

FIGURE 9-13

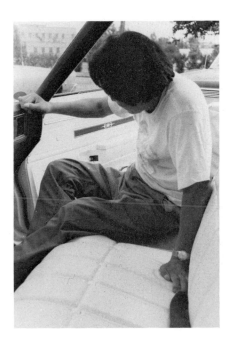 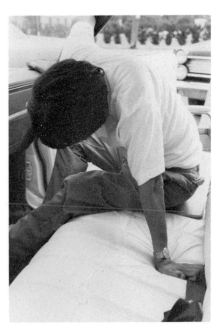 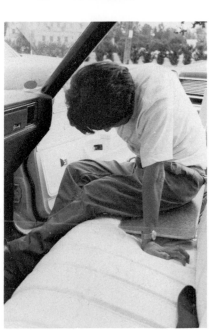

FIGURE 9-14

Method 2. (Fig. 9-14) The patient places his bridge board in position. He places one hand on the dashboard and one hand on the car seat and flexes his trunk forwards. This movement helps to pivot him as he pushes himself backwards out of the car.

Method 3. (Fig. 9-15) The patient leans away from the chair to place one end of the bridge board underneath him with the other end resting on the wheelchair. He places the hand furthest from the chair by his buttock and locks the elbow. The other hand is placed on the dashboard or the wheel to maintain balance and to assist him to twist his trunk away from the chair. He throws his weight over the locked arm and flexes the shoulder of that arm strongly. Simultaneously the shoulder of the arm nearest the chair is internally rotated bringing the elbow up, permitting strong elbow flexion and shoulder adduction to push the patient towards the chair. At the halfway point the hand near the chair may be moved to the door windowsill to gain new purchase.

Method 4. (Fig. 9-16). The patient places his bridge board in position and lifts his feet onto the footrests of the chair. Since his legs are blocked by the doorsill of the car, they act as a fulcrum to assist him to pivot out of the car. He flexes his trunk forward and places one hand on the chair wheel or back and the other on the car seat close to his buttock. He externally rotates the shoulder nearest the car and flexes and abducts it to push. His arm on the chair is internally rotated and adducted to pull him towards the chair.

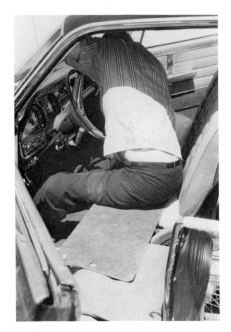

FIGURE 9-15

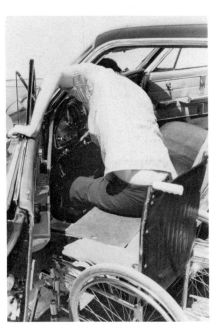
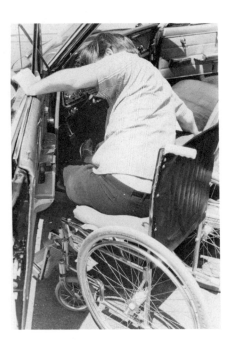

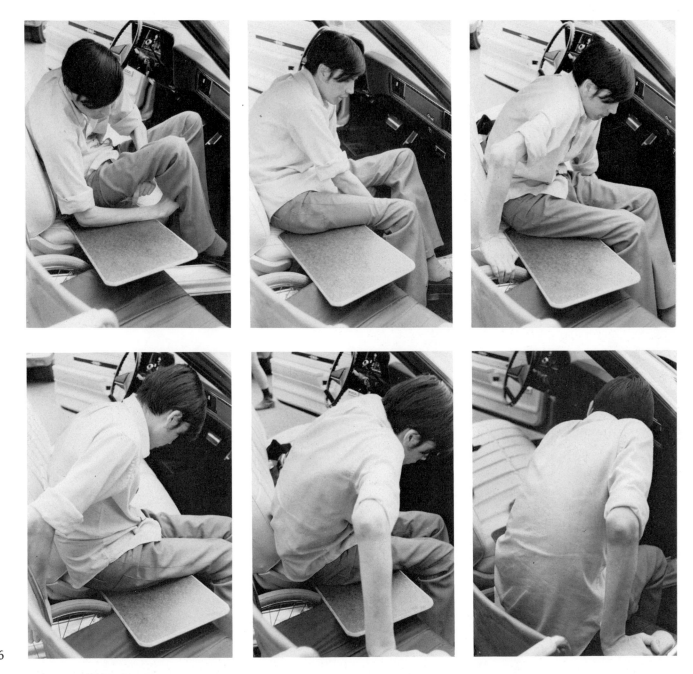

FIGURE 9-16

Method 5. (Fig. 9-17) The patient lifts both feet out of the car and places the forearm nearest the chair in the overhead strap. He leans away from the wheelchair and places his elbow on the carseat, so relieving some of the weight from his buttocks. A combination of a pull with the arm in the strap and a push with the arm on the car seat will twist and lever him towards the chair. He sits himself up by either

277

pulling on the strap or hooking a wrist around the wing window frame, the front door post, or the roof of the car. He completes his transfer by placing a hand against the wing window frame and the other against the side of the car seat. When he flexes his trunk and pushes with both arms, his buttocks are moved back onto the chair.

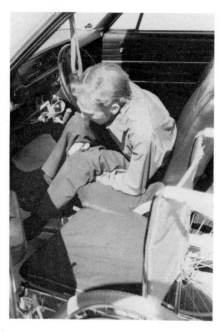
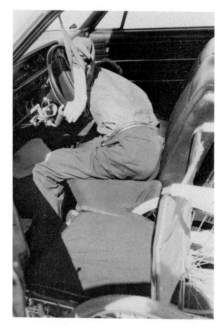
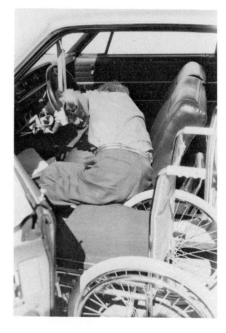
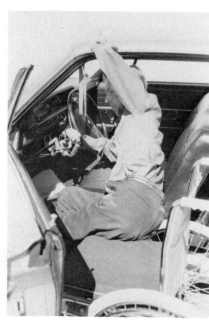
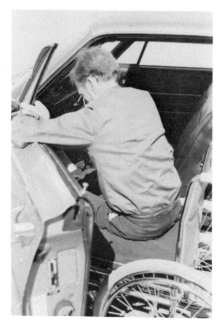
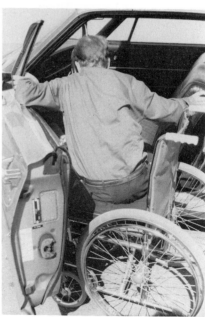

FIGURE 9-17

Foot Position

The feet may be lifted onto the footrests at the beginning or the end of the transfer, or one foot only may be lifted out before transfer. The latter is the most common method because it can help to lever the patient towards the chair by blocking the calf against the doorsill when the trunk is rotated. Balance may be easier in this position because of the wide base and sometimes the elimination of a position which could trigger spasm.

The patient who places both feet on the footrests before transfer may do so because of long legs which can be difficult to move under the controls when transferring. He may be a patient who has tight hamstrings or who has flexor spasms which could pull him forward off the seat of the chair if he leaves his feet inside the car.

LOADING THE WHEELCHAIR INTO THE CAR

It is almost impossible for a quadriplegic person to load a wheelchair into the back of a four-door car because of the interference of the centre post. Therefore, we give directions for loading the wheelchair behind the driver in a two-door car or beside the driver in a two- or four-door car.

Behind the Driver in a Two-Door Car

To facilitate loading and unloading the wheelchair, the well between the doorsill and the drive-shaft housing can be filled in with plywood to within ¾-inch of the top of the doorsill. The slight drop at the doorsill prevents the chair from rolling away when loading and unloading the chair.

The quadriplegic driver first removes the bridge board and places it and the cushion beside him. He then leans over and releases the wheelchair brake on the side nearest him, enabling him to swing the chair around so that it faces him. He now unlocks the other brake. He swings his footrests up and places his wrist under the chair seat and lifts it to fold the chair (Fig. 9-18). He lines the chair up with the gap between the car-seat back and the doorjamb. He leans over and hooks his wrist under the leg strap of the chair to lift the front wheels of the chair over the sill. In a car with a split-seat back, he may move over toward the other side and tip the seat back forward to allow more room for the wheelchair. In a car with electrically controlled seats he need only move them into the forward position. He leans towards the chair over the seat back and catches the leg strap again. By pulling and leaning back, he rolls the chair into the car. He then moves back into the driver's seat and shuts the door.

Beside the Driver in a Two- or Four-Door Car

The person who enters the car from the curb side may place his chair behind the front seat as described, or he may place it on the floor beside him. This technique is described here.

Having transferred into the car, the quadriplegic driver maintains balance with his right arm over the seat back while he hooks his left wrist under the wheelchair seat and raises it to fold the chair. He manoeuvres the chair so that it

FIGURE 9-18

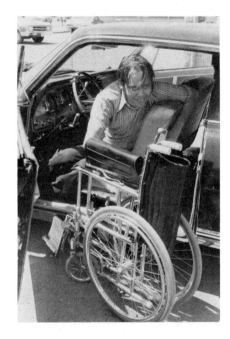

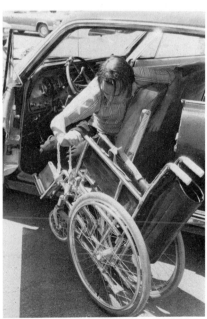

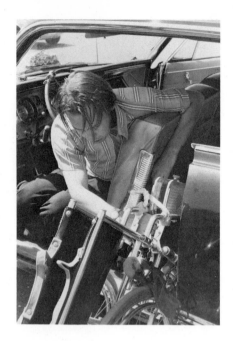
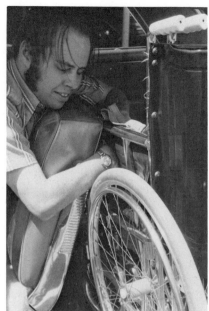
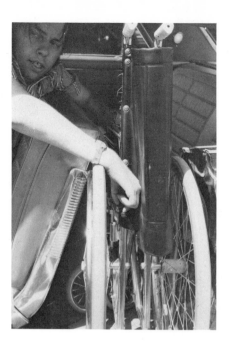

faces him (Fig. 9-19). He now releases the chair seat and disengages the brakes. He moves himself further into the car and reaches down with his right arm to the leg strap or chair-front upright to lift the front wheels of the chair onto the doorsill. He moves towards the driver's side and maintains balance with his left arm on the

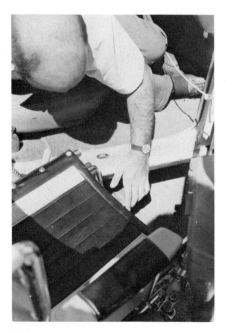
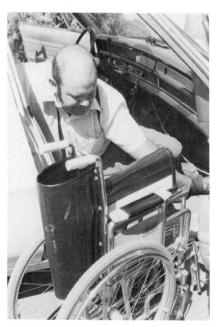
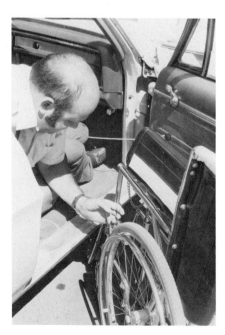

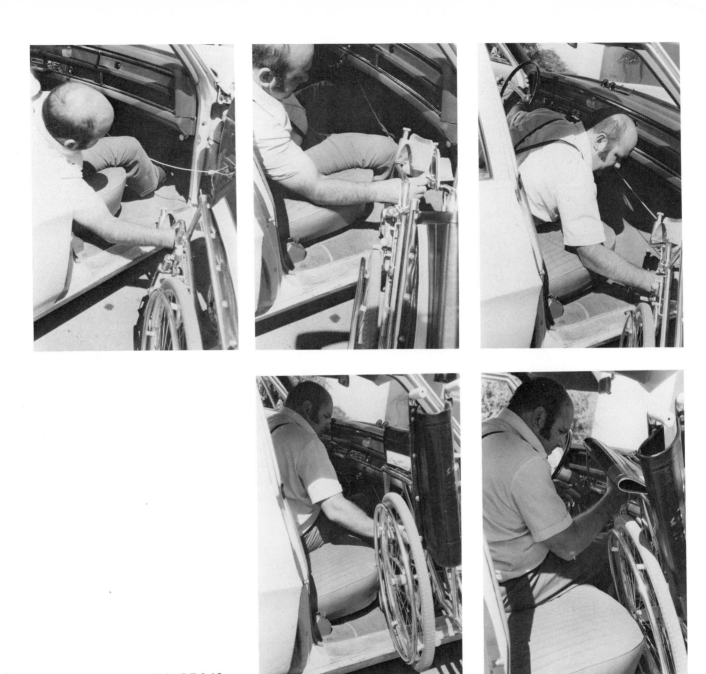

FIGURE 9-19

steering wheel or over the seat back. He then leans down to hook his forearm behind the front chair upright so that, when he pulls himself erect with his left arm and pulls on the chair with his right arm, the chair rolls into the car. A long cord, permanently fastened to the door and conveniently placed on the dashboard, will enable him to close the door.

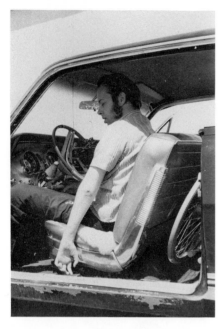 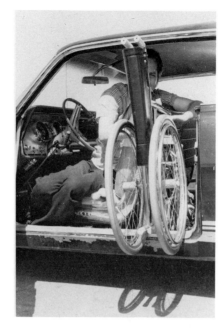 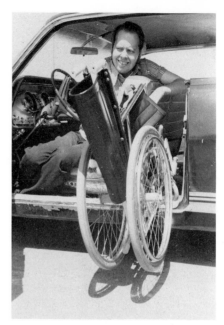

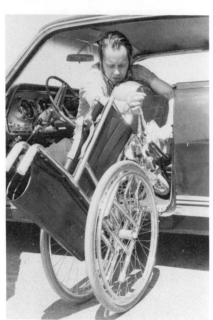 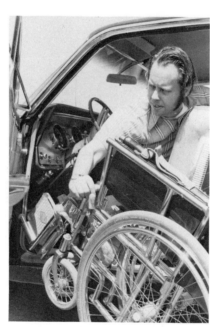 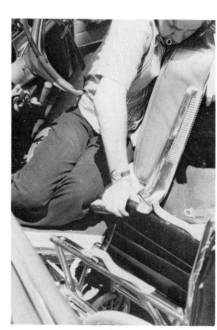

FIGURE 9-20

UNLOADING THE CHAIR

From the Two-Door Car

The driver opens the car door and slides onto the other seat in order to pull the seat back forwards or he moves an electrically operated seat forward (Fig. 9-20). He leans over the seat back and pushes the chair out carefully until the back wheels

282

are on the ground and the front castors are hooked over the doorsill. The chair remains in this position while he moves across towards the door. He reaches around the seat back and places his wrist under the closest seat rail. As he lifts the chair so that the castors clear the doorsill, the chair will start to open as it is rolled back. This lessens the danger of the chair tipping over. As he lowers the chair he swings the front towards himself. He pushes down on the seat rail nearest him, partly opening the chair, and then puts on the far brake while it is still within reach. This will not prevent his manoeuvering the chair, which he does by pushing again on the rail nearest him and jiggling the chair into position. He then applies the near brake and puts the cushion and bridge board in place.

From Beside the Driver

The person leans across and opens the door. He maintains balance with the arm near the chair over the back of the car seat, a position which allows him to push against the chair front with the other arm (Fig. 9-21). When the chair is balanced on the doorsill, he moves over towards the door. He now stabilizes himself by placing the arm near the driver's side on the dashboard or by hooking it through the steering wheel. The other arm controls the chair while the back wheels are lowered to the ground. He changes arms once again and places the arm near the chair over the car-seat back while the other arm lowers the front castors. The chair is opened by pushing down and jiggling a seat rail; it is worked into position for transfer. The changes of arm position are necessary to secure a strong and stable hugging action throughout the manoeuvre.

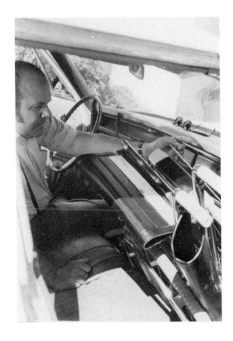
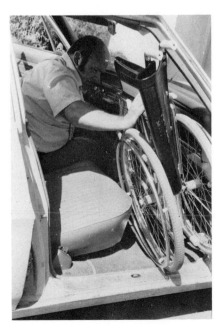
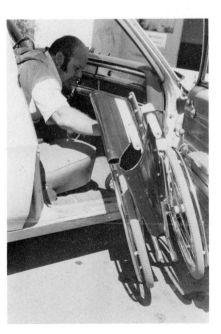

FIGURE 9-21

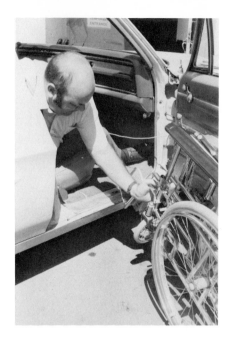

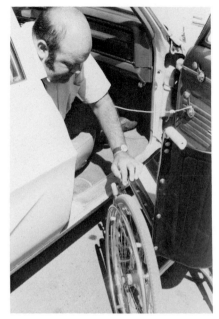

THE PATIENT WHO CANNOT LOAD HIS CHAIR

Two wheelchairs are a satisfactory solution for the patient who drives himself to work. One chair is used at home and one at the office. If there is a carport he can leave his chair in position and back up to it with the door open when he returns. If there is no carport there should be no problem in having the chair delivered to him

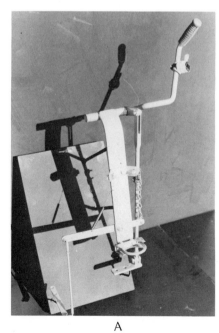

A

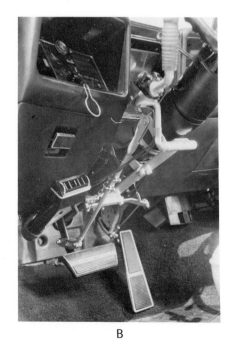

B

FIGURE 9-22. *A*, Control mounted in car; *B*, Close-up view of control.

284

on arrival. If the patient can afford only one chair, someone else must load and unload it for him.

DRIVING EQUIPMENT REQUIRED

Required equipment includes automatic transmission, power brakes, and power steering.

A hand-controlled throttle, brake, and dimmer switch on one lever are required. Many hand controls have been developed throughout the world for disabled individuals. A particularly satisfactory model for the quadriplegic driver has been designed by the Canadian Paraplegic Association, British Columbia Branch, and has been approved by the British Columbia Motor Vehicle Branch (Fig. 9-22). The simplicity of design involving few moving parts makes this a particularly safe and troublefree device. The special design provides maximum efficiency with minimum travel of the lever arm.

FIGURE 9-23. Steering wheel swivel and hand attachment.

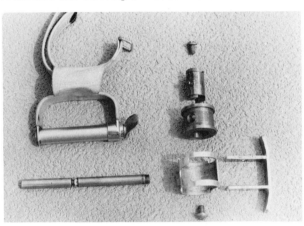
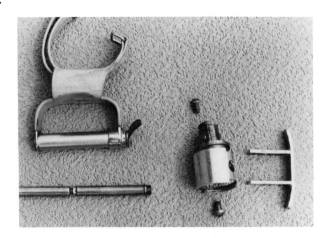
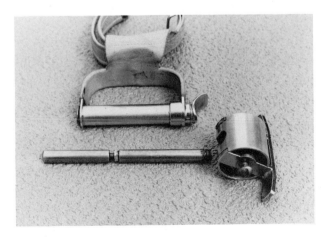
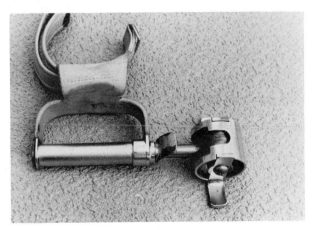

The action used is a rocking action on a vertical plane—back for throttle and forward for brake, since a push is the natural stopping reaction. The rocker action makes an ideal device for the quadriplegic driver because he can use elbow and shoulder flexion to apply his brakes. The hand does not slip off the lever because the angle never reaches the vertical when the brakes are fully on. The throttle is applied by shoulder extension and the weight of the hand and arm. If the patient has wrist flexion this is also used. Endurance on long drives is much enhanced by the relaxed position of the arm which maintains throttle by the use of gravity.

A steering-wheel swivel and hand attachment is an additional requirement. This quadriplegic driving attachment was designed by G. A. Taylor of the G. F. Strong Rehabilitation Centre, Vancouver, British Columbia, and is approved by the British Columbia Motor Vehicle Branch. The attachment is in two parts—a steering-wheel swivel and a hand attachment (Fig. 9-23). When the two are mated, the hand is locked to the wheel.

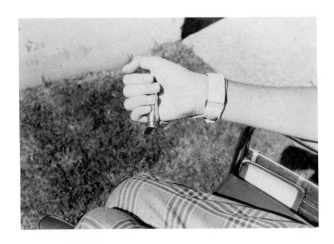

FIGURE 9-24. Hand attachment.

The wheel swivel is placed on the inner border of the wheel with tridon gear clamps. It is usually placed at one o'clock and then adjusted to the individual's needs. The hand attachment (Fig. 9-24) consists of a tube fastened to a dorsal splint, usually extending no further than the wrist. The splint is the only part of the attachment that must be individually fitted.

The wheel attachment is normally in the folded position so that it does not interfere with the transfers (Fig. 9-25). To lock the two parts together the stem is partially raised and the tube slipped over it until the flange on the tube matches the slot in the wheel attachment (Fig. 9-26). The stem is then swung up to a right angle to the wheel. It is now locked. To release the lock, the plunger on top of the stem must be pushed down with the other hand, the forehead, or the chin (Fig. 9-27).

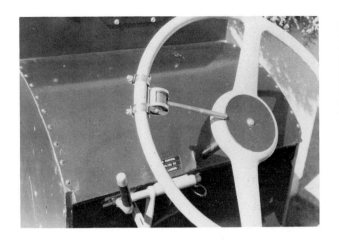
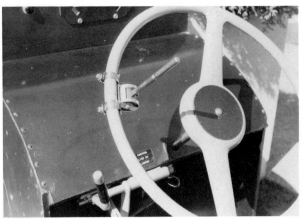

A, Folded

B, Unfolded

FIGURE 9-25. Wheel attachment.

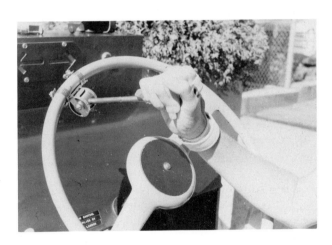
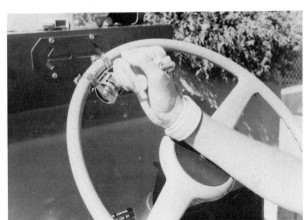

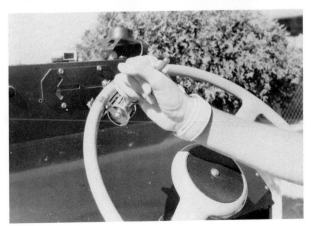

FIGURE 9-26. Engaging the swivel and attachment.

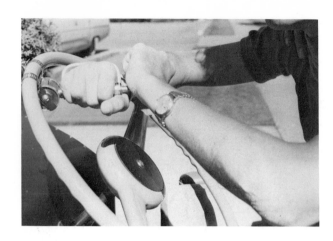

FIGURE 9-27. Disengaging the swivel and attachment.

OPTIONAL EQUIPMENT

Additional equipment, which will provide easier transfer and ease in driving, include electrically operated windows, extension lever on ignition key and control knobs, nylon seat covers, side mirrors, and electrically adjustable seat.

MODIFICATIONS WHICH MAY BE NECESSARY

Adjustment of the seat position is important. Generally a quadriplegic driver will handle the controls best when the seat is in the forward position. However, care must be taken that the steering attachment is not so close that it will catch on clothing. The tilt of the seat is usually fairly upright, as in the wheelchair. The seat may require raising so that greater mechanical advantage is obtained when turning the steering wheel. This will aid in turning through the possible dead spot that sometimes occurs near eleven o'clock. All the positioning may be tried out using cushions initially in a car with no electrical adjustment for the seats, but once the optimum position is decided the seat should be permanently adjusted by a mechanic.

The armrest on the door frequently is used by the driver as a fulcrum to gain leverage when managing the controls. It is possible that the armrest may require repositioning.

It is essential that the quadriplegic driver be stabilized in his driving position or he will lose leverage on both controls and steering wheel. The combination seat and over the shoulder safety belt will often suffice (Fig. 9-28A), but if the patient still loses balance a shoulder and seat combination may be used with one additional belt. This belt runs from the door post, around the driver below his arm pits, and back to the door post (Fig. 9-28B). This enables him to lean forward but prevents any lateral movement to the right. Sometimes a thumb loop must be fastened to the belt near the buckles to permit the driver's fastening his belt. A push button type buckle is easily released.

The steering attachment can be moved to various places on the wheel to increase the comfort of the driver and to facilitate the turning of the steering wheel.

The throttle and brake can be set forwards or backwards, and the range increased or decreased. The control lever may have to be slightly repositioned to provide more comfort.

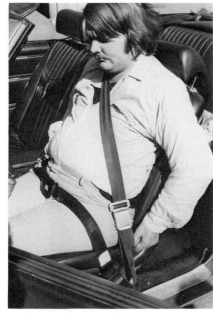
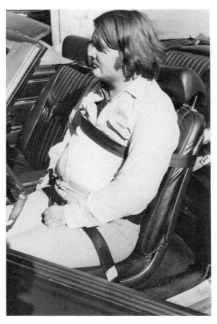
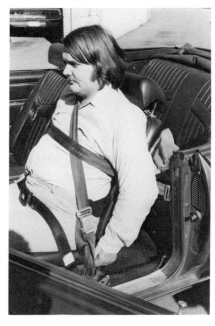

FIGURE 9-28

A   B

DRIVER TRAINING

The ability to drive, both for transportation to work and for recreation, is a most valuable skill for a quadriplegic patient. This ability and the availability of a car can make employment possible, where, without independent transportation, a job may be out of the question.

The quadriplegic driver has equality on the road both in skill and control of his car. This is shown in a recent survey in one area where 90 per cent of the paraplegic and quadriplegic drivers were claim-free and 83 per cent were

MARKS	QUADRIPLEGICS		GENERAL PUBLIC	
	Number	%	Number	%
FAIL	2	8.3	24245	23
70% - 79%	9	35	43429	40
80% - 84%	7	26.66	16701	16.6
85% - 89%	4	15	12752	11.6
90% - 100%	4	15	8826	8.3

289

conviction-free for the last three years. Of this group, 14 per cent were quadriplegic drivers. This compares with 41.69 per cent claim-free of the general public.

A comparison between the driver examination results of quadriplegic drivers and those of the general public in Vancouver, British Columbia, Canada, is shown, although there is, of course, a very large difference in numbers compared. The marks ranged from 71 per cent to 94 per cent, averaging 78.08 per cent. The sample of 26 was taken at random from 41 examinations.

Thorough training by a qualified instructor contributes greatly to these results. For this reason a commercial driving school should be utilized for driver training if at all possible. The driving school selected should have a car equipped with power steering and power brakes. Hand controls should be easily removable so that the car is available for all drivers, since it is unlikely that the car will be totally utilized by drivers requiring hand controls. The quadriplegic student often requires two-hour sessions of driver training because adjusting the position of the driver and his controls takes time initially. An orientation programme should be made available to the instructor since some familiarity with the disability can be of great help to him.

10
Housing

Houses are seldom built with a wheelchair in mind; therefore, modifications may be necessary. Sometimes the best and least expensive solution is to relocate in a more suitable dwelling. Many books, pamphlets, and building codes refer to wheelchair housing. Useful information will be found in "Housing the Disabled" by Michael Pine, available from the Central Mortgage and Housing Corporation of Canada, Ottawa. This chapter concerns points with particular reference to the quadriplegic patient's needs.

OUTSIDE THE HOUSE

It is necessary to have smooth level pathways at least 36 inches wide from the car to the house entry, and it is desirable to have a hard-surfaced area for recreation. Sheltered access to the house directly from the basement, garage, or carport adjoining the house is most suitable for a quadriplegic patient's use.

There must be sufficient room to provide wheelchair space alongside the car for transfer and for putting the wheelchair into the car. The type of garage door that opens and closes by radio beam is ideal, but an overhead door that is operated by electric motor and pushbottom may be adapted. If there is a garden, a pathway may be constructed to reach it. If gardening is a particular interest, planters of wheelchair height may meet this interest.

Ramps should be constructed of nonskid material. A grade of slope which can be managed by the individual must be worked out carefully. Quadriplegic patients generally are not able to handle more than a minimal grade. There are commercial hill holders available to assist the wheelchair user. Ramps must be at least 36 inches wide and should have wheel guides at either side to prevent the wheels from running off the ramp. There must be a level area at the top to allow turning and opening of doors. Sometimes it is necessary to bridge the gap between the porch and the sidewalk or pathway where there is a sunken area (Fig. 10-1). This bridge should have guard rails.

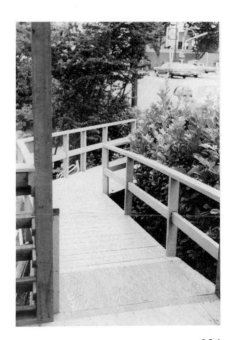

FIGURE 10-1

ESCALATORS OR ELEVATORS

There are several types of escalators and elevators that may be used inside or outside the house.

The counterbalanced elevator is the most economical because it can be built by a handyman. However, this elevator is difficult for a quadriplegic patient to operate and is recommended only for the dependent patient with a helper. The superstructure required may detract from the appearance of the house.

The electrically powered escalator may be built over stairs while still allowing the stairs to be used (Fig. 10-2). The track substitutes for the balustrade. These escalators are commercially available. Needless to say, a power failure will put the elevator out of use.

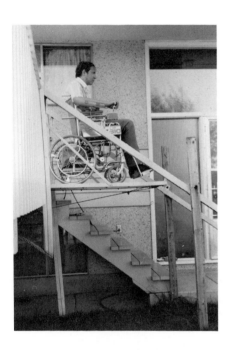 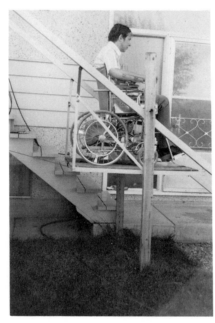 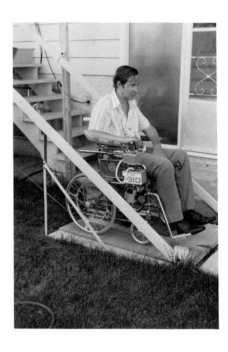

FIGURE 10-2

An electrically powered elevator may be built into a stairwell shaft or other waste space inside or outside the house (Figs. 10-3 and 10-4). These are widely available commercially.

A water-powered elevator may be built fairly economically by a handyman in areas where freezing is not a problem. The elevator can only be installed outside because of the depth of the shaft required for the piston. This is a very smooth, quiet elevator.

The concrete path should be level with the surface of an elevator so that there is no lip to wheel over.

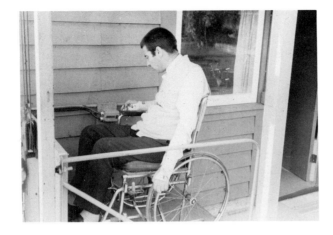

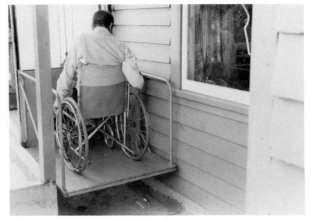

FIGURE 10-3. Built-in electrically powered elevator.

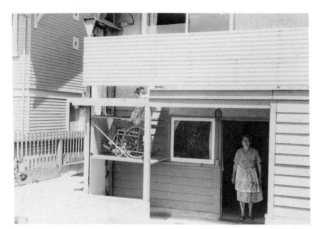

FIGURE 10-4. Transportable electric/hydraulic elevator.

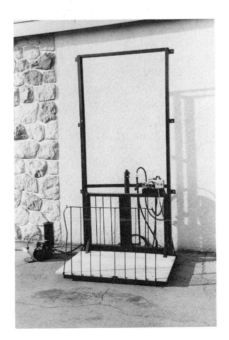

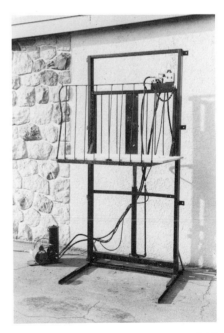

HOUSE ENTRY

Many quadriplegic patients cannot wheel over small obstacles such as doorsills. These can be eliminated where there is a covered porch. There should be room for turning outside the door to permit closing of the door.

INSIDE THE HOUSE

DOORS

Doors should be a minimum of 30 inches wide for a direct approach. Angled approaches may require a wider doorway. Door knobs may be exchanged for lever handles, which are easier to operate. A handle 12 inches from the hinge side of the door, wide enough to insert a wrist, will aid in closing the door. Alternatively a looped rope can be used to pull the door shut. Folding or sliding doors with a large handle are easy to open and close.

FLOOR SURFACES

Slip mats and deep pile rugs are obstacles and should be removed. Wood or linoleum floor surfaces are the easiest to wheel on, followed by indoor-outdoor carpeting since this has a very short pile. The deeper the pile of a carpet the harder it is to push the chair over it.

HALLWAYS AND CORRIDORS

Corridors should be wide enough to allow the wheelchair to turn around and approach doors directly. Areas of the walls and door jambs that may be scraped by the wheelchair may be covered with a protective material.

FURNITURE

An adequate passageway should be left between pieces of furniture so that the wheelchair can be easily manoeuvred. One chair may be removed from dining and family areas to provide wheelchair space and avoid conspicuous furniture moving each time the room is used. Dining tables should be high enough to clear the patient's knees. A wheelchair tray will be useful for carrying things, particularly hot drinks, and as an occasional table and desk.

WINDOWS

Because temperature changes plague the quadriplegic patient so much, he should be able to control the windows or temperature control independently, particularly in his bedroom. The easiest to manage is the swing-out window with a lever or crank control.

BEDROOM

There must be room for the patient to manoeuvre easily into position for bed transfers and to gain easy access to his clothes cupboard and chest of drawers. The clothes rail must be lowered to within reach. Drawer pulls may be adapted by adding a loop of strong material such as webbing, leather, or tape. A large drawer may have a strap fastened between the two pulls. This strap should not be so loose that it can be caught in the drawer below. Ideally the drawer pulls may be changed to metal loop handles.

BATHROOM

The placement of bathroom fixtures frequently necessitates that plumbing be changed to accommodate a wheelchair. This may be a minor change such as pivotting the toilet a quarter turn on its mount, or it may involve relocating fixtures or replanning the bathroom.

Often it is preferable and cheaper to build an additional bathroom. Since a quadriplegic patient may spend some time in the bathroom, a second bathroom may be a great asset in a family home. A bathroom should have adequate turning space for the wheelchair. The placement of plumbing will depend upon the method of transfer used by the patient. Due consideration is given to the layout of the individual's bathroom when the method of transfer is worked out; for instance, if before his return home the patient can transfer equally well from the left or right side of the toilet, the transfer appropriate in his own bathroom would be perfected. If a wheelchair shower is used it should be incorporated into the bathroom if possible. The bottom of the sink and drainpipe should be insulated to prevent possible burns to knees. Overhead bars and special fixtures have been discussed in the Chapters 4 and 5. An additional fixture is a large and conveniently situated cupboard for storing equipment.

KITCHEN

Some quadriplegic patients may wish to cook occasional snacks or complete meals. Many articles have been written about kitchen layout for wheelchair users; these directions can be conveniently followed for quadriplegic patients with some minor changes since the restrictions of reach and grasp must be taken into consideration. A useful reference book is "Planning Kitchens for Handicapped Homemakers" by Virginia Hart Wheeler.

The patient's existing kitchen plan should be drawn up to see whether changes will be required. Planning may be facilitated by using a board covered with fluffy velcro and by using scale cutouts of contrasting colour hook velcro to represent counter tops, appliances, etc. Major alterations may be necessary if the patient is to be the homemaker, but if another person is to be the major homemaker these alterations may be modified for the convenience of both. Wheeling and turning must be cut to a minimum by thoughtful design of the kitchen, particularly for the patient who uses a flexor-hinge splint since wheeling is usually difficult when wearing a handsplint.

A cart or trolley on wheels may be used beside the patient to bring more counterspace close to him and to ensure that he can work at a convenient height. If he uses electrical appliances on this, he must be sure that he unplugs the electric cord before pushing the trolley away. A pullout board may serve the same purpose as the trolley and may be used in addition to it. Areas of counter or sink may be opened so that the patient's knees can be placed under, allowing him to reach a larger area of counter, overhead cupboards, and drawers beneath the counter beside him. A wheelchair tray may be of great value as a convenient working surface and for transporting dishes, etc., particularly if they are hot.

Refrigerator and stove doors must be within reach and easily opened and closed. They may require adapted loop or lever handles (Fig. 10-5). The most frequently used shelves should be on a level with a pullout shelf beside the appliance or with the wheelchair tray so that heavier objects may be slid out rather than lifted. This may mean that a wall oven will be more convenient than a floor model range, particularly if it is lowered so that the centre shelf is level with the counter. Stove and appliance switches must be within reach and easily pressed or turned without reaching over a hot burner. The switches may be adapted or changed for easy handling. A stick with a T-handle may be used to reach back controls safely. The other end of the stick may be adapted for the controls.

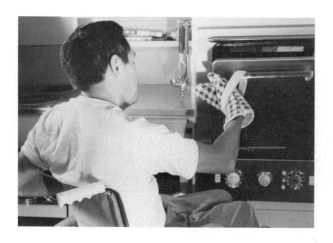

FIGURE 10-5

Small electrical appliances such as an electric frying pan or broiler are easily placed at a convenient working height and may be used as a substitute for range top or oven. Taps should be lever type and within reach. A hose for filling pans with water to avoid lifting them will probably be useful.

A pullout board may have a hole cut in it just smaller than the rim of a mixing bowl (Fig. 10-6). This stabilizes the bowl and may lower it to a more convenient working height. Electrical appliances such as can opener, knife, open grill toaster, mixer, and dish washer may be indicated.

The cook who cannot distinguish hot or cold must take great care when handling hot utensils. Some quadriplegic patients seem more sensitive to heat than is normal and blister after touching almost tepid objects. Oven mitts should be worn when handling hot objects and should be checked often for worn spots and wet areas. They may be adapted to be worn over a flexor-hinge splint. This is done by splitting them longitudinally over the leverage mechanism and rebinding the edges.

Casseroles may be pulled out of the oven by pulling out the oven shelf with a hook or oven mitt (Fig. 10-7) and sliding the casserole straight onto a shelf, wagon, or wheelchair tray level with the oven shelf. A baker's peel, a wooden paddle with

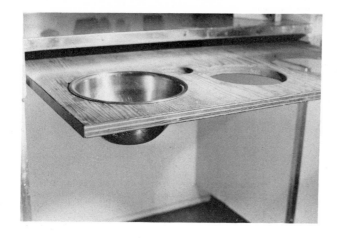

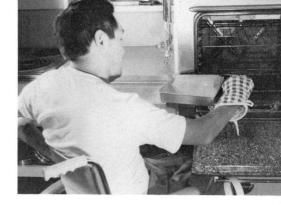

FIGURE 10-6   FIGURE 10-7

handles which can be slipped under the casserole may be used to slide it onto the adjacent surface.

Pots and pans should have large handles, double handles, bail handles, or loop handles. A small bailer or ladle should be used to substitute for pouring when the pot cannot be lifted. Vegetables that must be drained can be cooked in a sieve, ready to be lifted out of the pot. Nonstick type pans are useful because many quadriplegics are unable to stir fast enough to prevent sticking.

A cutting board with galvanized nails protruding up through it may be used to impale vegetables, etc., freeing both hands (Fig. 10-8). The board is held in place with suction cups or a nonslip pad. A small rim on two sides of the board may be useful for wedging food, for instance, as when buttering bread.

Another type of functional cutting board may be made by drilling the tip of a sharp knife and bolting it to the cutting board between two corner brackets. This forms a fulcrum so that very little pressure is required to slice food (Fig. 10-9).

A nonslip pad may be used when opening jars or stabilizing bowls (Fig. 10-10). Utensils may be adapted by padding handles or by providing velcro D-ring holders with large pockets. Used utensils or sharp knives may be placed in the pocket safely by folding a paper towel over the working end of the utensil (Fig. 10-11).

Eggs may be broken open by dropping them from about 12 inches above the pan (Fig. 10-12) and picking out the eggshell. A sharp tap with a knife on the side of the egg will cut the shell sufficiently to allow the knife tip to be inserted (Fig. 10-13). The shell may be levered open slowly so that, if wished, the yolk may be separated.

Tin cans, etc. can be reached and lifted with one hand if a magnet with a loop handle is used (Fig. 10-14). This may be useful where storage space within easy reach is at a premium.

Further reference is contained in "Mealtime Manual for the Aged and Handicapped," The Institute of Physical Medicine, New York University Medical Center.

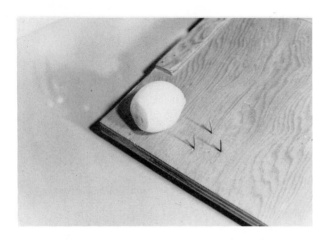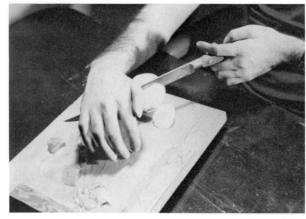

FIGURE 10-8

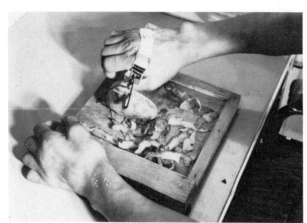

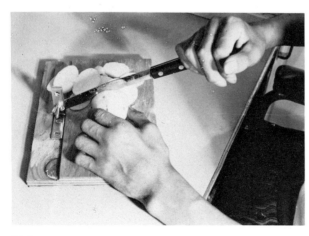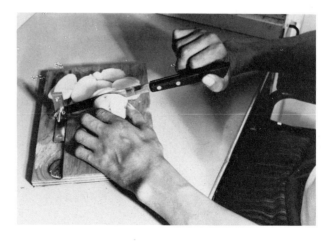

FIGURE 10-9

298

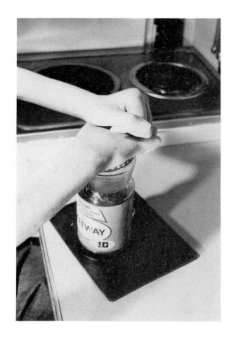

FIGURE 10-10

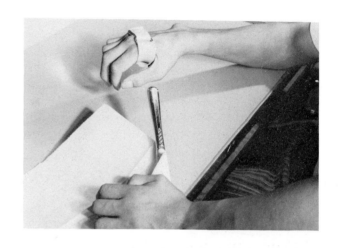

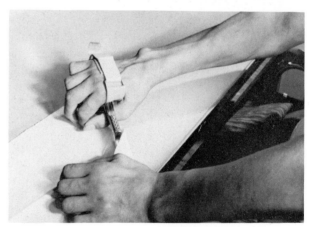

FIGURE 10-11

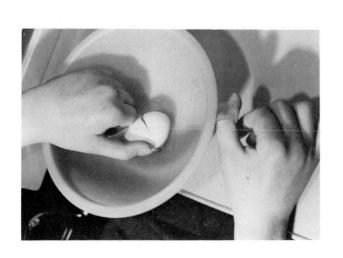

FIGURE 10-12

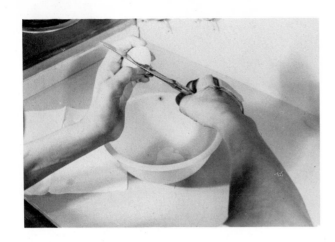 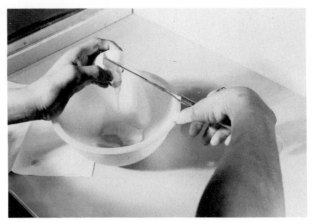

FIGURE 10-13

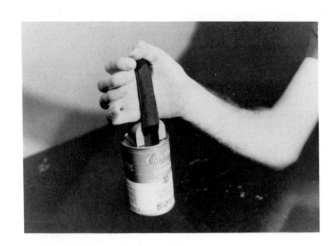

FIGURE 10-14

11

Vocation and Recreation

VOCATION

Vocational placement and counselling is a specialized field. This section of the chapter, therefore, is intended only to point out some basic requirements and to show that there are opportunities of employment for the quadriplegic. The types of jobs available vary considerably with the locale. Vocational placement of the patient is dependent upon the following:

Motivation
Intelligence and personality
Physical assets and limitations, i.e.
    Legible writing and/or typing
    Mobility—automobile and wheelchair
    Independence or minimal dependence during working day
Previous job experience
Community resources, i.e.
    Counselling
    Placement services
    Educational facilities
    On-job training facilities
Family financial resources, i.e.
    Self-employment
    Higher education
Jobs available in given area
Physical layout of and access to building

Listed below are some examples of jobs that were held by traumatic quadriplegics when a brief informal survey was carried out in Vancouver, British Columbia. Canada.

Coordinator   Stock Security Salesman
Cablevision Services   Librarian (Industrial)

Aerial Map Reader
Kardex Stock Controller
Dispatcher Automobile Association
Radiologist
Proprietor and Manager Secretarial Business
Hospital Manager
Fishboat Skipper (adapted chair for bridge)
Executive Director, Association
Director Finance Company
University Student
Aviation Engineer

Sales Clerk (heavy equipment)
Office Clerk (prison)
Coordinator Cablevision Installation
PBX Operator
Grocery Store Owner, Laundromat Owner and Manager
Public Relations Man and Concessionaire

RECREATION

The importance of recreation is well known and should not need re-emphasis. However, a list follows, containing some of the known recreational activities of quadriplegic persons, as a rough guide of possibilities. The conceivable activities are so numerous they can't all be listed.

SOME RECREATIONAL ACTIVITIES PARTICIPATED IN BY QUADRIPLEGICS

Sports Involvement	Personal Hobbies	Group Involvement	Social Activities
W/Chair volleyball	Driving	Sports:	Church groups
W/Chair table tennis	Travelling	Refereeing	Discussion groups
W/Chair track and field	Playing cards	Coaching	Service clubs
Swimming	Checkers	Judging	Hobby clubs:
	Chess	Time Keeping	Gardening
(The above are also	Collecting	Score keeping	Photography
recognized Olympic	Ham radio	Starting	Stamp collecting
sports)	Model building	Tournament official	Archery, etc.
	Model road racing		
	Astronomy	Religious activities	Most social functions
Driving (car rallies)	Ornithology	Politics	and parties
Flying	Gardening	Organizing	Visiting and entertaining
Fishing	Adult education	Volunteer work	Theatre
Camping	Animal breeding	Cubs, Scouts, Y.M.C.A.	Spectator sports
Boating (towing	Watching T.V.	Boys Club, Red Cross,	Pen pals
Water skiers, etc.)	Reading	etc.	
Helming sail boat	Writing	Drama (directing, etc.)	
Sporting rifle	Photography	Tutoring	
Skeet shooting	Cooking	Public speaking	
Table shuffleboard	Music	Singing	
Billiards	Tape recording		
	Lapidary		
	Weaving		
	Printing		
	Mosaic tile work		
	Leather work		
	Carpentry		
	Wood carving		
	Ceramics		
	Painting		

ADAPTIONS WHICH MAY BE REQUIRED FOR SOME RECREATIONAL EQUIPMENT

Table Tennis. A table tennis paddle may be held by bandaging the hand around the handle with an elastic bandage, or it may be held as in Figure 11-1 with masking tape. Both methods allow the paddle to be adjusted while being held firmly.

Archery. This splint for holding and releasing a bow string is simple and has a smooth release action. Two loops of fine shock cord are attached to a metal hand splint with a trigger-shaped projection. The larger loop is placed over the bow string and the smaller loop is pushed through the large loop and over the trigger (Fig. 11-2A). A small movement of the hand (Fig. 11-2B) will release the bow string (Fig. 11-2C).

Fishing. A metal thumb loop may be required in the reel handle and the tension control or the brake may require enlarging for easier handling. A rod holder may also be needed.

Sporting rifle. The quadriplegic marksman may be at no disadvantage competing against able-bodied marksmen in sporting rifle shooting but is at some disadvantage in skeet shooting because he cannot turn far enough to follow the complete arc of the target. (A gold shield has been won by the marksman who supplied this information.)

Sailing. Several quadriplegic sailors helm their boats, but they require a crew.

Flying. At least one make of small plane, the Aercoupe, has been flown by quadriplegic pilots. Quadriplegic pilots have been licenced by the Canadian Department of Transport.

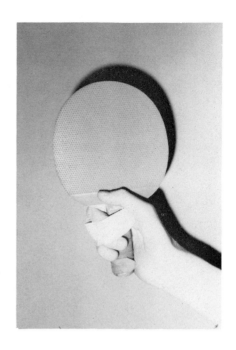

FIGURE 11-1

A

B

C

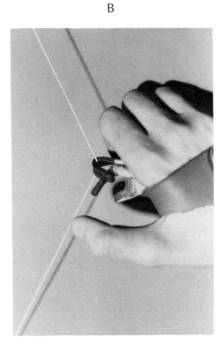

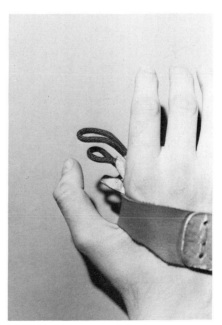

FIGURE 11-2

303

Standing. Standing in braces can be regarded as a recreational exercise for some low-lesion quadriplegic patients (Fig. 11-3). Mental and physical benefits are derived from the change of posture. The braces, with sole plates and anterior and posterior stops, are the type used by paraplegics. A standing table may be used instead of parallel bars so that study, reading, or other hobbies may be carried out at the same time.

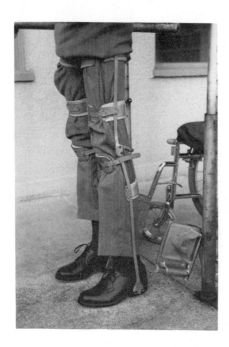 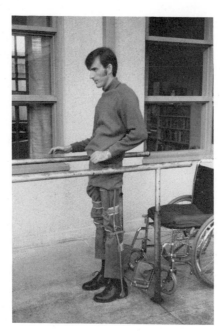 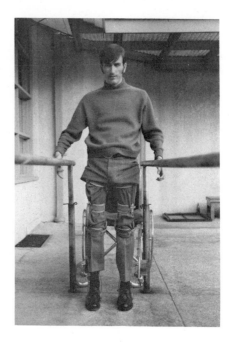

FIGURE 11-3

Radio and Record Players, etc. Knobs or switches of radios, record players, television, etc. may require adaption. Some plastic knobs can be drilled to take a short length of metal rod to add leverage.

Photography. A cable release may be required for the shutter mechanism and this may require adaption.

Card Playing. Card holders may be purchased or made. Figure 11-4A shows a card holder that may be used to turn cards face up with the use of hand or mouthstick. Figure 11-4B shows a small box turned upside down with the cards held between cover and box. Figure 11-4C shows a board with diagonal saw cuts and a commercially available plastic card holder fastened to a homemade base. Card shufflers may also be purchased.

Cribbage, etc. A large size crib board with ¼-inch-diameter pegs is easier to manage than standard boards (Fig. 11-5). Large chessmen, adapted checkers, etc. may enable the patient to make moves more easily.

304

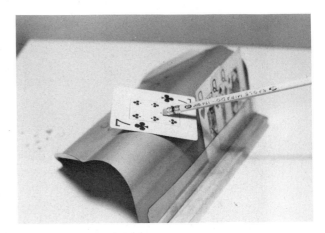

A

FIGURE 11-4

FIGURE 11-4

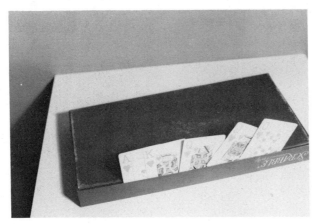

B

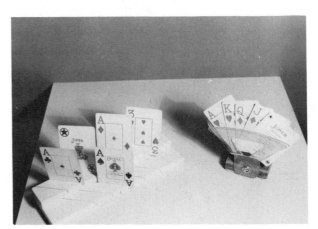

C

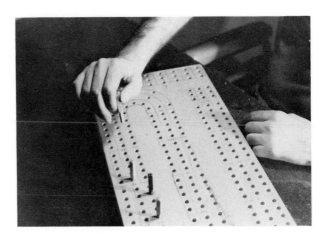

FIGURE 11-5

Reading. A reading stand may be bought or made. If a mouthstick or headstick is used to turn the pages, it is often necessary to stretch an elastic over the pages which have not been read. If the stand is nearly vertical other elastic strips are used to retain the book cover in position (Fig. 11-6A). The type of swingaway clip used on a music stand may be attached to a reading stand to keep the pages down.

If a stand is used in bed, the book will be facing downward (Fig. 11-6B). In this case both the elastic and the music clips will be required. If the patient uses an overhead bar, a book holder may be suspended from it, and two legs may be added to rest on the bed to adjust the angle and stabilize the stand. If a page turner is required, the eraser end of a pencil may be used, or a wad of electrical and moisture insulator gum may be pushed onto a suitable length of dowelling.

Playing Musical Instruments. Instruments which do not require finger dexterity can be played satisfactorily; the trombone and harmonica, or mouth organ, are examples. In some cases the instrument must be adapted for holding.

Camping. Some quadriplegic patients will participate with their families in camping. Trailers may be custom built or modified, providing access by elevator and room to move around within the trailer. Special attention will be required to provide adequate bathroom facilities.

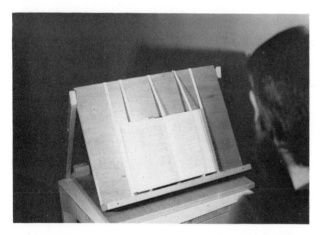

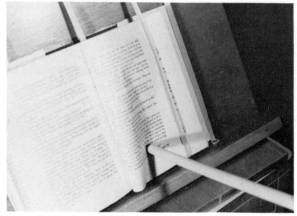

A

FIGURE 11-6

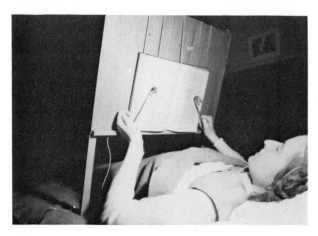

B

12 *Management*
of the Dependent Patient

Easy transfer methods should be used for the protection of both the patient and staff before the patient has learned to transfer himself. Later these methods will make nursing care easier for those patients who are not able to attain full independence or make it possible for some of these patients to be cared for at home.

ADJUSTING POSITIONS IN THE WHEELCHAIR

The patient must be positioned in the wheelchair in a posture which will allow him to maintain balance, with maximum mobility and comfort (see Chapter 2). The front castors of the wheelchair should be turned forward while positioning the patient. This lengthens the wheel base and prevents the wheelchair from tipping forward. The brakes must be applied to prevent the chair from moving.

MOVING THE PATIENT FORWARD

Method 1.   Apply the brakes and swing the front castors forward. Grasp the patient's slacks or skirt behind the knees, so making sure they will be pulled simultaneously to avoid wrinkling. Place a foot against the front bumper and lean back to pull the buttocks forward (Fig. 12-1).

Method 2.   Small adjustments forward and adjustments to square the patient in the chair may be made by pulling the patient from behind his knee with one hand and pushing against the chair seat beside the knee with the other hand (Fig. 12-2). There is little strain on the back because mainly the arms are used.

Method 3.   Sometimes it is desirable to move the patient forward while standing behind the chair. The helper places his hands, palm up under the buttocks. This places the elbows against the back of the chair for leverage. Flexion of the elbows will now move the patient forward (Fig. 12-3). The helper's arms may be placed over the upper arms of the patient first if the patient requires stabilization.

Method 4.   A patient may be moved forward slightly if the helper places a foot well under the chair so that his thigh can be used to push against the bottom of the chair back. The helper holds the patient under the arms to pull back slightly and to maintain the patient's balance (Fig. 12-4).

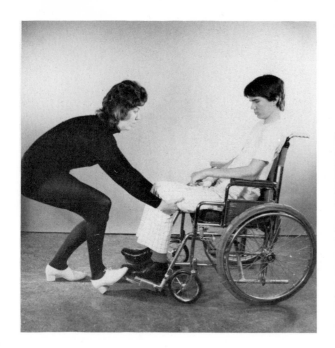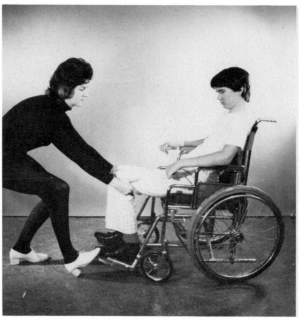

FIGURE 12-1

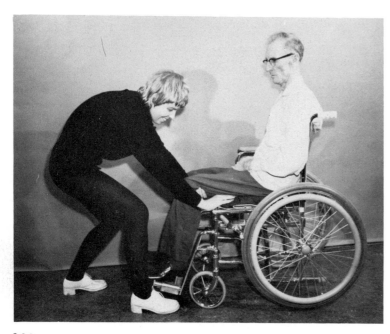

FIGURE 12-2

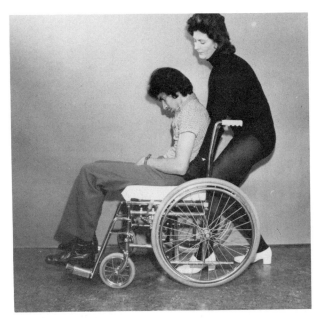

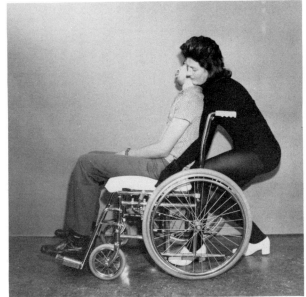

FIGURE 12-3

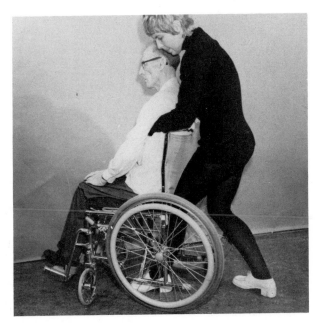

FIGURE 12-4

MOVING THE PATIENT BACKWARD

Method 1. (Fig. 12-5). Minimum effort for the maximum movement is expended in this method. The helper stands behind the chair with her arms underneath the patient's upper arms while the patient remains leaning back in the chair; the patient's hands are placed one on top of the other over the lower abdomen. The helper's hands are placed over the patient's hands and the patient's trunk is flexed forward. The forward flexion is controlled by the adduction of the helper's arms. The forearms are now placed below the patient's ribcage. By adducting the arms and straightening the elbows the patient is levered back into the chair. The ribcage provides a fulcrum and the pubis symphysis provides the point of leverage. When a large patient is moved, one hand may be positioned on the patient's hands and his trunk flexed forward before positioning the second hand.

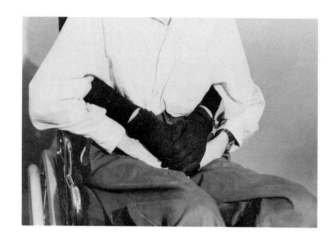

FIGURE 12-5

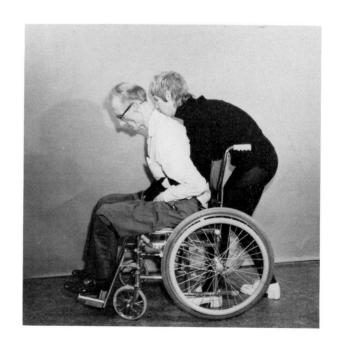

310

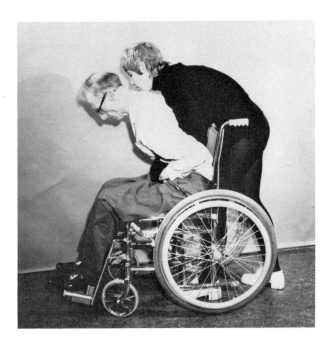
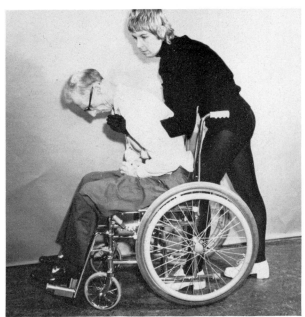

Method 2. The very heavy patient may require two people to move him (Fig. 12-6). One person stands behind the chair and the other in front. The person in front prevents the patient from sliding further forward by squeezing the patient's knees between her own. The front assistant now pulls the patient's trunk forward into flexion and holds him in this position. The assistant behind the chair grasps the slacks at the outside seams anterior to the hip joints and, with a combined pull and lift, moves the patient back in the chair.

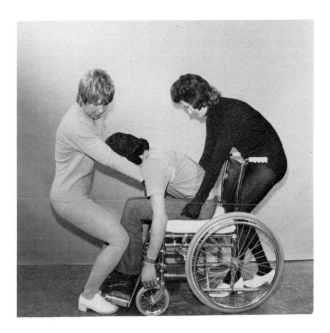
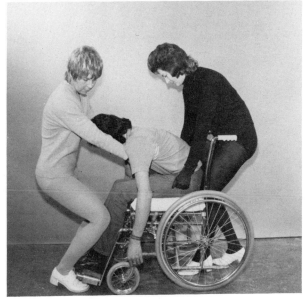

FIGURE 12-6

Method 3. The assistant stands in front of the patient and stabilizes the knees between her own. She places her palms against both sides of the patient's upper rib cage. The assistant abducts her shoulders so that her elbows protrude, enabling the patient to place his arms over the assistant's elbows. The patient flexes his elbows as strongly as possible and hugs with his shoulders, thus helping the assistant. The patient's trunk is pulled forward and simultaneously the assistant flexes her knees, thus using body weight to move the patient back into the chair (Fig. 12-7).

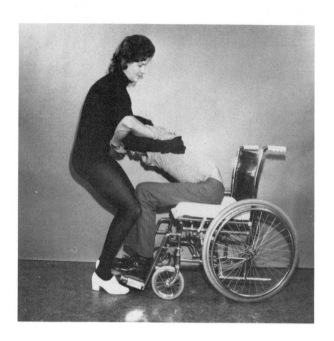 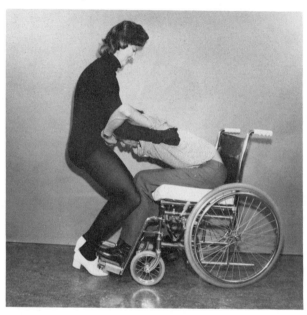

FIGURE 12-7

Method 4. The assistant stands in front of the chair and stabilizes the patient's knees with her own. She slips her hands over the patient's shoulders and grasps the patient's upper arms close to the axillae. The assistant must straighten her arms at this point or she will lose most of her leverage. The assistant rocks her weight back and flexes her knees simultaneously, moving the patient back into the chair (Fig. 12-8). This method is most suitable when managing a heavy patient or a patient with very weak upper extremities. A shorter assistant may use the same method but slip her hands under the patient's axillae from the front.

A patient may be positioned and centered by movement of the helper's knees in this or the previous method.

Method 5. Two assistants may be necessary when a patient has been placed in an easy chair or in a high-backed or old-fashioned wheelchair (Fig. 12-9). They stand one on each side and in front of the patient, the outside foot forward and the knees flexed. The inside hand is placed under the patient's axilla, grasping the upper arm; the outside hand is placed under the patient's midthigh and the assistant's elbow rests on her own knee. The patient is pulled forward with the inside hands at the same time that he is pushed back with the outside hands. This must be done by both assistants simultaneously using a preplanned signal.

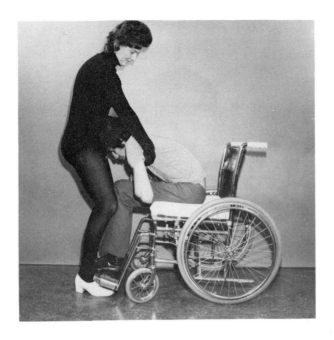

FIGURE 12-8

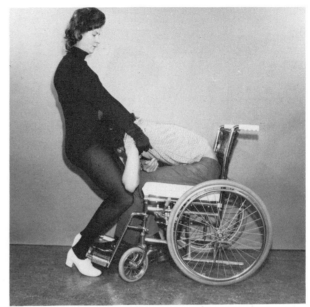

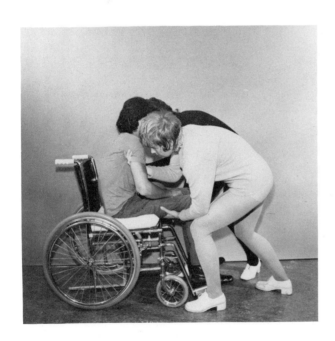

FIGURE 12-9

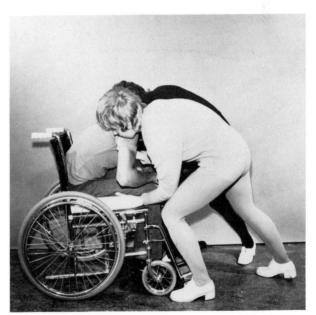

Method 6. There is an easy way to retrieve a patient who has slid forward so far that he cannot be sat upright on the seat of the chair. The assistant tilts the chair far back by stepping on the tipping lever and pulling back on the pushing handle (Fig. 12-10). The patient will slide back into the chair far enough to make one of the previous methods possible.

313

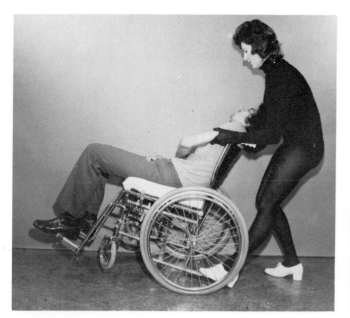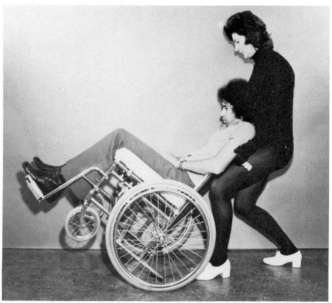

FIGURE 12-10

Method 7. If the chair is in such a location that it cannot be tipped back or, if the patient must be retrieved immediately, he must be pulled up from behind (Fig. 12-11). The belt may be grasped or, if there is no belt, the wrists may be grasped by reaching under the axillae. Because a pull in this position is not easy, the patient should be pulled back just far enough for one of the other methods to be used to position him.

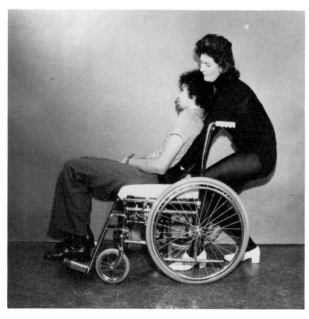

FIGURE 12-11

Method 8. Two assistants may stand one on either side of the patient facing in the same direction as the patient. The hand closest to the patient is placed underneath the patient's axilla from behind and over the patient's forearm near the elbow. This is a flat hand hold with the thumb aligned with the fingers. The other hand is placed under the thigh near the knee. The patient is levered back into the chair as both assistants lift, straightening their arms (Fig. 12-12).

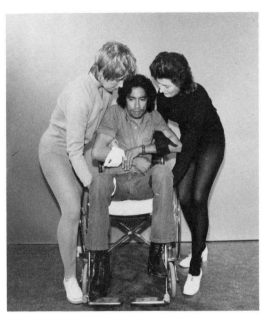 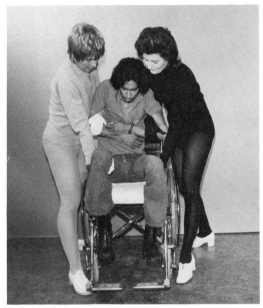

FIGURE 12-12

MOVING THE PATIENT SIDEWAYS

Method 1. The patient's trunk may be flexed sideways before grasping the slacks at the hip. The patient should be leaned away from the proposed direction of travel (Fig. 12-13). The patient may help to maintain his balance by flexing his elbow around the pushing handle on the side he is moving towards.

Method 2. The helper may stand behind the chair and grasp the slacks just forward of the hip. The other hand is placed on the opposite side of the patient, on the cushion by the trochanter. By the helper's pulling up on the slacks and pushing down on the cushion not only will the patient slide over but his slacks will be unwrinkled beneath him (Fig. 12-14). If the assistant's grip is not adequate, an object such as a cigarette lighter may be placed in the patient's pocket and the slacks may be grasped around it.

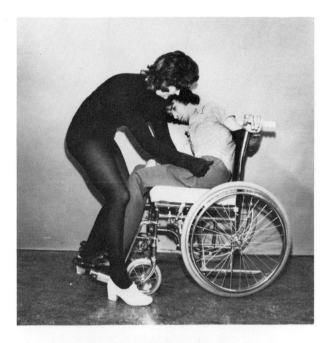

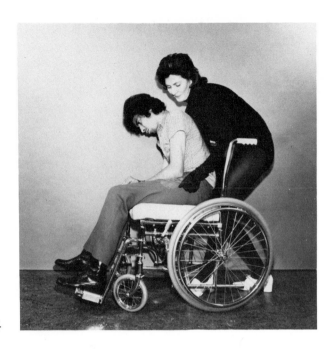

FIGURE 12-13

FIGURE 12-14

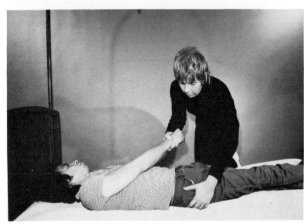

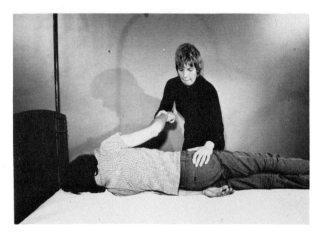

FIGURE 12-15

316

MOVING THE PATIENT IN THE BED

TURNING THE PATIENT

Supine to Prone

Method 1. (Fig. 12-15) The helper places the patient's near arm under his buttock palm up and crosses the far leg over the near one. She grasps the patient's far arm with one hand and his thigh with the other. A pull will roll the patient over.

Method 2. A patient may be turned with greater control and increased mechanical advantage using this method (Fig. 12-16). The patient's far hand is placed palm up under the buttock, and his near leg is crossed over the far one. The helper places one hand under the near leg and over the far leg, placing the crook of her elbow under the near buttock. The helper's other arm is placed under the near shoulder and the hand is placed on the far shoulder. When the helper's arms are straightened the patient is levered over.

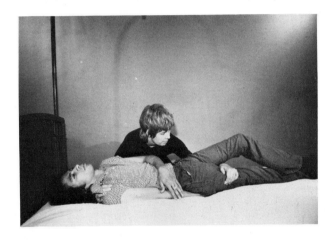
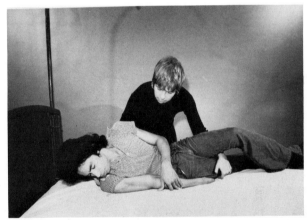
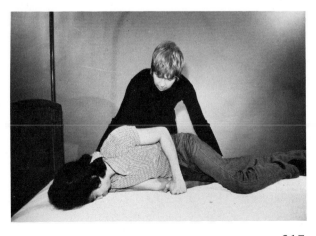

FIGURE 12-16

Prone to Supine

Method 1. (Fig. 12-17) The patient's head is turned towards the helper, and his far hand, palm up, is placed under the thigh as far under as possible. The near leg is crossed over the far leg. The helper reaches under the near thigh and grasps the patient's hand. Pulling on the hand and pushing on the pelvis will roll the patient over.

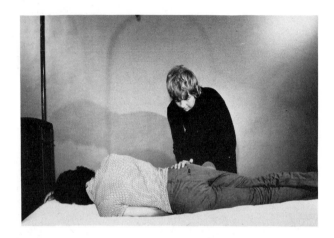
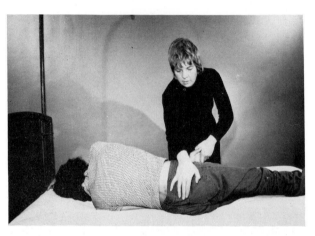
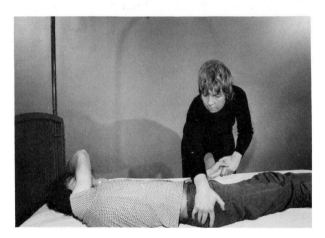

FIGURE 12-17

Method 2. (Fig. 12-18) The patient's head is turned towards the helper, and his far hand, palm up, is placed beneath his thigh as far under as possible. The near leg may be crossed over the far leg. The helper places an arm under the near thigh with the hand over the far thigh. The other arm is placed under the patient's axilla from the direction of the foot of the bed. The helper's arm continues through, placing her arm behind the patient's neck and onto his far shoulder. When the helper's arms are straightened the patient is levered over. If, at the same time, the helper pulls, the patient may be positioned in the centre of the bed.

318

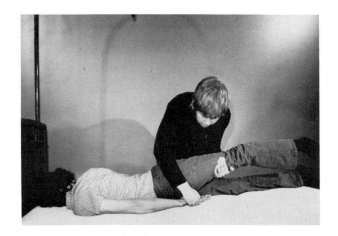
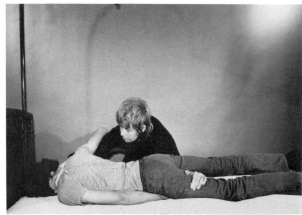

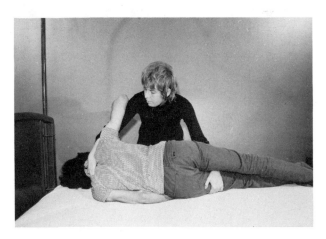
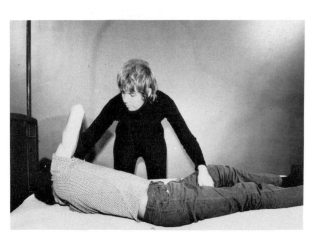

FIGURE 12-18

Method 3. (Fig. 12-19) Two people may turn a very heavy patient. His head is turned towards the helpers and his far hand is tucked palm up under him to midline. This arm must be straight, thus eliminating any blocking by a flexed elbow and ensuring that the arm will not be hurt. The helper near the head places one arm under the patient's axilla from the direction of the foot of the bed. This arm is continued through over the back of the neck and onto the far shoulder. The other hand rests on the patient's far shoulder blade to tuck it under as he is levered over. The second helper places the hand nearer the head of the bed under the patient's hip and the second hand is placed under the near leg and over the far leg at midthigh level. The helpers pull simultaneously, an action which will not only turn the patient but also position him at any point wished on the bed.

319

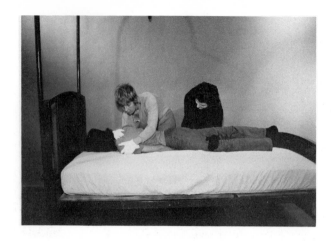
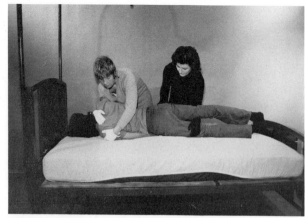
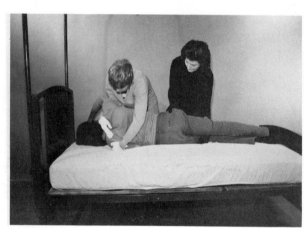
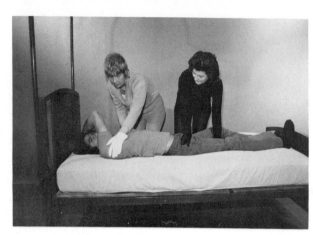

FIGURE 12-19

MOVING ACROSS THE BED

Method 1. (Fig. 12-20) The helper stands by the side of the bed farthest away from the patient. She grasps the slacks near the trochanter and the patient's upper arm near the axilla. The helper leans back with elbows extended to pull the patient over.

Method 2. The helper stands by the side of the bed farthest from the patient with a knee against the side of the bed or on the mattress. She slides one arm under the patient's upper thighs and one arm under the patient's shoulders. Cupping both hands the helper leans back to slide the patient over (Fig. 12-21). This method may be used for a very heavy patient, moving first the shoulders, then the buttocks, and then the legs.

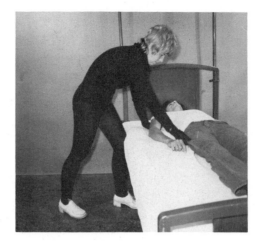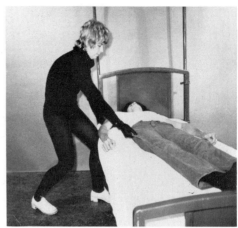

FIGURE 12-20

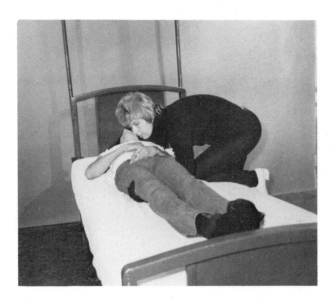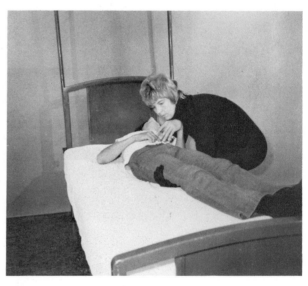

FIGURE 12-21

Method 3. Momentum can be used very effectively in moving the patient. The helper maintains the patient's sitting balance with one hand and grasps the slacks at the hip joint with the other hand. A rhythmical bouncing combined with a pull will allow the patient to be moved as his buttocks clear the mattress (Fig. 12-22).

MOVING DOWN THE BED

The helper moves to the foot of the bed and grasps the patient's ankles, including the slacks. The helper leans back with one knee braced against the foot of the bed and with straight arms pulls the patient into position (Fig. 12-23).

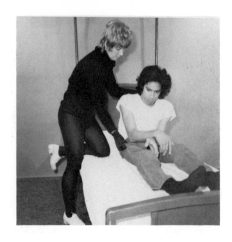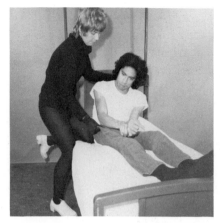

FIGURE 12-22

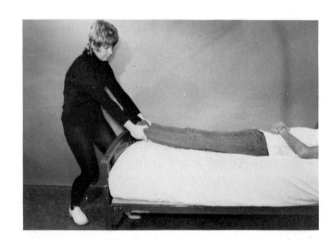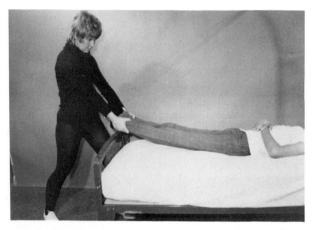

FIGURE 12-23

MOVING UP THE BED

Method 1. (Fig. 12-24) The helper moves to a position behind the head of the bed. Using a knee to stabilize herself against the head of the bed, the helper grasps the patient's upper arms and leans back to slide the patient up the bed.

Method 2. (Fig. 12-25) The patient is placed in long sitting on the bed. The helper kneels on one or both knees behind the patient. The slacks are grasped at the hips or the hands are placed under the buttocks if no slacks are worn. In this position the patient is fully stabilized. The patient may be pressed down into the mattress, thus giving a bouncing assistance from the mattress springs. In rhythm with the bouncing the helper sits back on her heel, thus moving the patient back with a minimum of friction.

Method 3. (Fig. 12-26) The helper stands beside the bed facing the head and places a knee on the bed. She slides her hands palm down under the patient's axillae and then clenches her fingers. The patient is asked to adduct his arms. The helper rocks forward on her knee and flexes her wrists while pressing down into

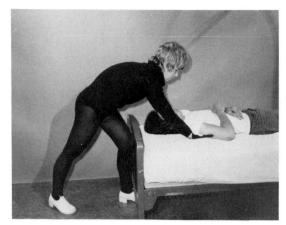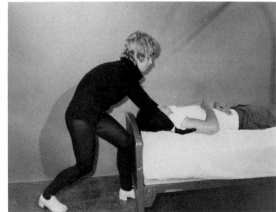

FIGURE 12-24

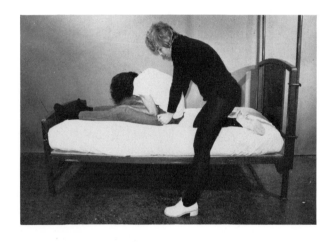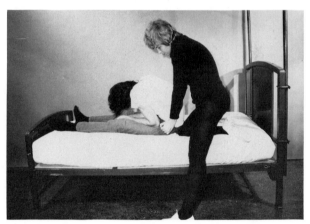

FIGURE 12-25

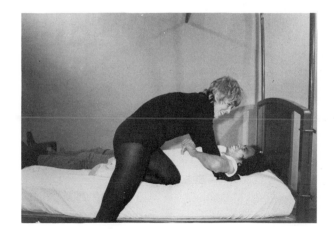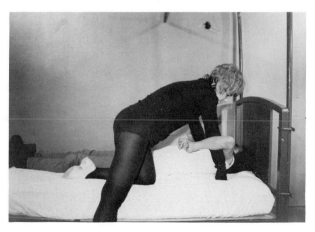

FIGURE 12-26

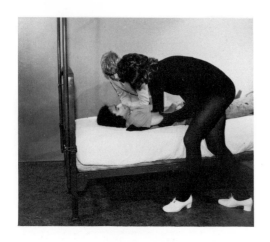

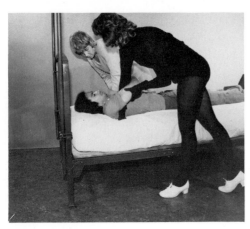

FIGURE 12-27

the mattress. The leverage obtained by this method moves the patient a short distance but with relative ease.

Method 4. (Fig. 12-27) A method similar to Method 3 may be used by two helpers, who place the hands nearest to the bed under the patient's axillae. The fingers are clenched and pressed into the mattress. The far hands are used to hold the patient's elbows to his sides. By flexing the wrists and rocking forward, the helpers will move the patient up the bed.

Method 5. (Fig. 12-28) The patient is placed in long sitting and the two helpers stand on either side facing the head of the bed. Each places one knee on the bed at the level of the patient's hips. The helpers' shoulders are placed under the patient's axillae with his arms resting on the helpers' backs. The helpers' outside hands are placed on the bed towards the head and with the elbows locked. The inside hands are placed under the patient's upper thighs from the medial sides. The helpers rock forward together onto their knees and locked arms, thus lifting and moving the patient up the bed.

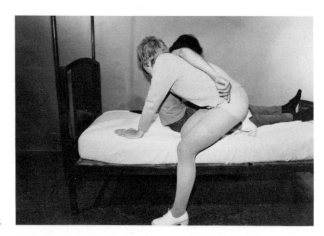

FIGURE 12-28

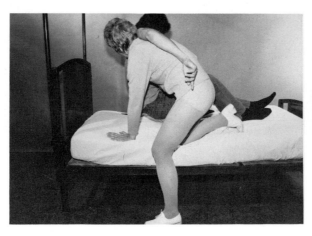

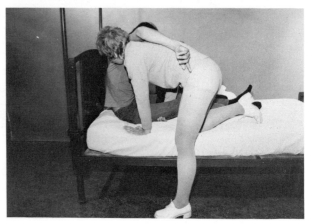

SITTING THE PATIENT UP IN BED

Method 1. (Fig. 12-29) To sit the patient on the edge of the bed the helper moves the patient's buttocks towards the side of the bed and then swings the patient's legs over the edge. Standing facing the patient, she then blocks the patient's knees with her own. The helper grasps the patient's wrists and leans back to rock the patient into a sitting position.

Method 2. (Fig. 12-30) To sit the patient on the side of the bed the helper stands by the bed facing the patient with the knee nearest the head resting on the bed. The helper slides one hand under the patient's knees and flexes his knees and hips. She slides the other hand under the patient's far shoulder, supporting his head in the crook of her elbow. The patient is rocked back and then forward and is pivotted so that his feet are swung to the floor as he is placed in the sitting position.

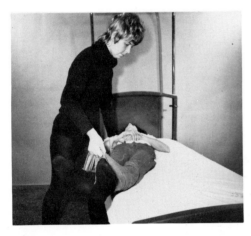 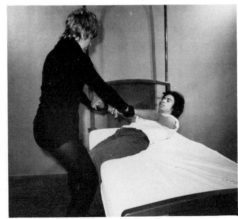 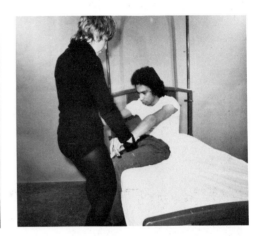

FIGURE 12-29

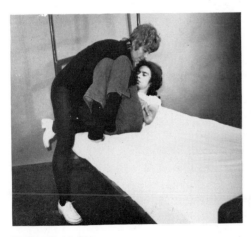 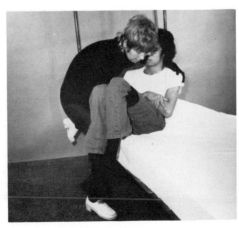 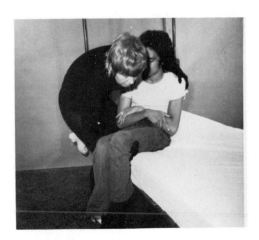

FIGURE 12-30

Method 3. (Fig. 12-31) The helper stands by the patient's shoulders and slides the hand near the top of the bed under the patient's far shoulder. The patient's head rests in the crook of the helper's elbow. The helper leans forward to raise the

325

patient's head and places a knee on the bed under the patient's head. The helper's other hand is placed under the patient's other shoulder. By rocking forward the patient will be placed in a long-sitting position. As the patient nears the upright position the helper's hands are slid over the shoulders so that forward momentum can be controlled.

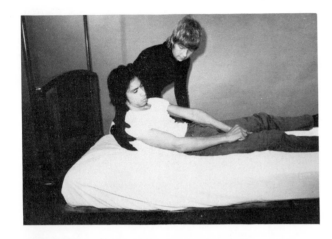

FIGURE 12-31

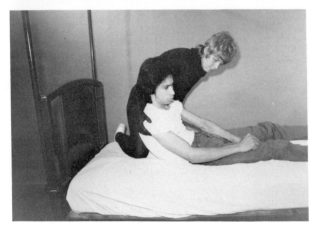

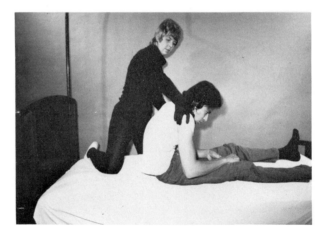

TRANSFERRING

ONTO THE BED FROM COMMODE OR WHEELCHAIR

The bed should be equipped with a nylon contour sheet, plywood boards, and a firm mattress. The bed should be the same height as the wheelchair cushion. The chair usually is positioned at 30° to the bed facing the foot and locked to the bed. The front castors should be swung forward to give maximum stability, and the brakes must be applied. The armrest by the bed should be removed. If a bridge board is necessary it should be positioned at this time. Talcum powder on the bridge board will facilitate sliding.

326

Method 1.   Some patients can take part of their weight by having their arms placed in an overhead strap (Fig. 12-32). The helper places one arm under the patient's knees and one by the trochanter while standing close to the patient. She pulls the patient forward, thus clearing his buttocks from the chair seat, and swings him onto the bed. The hand by the trochanter guides the direction of travel.

FIGURE 12-32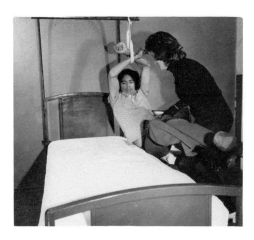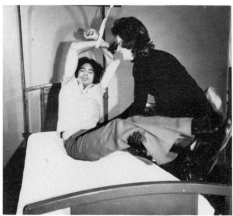

Method 2.   (Fig. 12-33) The helper moves the patient forward in the chair and stands with the outside foot inside the footrests to stabilize the patient's thigh against her own. The patient's trunk is flexed far forward onto his knees. The helper reaches over and grasps the slacks in front of the hips. This places one arm against the patient's shoulder blade, thus adding an extra fulcrum. By rocking back and pivotting towards the bed the patient's buttocks are very easily lifted onto the bed. To lay the patient down one hand can now be placed under the patient's knees and another on his far shoulder, so supporting the patient's head on the helper's forearm. As the patient is pivotted, his legs are lifted and his trunk is lowered. In pivotting type transfers it is advantageous to rock the patient in place to get the feel of the weight distribution, to add momentum, and to reassure the patient.

Method 3.   (Fig. 12-34) The helper stands with the outside foot inside the footrests and stabilizes the patient's knees against her own. The helper places her palms on either side of the patient's rib cage and abducts her shoulders so that her elbows protrude. The patient places his arms over the helper's elbows and hugs strongly. The helper rocks back and pivots, thus raising the patient's buttocks and swinging him over onto the bed.

Method 4.   (Fig. 12-35) The patient's buttocks are pulled forward in the chair and his legs are lifted onto the bed. His forearms are placed in an overhead sling. The helper now moves to the other side of the bed. She puts one knee on the bed and grasps the belt or slacks. The other hand pushes on the bed while the patient is pulled across the bridge board towards the helper. Some helpers may have to kneel on the bed in order to reach the belt comfortably.

Method 5.   (Fig. 12-36) The area between the wheelchair cushion and the bed is padded with a pillow. The patient's buttocks are moved forward in the chair and his feet are placed on the bed, preferably with the outside leg crossed over.

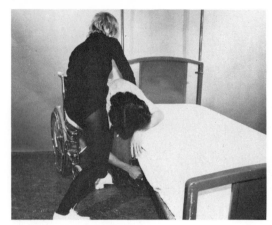

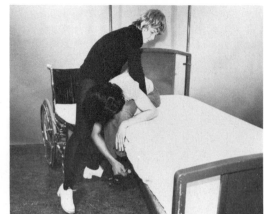

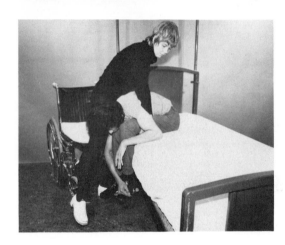

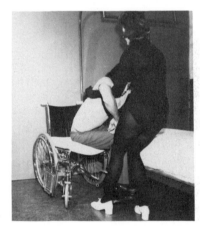

FIGURE 12-33

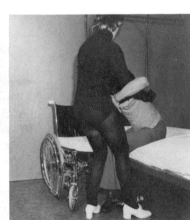

FIGURE 12-34

FIGURE 12-35

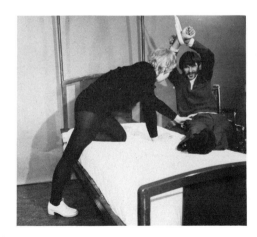

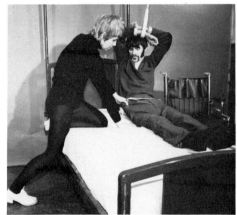

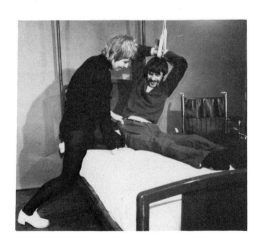

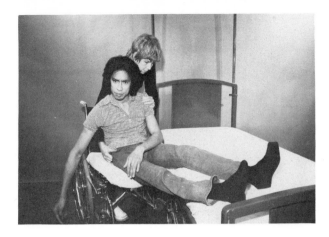
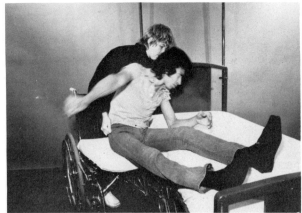

FIGURE 12-36

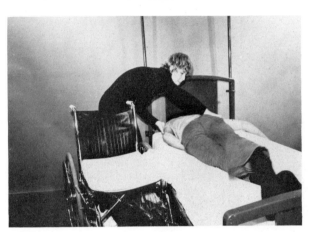

The helper moves to the rear of the chair and grasps the patient's slacks by the trochanter with her outside hand. She now steps close to the bed so that this arm rests across the patient's back. The other hand controls the shoulder nearest the bed. When the helper's outside arm is straightened and she pivots towards the bed, the patient is rolled onto the bed. The speed is controlled by the hand on the patient's inside shoulder. The patient may assist by swinging his arms towards the bed in synchronization with the helper's movement. A foot retainer board will be necessary if the patient's legs tend to slide off the bed during this transfer.

Method 6. (Fig. 12-37) The patient is placed facing the bed and his feet are lifted onto the mattress. The leg rests are swung away and then the chair is pushed up to the bed, leaving no gap between bed and cushion. The brakes are now applied. The helper goes to the opposite side of the bed facing the patient. The helper abducts the patient's legs to provide lateral stability and grasps the patient's wrists, pulling his trunk forward into flexion. The patient's hands are placed on his ankles. The helper grasps the patient's hands and ankles together and placing one knee on the bed she rocks back, thus pulling the patient onto the bed. The patient is placed lengthwise on the bed by swinging the feet towards the foot of the bed.

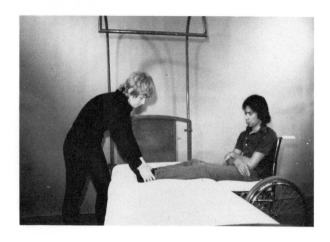
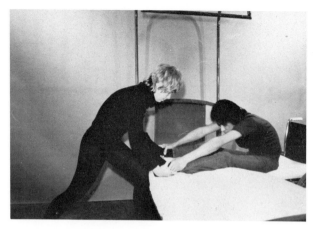
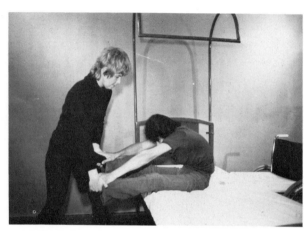
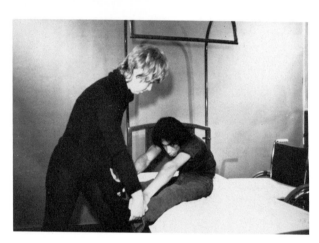

FIGURE 12-37

Method 7. (Fig. 12-38) The chair is wheeled backwards to contact the bed about two-thirds of the way up. The brakes should *not* be applied. The patient's head must be supported while the wheelchair is tipped back. The hips are grasped and lifted towards the bed. The feet are now placed on a leg strap before lifting the hips again. Just before the patient's buttocks are free of the wheelchair back, his feet are moved to the seat. The helper now moves to the other side of the bed to pull him further back, holding under one arm, and supporting his head. The patient's knees are lifted into flexion, releasing the chair and allowing it to fall onto four wheels. The helper's arm nearest the foot of the bed is slipped right under the patient's knees, and the other arm still supports the patient's head while holding the shoulder. He is now easily swivelled into position.

Method 8. A track may be attached to an overhead bar, an A frame, or to the ceiling and used in conjunction with a mechanical hoist or block and tackle. Slings (see Appendix), one under the thighs and one behind the back are attached to one another near the hips by means of an adjustable strap and hooks (Fig. 12-39A). The four ends of the slings are equipped with snap hooks and the hooks are clipped onto chains, which are held apart above head level by means of a

330

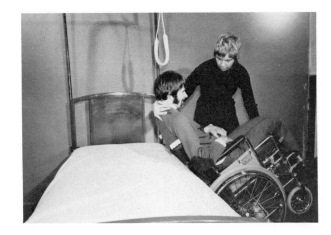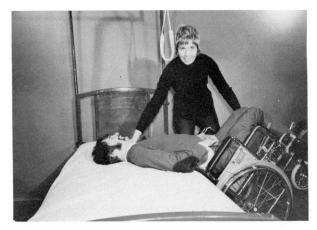

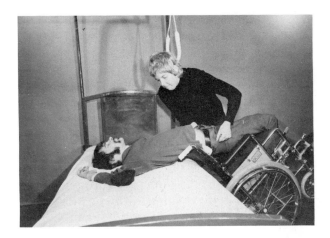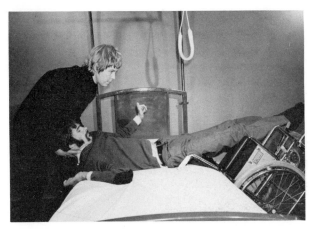

FIGURE 12-38

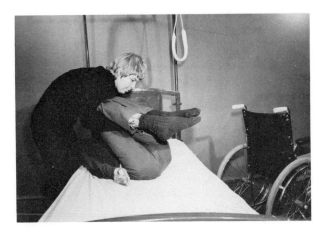

spreader bar. The centre of the spreader bar is attached to the lifting mechanism (Fig. 12-39B).

The sling at the back may be stiffened so that when the patient is flexed forward in the chair it may be dropped into position without collapsing behind him. The

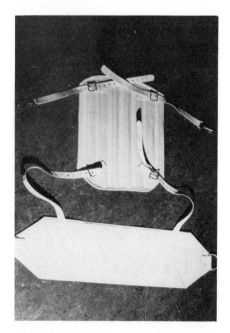

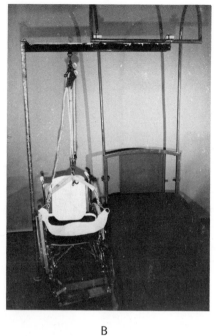

FIGURE 12-39

A B

other sling may be placed in position under his thighs by lifting his legs only and is hooked to the back sling at each side. The slings are now hooked onto the suspended chains so that when the lifting mechanism is operated the patient is in a comfortable sitting position. When the patient's buttocks are clear of all obstacles the mechanism may be moved along the track and the patient lowered to the bed (Fig. 12-40). This sling can be positioned without lifting the patient and is easily

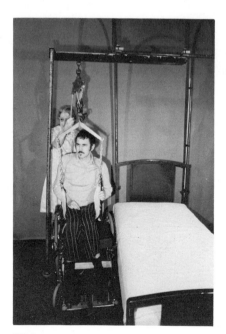

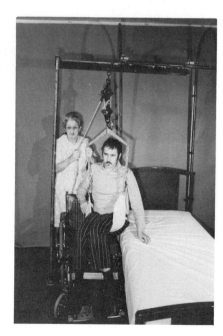

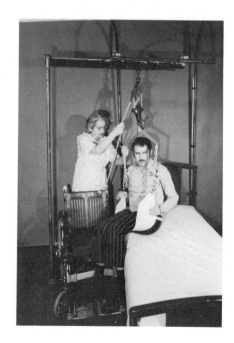

FIGURE 12-40

adjustable to the individual patient. These mechanisms are versatile in that they may be moved to another track, i.e. in the bathroom.

Hydraulic patient lifters are available on the commercial market and operate well, but they may be bulky to store and manoeuvre in a small house. They may be used in all patient transfers, including the car, and may be used to position the patient in the bed.

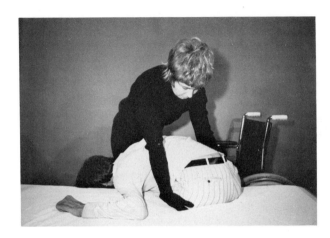
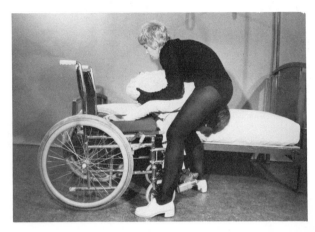
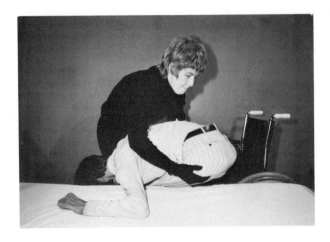
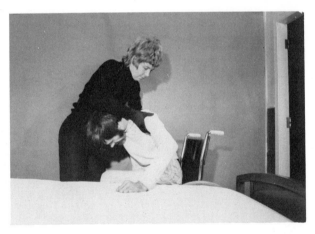

FIGURE 12-41

FROM THE BED

Method 1.   (Fig. 12-41) The helper places the patient's feet on the footrests so they are free to turn as he is pivotted. He now flexes the patient's trunk forward so that his trunk rests on his thighs. The helper places one foot beside the footrest on the outside to block the chair and to position herself correctly. The patient's thigh is blocked and controlled by the helper's inside knee as the patient is rocked onto the chair.

Method 2.   (Fig. 12-42) The patient's forearms are placed in an overhead sling. The helper stands beside the patient and lifts his legs with one arm under his thighs. The other hand is placed behind and under one buttock to guide and swing him forward from the bed and back onto the chair. The patient who can hold his weight will maintain and perhaps improve his strength; therefore, this method is used sometimes for preparing patients for learning independent transfers.

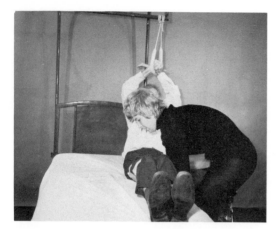
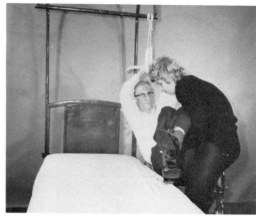

FIGURE 12-42

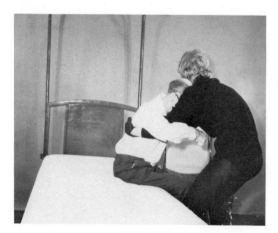

FIGURE 12-43

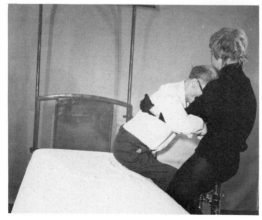
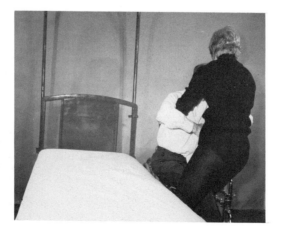

Method 3. (Fig. 12-43) The helper stands in front of the patient and blocks the patient's knees with her own. She places her palms against the patient's rib cage. The patient puts his arms on the helper's elbows and hugs to assist holding. The helper rocks back to pivot the patient onto the chair. The chair should be hooked to the bed to prevent it from swinging away as the patient is pivotted.

Method 4. (Fig. 12-44) The patient's forearms are placed in an overhead strap so that he can take some of his weight. The helper holds him by the belt or pants by the trochanter to swing and slide him into the chair over a bridge board.

Method 5. (Fig. 12-45) The helper swings the footrests back and butts the chair against the bed facing it. The patient is sat up, and his trunk is flexed forward. The helper holds the patient under the upper thigh and bounces the patient to shift him back into the chair. This is an excellent method for the very flaccid patient who can lie forward on his legs.

Method 6. (Fig. 12-46) The patient is in side-lying facing away from the chair, in a jack-knife position. The patient's belt is grasped to lift and slide his buttocks into the chair seat. The helper's knee is placed against the bed to hold the patient's legs in position and to provide a fulcrum when rolling the patient up to sit.

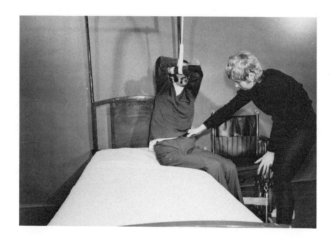
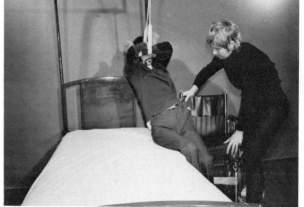

FIGURE 12-44

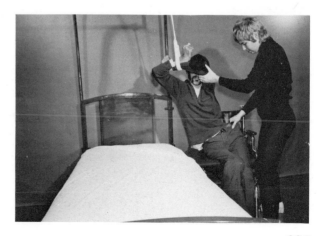

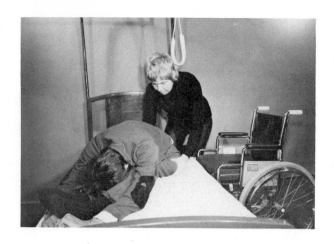
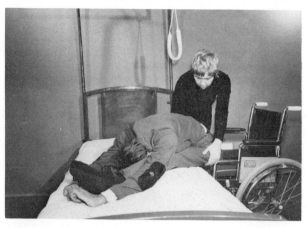

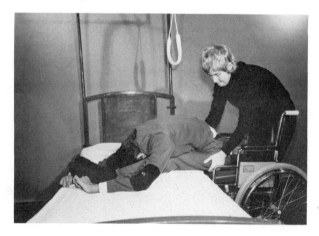
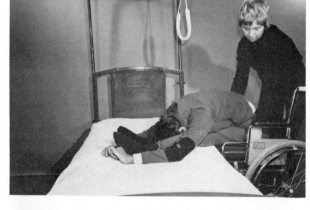

FIGURE 12-45

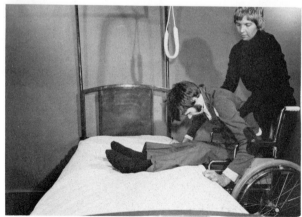

Method 7. (Fig. 12-47) The helper holds the patient's far wrist and his slacks at the ankles. She synchronizes her pull on the arm and swing of the legs to pivot the patient at his buttocks. She now hooks the patient's legs over the back of the chair. The helper pushes the wheelchair handles down onto the mattress and

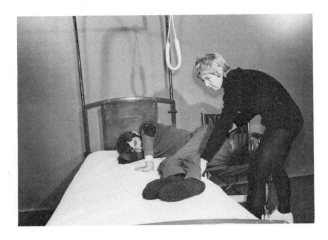
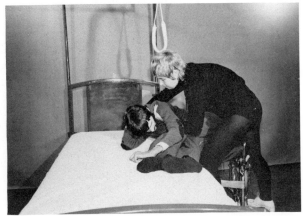

FIGURE 12-46

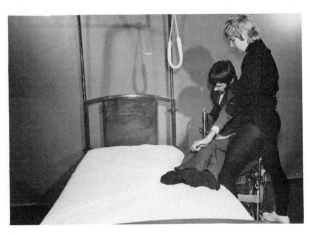

straightens the patient's legs to rest over the edge of the seat. She pulls the patient's legs forward alternately to pull his buttocks into the chair. As the patient slides into the chair the slacks are pulled to ensure that they are not tight at the groin. The helper slips an arm under the neck to the far shoulder and sits the patient up while controlling the chair position with her hand on the pushing handle. Throughout this transfer, the wheelchair brakes are not applied so that the wheelchair can be tipped. The pushing handles digging into the mattress will stabilize the wheelchair when there is weight in the chair.

FLOOR TO WHEELCHAIR

Method 1. (Fig 12-48) The chair is tipped back with the pushing handles on the floor by the patient's feet. The patient's legs are lifted and the chair is slid towards the patient's buttocks until his ankles rest on the edge of the chair seat. The helper now moves around to the front of the chair and grasps the patient's ankles and slacks together. The helper also places one knee on the cross bars to block the chair and keep the chair open. By leaning back with straight arms, the patient's buttocks are lifted and pulled into the chair. His feet may now be placed on the footrests. The helper now moves to the rear of the chair. She squats by the

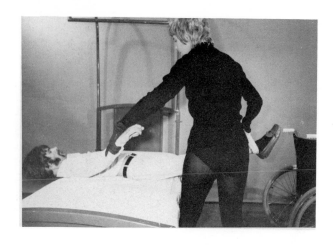
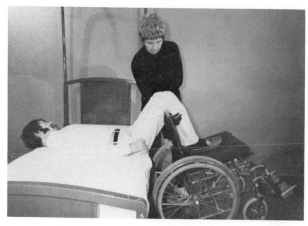

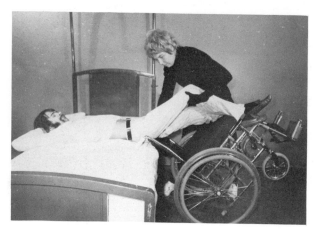
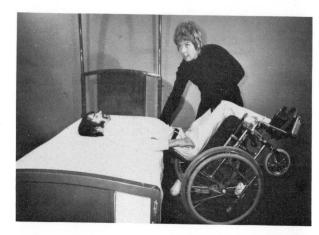

FIGURE 12-47

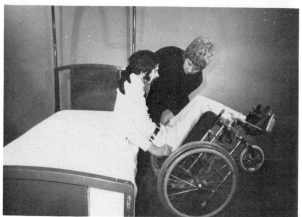

patient's head and places one hand under his neck and one under the pushing handle. The chair is righted as the helper stands. As the chair nears the upright position the helper's hand is moved from the patient's neck to the front of his shoulder in order to steady him.

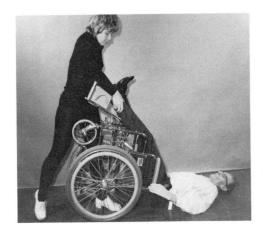
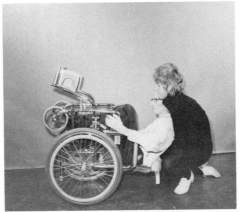
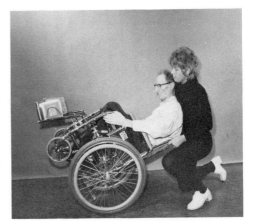

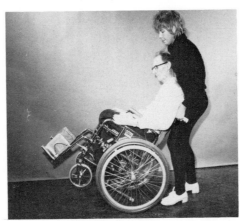
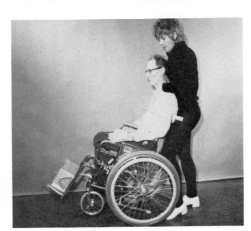

FIGURE 12-48

Method 2. (Fig. 12-49) Method 1 is easier with two helpers, one on either side of the patient, working as a synchronized team. In this case, the patient's head is supported with the helpers' inside arms while the outside hands lift the pushing handles.

Method 3. (Fig. 12-50) The helpers squat one on either side of the patient, facing his feet, and bring the patient to the sitting position. The hand closest to the patient is placed underneath the patient's axilla from behind and over the patient's forearm near the elbow. This is a flat hand hold with the thumb aligned with the fingers. The other hand is placed under the patient's thigh near his knees. Both assistants stand to lift, keeping their arms straight. This method permits each helper to maintain balance even though movements may not be in perfect unison.

ONTO THE TOILET

The chair should be backed in alongside the toilet at approximately 40°. This angle may be increased to 90° if the size of room demands this approach. A toilet seat raised to the height of the compressed wheelchair cushion top and a footstool to compensate for this increased height will facilitate transfer. For all transfers, the arm of the chair near the toilet is removed and the brakes are locked. The castors are turned forward.

339

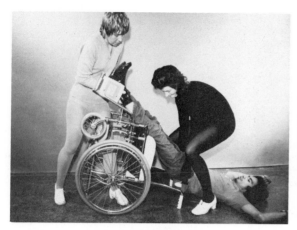
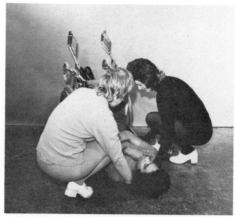

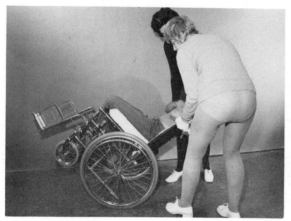
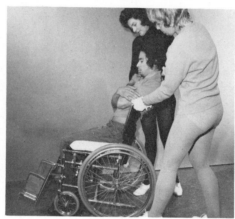

FIGURE 12-49

FIGURE 12-50

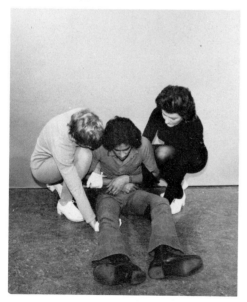
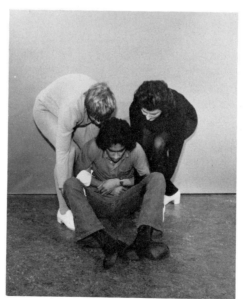
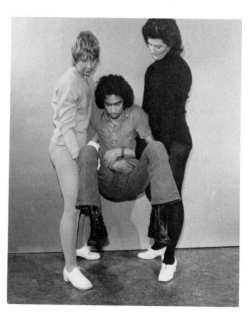

Method 1.   Some patients can lift part of their own weight by having their arms placed in an overhead strap centered over the toilet (Fig. 12-51). Standing close to the patient, the helper places one arm under the patient's knees and one by a hip. She pulls the patient forward, thus clearing his buttocks from the chair seat, and swings him onto the toilet. The patient who cannot lift as he reaches the toilet must be lifted slightly by the helper to avoid grazing the buttocks against the toilet seat.

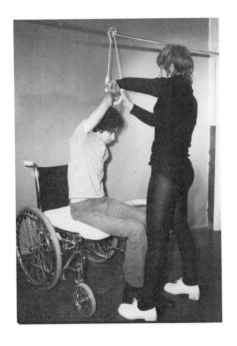 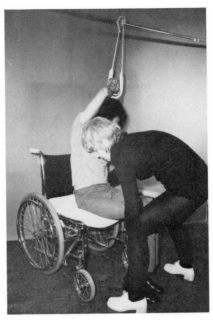 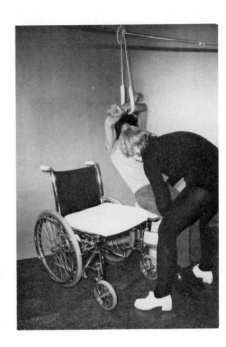

FIGURE 12-51

Method 2.   (Fig. 12-52) The helper stands with the foot furthest from the toilet inside the footrests and stabilizes the patient's knees between her own. The patient's trunk is flexed far forward onto his thighs and away from the direction of travel. The helper reaches over and slides her hands, palm up, under the upper thigh just below the crease of the patient's buttocks. The helper rocks back and pivots towards the toilet to position the patient. Care must be taken to ensure that the buttocks are not parted during this manoeuvre to prevent the possibility of a natal cleft split.

Method 3.   (Fig. 12-53) The helper stands with the outside foot inside the footrests and stabilizes the patient's knees between her own. The helper places her palms on either side of the patient's rib cage and abducts her shoulders so that her elbows protrude. The patient places his arms over the helper's elbows and hugs. The helper rocks back and pivots, placing the patient on the toilet. Any further positioning required may be obtained by repeating the procedure.

FROM TOILET TO CHAIR

Method 1.   (Fig. 12-54) The helper stands in front of the chair and blocks the patient's thighs with a knee. The patient is flexed far forward, transferring most

341

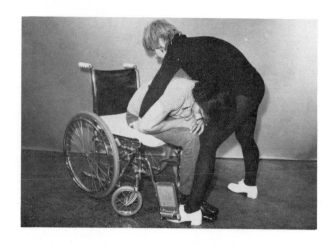

FIGURE 12-52

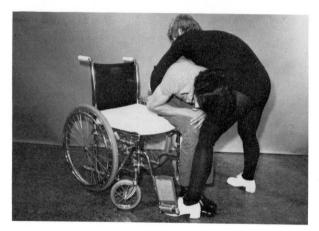

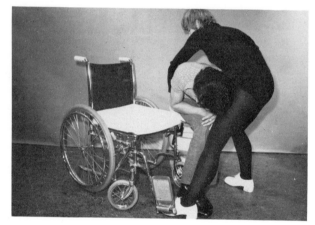

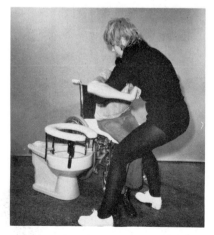

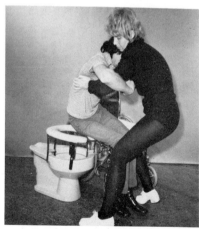

FIGURE 12-53

of his weight to his feet. The helper slides both hands under the patient's thighs just forward of the hips. The patient is levered over as the helper rocks back and pivots.

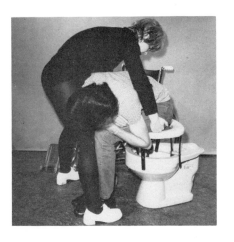
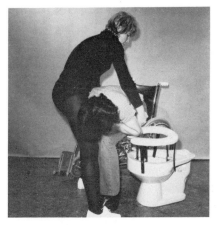
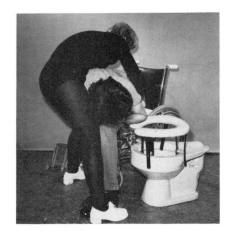

FIGURE 12-54

Method 2. (Fig. 12-55) The patient's forearms are placed in an overhead sling, which is then centered over the wheelchair seat. The helper stands in front of the patient and lifts his legs with one arm under his thighs. The other hand is placed behind and under one buttock to guide and swing him forward from the toilet and back onto the chair. This method is not useful if the patient's trunk elongates excessively when he holds his weight.

Method 3. (Fig. 12-56) The helper stands in front of the patient and blocks the patient's knees with her own. She places her palms against the patient's rib cage. The patient puts his arms over the helper's elbows and hugs to assist holding. The helper rocks back to pivot the patient onto the chair.

Method 4. (Fig. 12-57) Hoists used in conjunction with overhead tracks or commercial hydraulic hoists may be practical. The slings do not require a cut out, even for women, if the two-sling method is used.

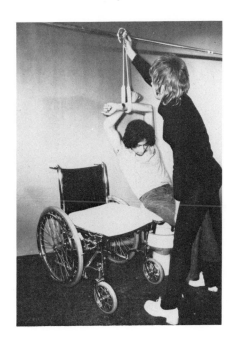
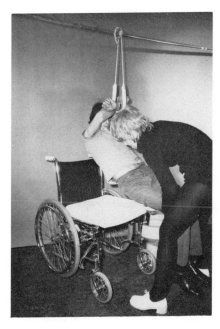
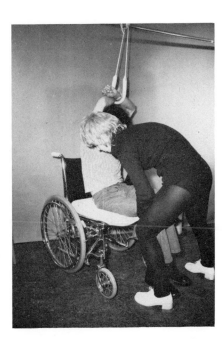

FIGURE 12-55

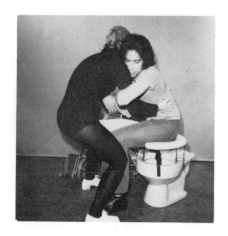 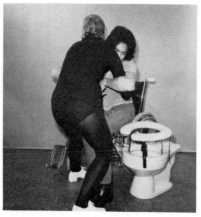

FIGURE 12-56

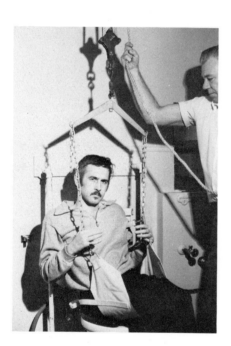 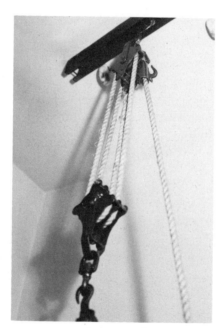 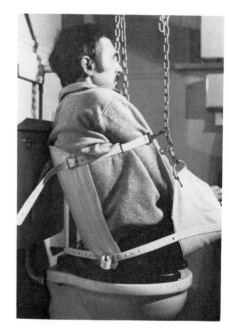

FIGURE 12-57

PICK UP AND CARRY BY ONE HELPER

This technique will be governed by the size of the patient and the strength and experience of the helper. The right-handed helper should stand on the patient's left side and remove the armrest. The patient's feet are moved to the far footrest, and the near footrest is folded up or swung away. The helper now places his right foot between the footrests with his knee close to the chair seat. The patient's right arm is placed over the helper's left shoulder, and the helper's left arm is slipped behind the patient to grasp his belt or his slacks at the hip. The right arm is placed well under the patient's thighs. The patient is now pulled in towards the helper, thus allowing a direct lift (Fig. 12-58).

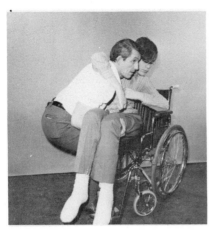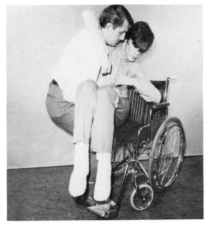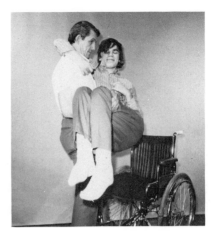

FIGURE 12-58

To lower the patient into the chair, the helper steps in very close before flexing his knees. A swinging motion is effective in placing the patient (Fig. 12-59). It should be noted that this technique is hardest to learn and should be practised with a light weight person.

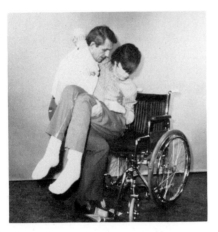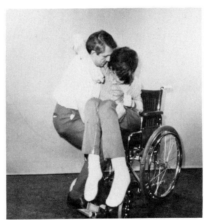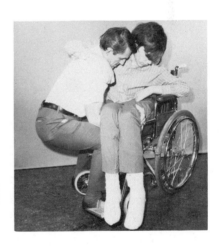

FIGURE 12-59

RESTING POSITION

There is a quick method of semi-reclining a patient in his chair without transferring him to a bed. Pillows are placed halfway down the bed. Then the chair is backed to the bed and tipped so that the patient's head rests on the pillows and the pushing handles rest on the mattress (Fig. 12-60). The brakes may now be applied for additional safety. This method should only be used when the bed is immobile. This resting position can be very useful when the patient is becoming conditioned to the upright position. It is also useful to relieve the weight from the patient's buttocks.

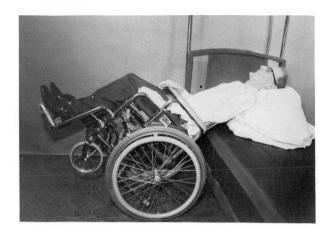

FIGURE 12-60

BATHING

Thorough cleanliness is essential for skin care. Because the dependent patient may be unable to check water temperature himself, the helper must be certain that the temperature is safe.

A shower seat for the bathtub or shower has been described for the use of the independent patient in Chapter 5. This may also be used in the management of the dependent patient. A wheel-in shower, also described in Chapter 5, may be practical. The drive wheels are unnecessary and a commode with castors will suffice since help is readily available.

An overhead track hoist may be used. This can be installed over the toilet and tub so that the patient may be transferred directly from toilet to tub. Commercial hoists are available. These can be placed in a floor flange, which is purchased as an extra especially for bathtub transfers.

Two people may safely lift a patient in and out of a bathtub (Fig. 12-61). The helper behind the patient places his hands under the patient's axillae and over his wrists using a flat hand hold. The front helper bends his knees to pick up the

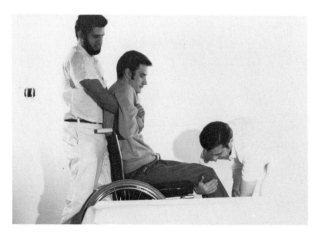

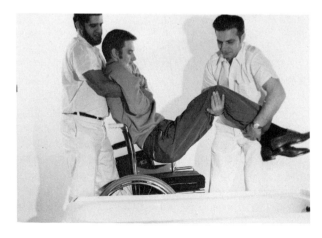

FIGURE 12-61

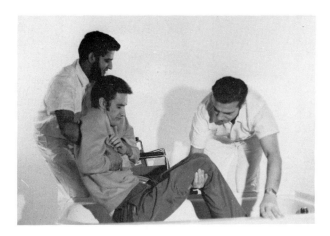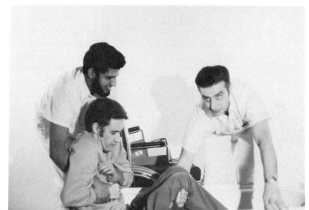

patient's legs, with one arm under both knees and the other at his ankles. The helper behind the patient swivels and holds while the helper in front swings the patient forward. This will lift the patient's buttocks up enough to clear the wheel and the bathtub edge. As the patient is lowered into the tub the helper at the front supports his weight by placing a hand on the edge of the bathtub. This relieves any undue strain on his back. The rear helper must bend his knees to lower the patient into the tub. In this lift the rear helper holds most of the weight but need not move a great deal. The front helper moves a good deal but takes less weight, thus protecting both helpers' backs.

The lift out of the tub is an exact reversal of the lift into the tub. For safety the patient should be towel dried before the lift is attempted.

Bedbaths may be a solution to the bathing problem.

CAR TRANSFERS

WHEELCHAIR TO CAR

The car seat is moved as far back as possible before the patient's buttocks are pulled forward in the chair and his feet are placed inside the car. The chair is now pushed forward close to the car seat and at an angle so that the rear wheel is not in the way (Fig. 12-62). The patient's knees should now be in flexion. The bridge board is positioned under the patient's buttocks, bridging the gap from the chair to the car. Any of the following methods may be used to transfer him to the car.

Method 1. (Fig. 12-63) The helper gets into the car on the driver's side. She may kneel on the seat facing the patient, kneel with one knee on the seat and one foot braced on the floor, or sit facing the patient. The helper checks that the patient's knees are still flexed, or the legs will lock and prevent the patient from moving. She now grasps the patient by the shoulders and flexes the patient's upper trunk forward and away from the direction of travel. She grasps the belt or slacks with the other hand and leans back, pulling the patient across the bridge board and into the car. The feet are now repositioned for comfort and stability.

347

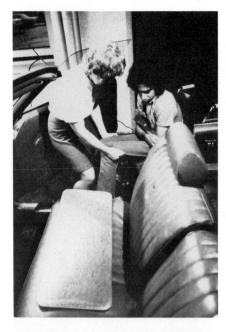
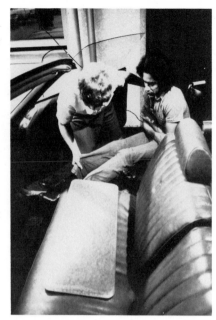
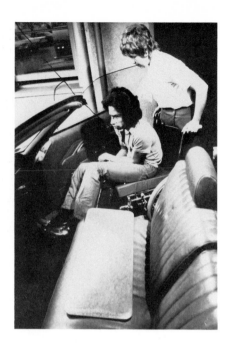

FIGURE 12-62

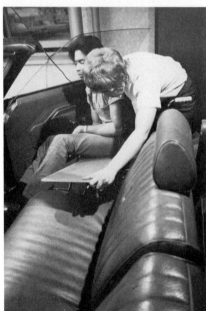

Method 2. (Fig. 12-64) The helper remains behind the chair and flexes the patient's trunk forward. She holds the patient's slacks by the hips and slides him over the bridge board by pulling with the arm near the car, and pushing with the other.

Method 3. (Fig. 12-65) The patient sits on a soft wide canvas belt with nylon sewn underneath. A buckle and strap are sewn to the ends of the belt so that it may be fastened around his hips. Webbing straps may be slipped through D-rings sewn to the belt near the patient's trochanters, providing a convenient hand hold. The belt provides a good sliding surface. The patient may be pulled into the car easily over a bridge board.

Method 4. The patient is positioned as in the previous methods. He sits on the wide canvas belt with nylon sewn to the underside (Fig. 12-66A). A pulley or a block and tackle is used. The pulley is attached to the inside of the driver's door and one end of the rope is hooked to the D-ring on the canvas sling. The helper stands beside the patient and guides the patient by the shoulder as she pulls on the rope (Fig. 12-66B). At the same time the helper flexes the patient's trunk forward and away from the direction of travel. Very little effort is required to slide the patient over the bridge board into the car.

A commercial hydraulic car top hoist may be utilized (Fig. 12-67). Other commercial hoists are mounted just inside the car and may be used to load the patient and then the chair.

348

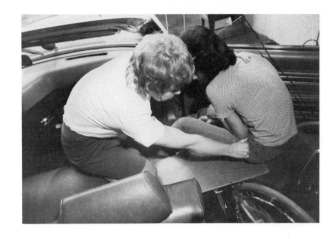
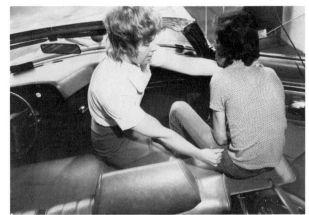

FIGURE 12-63

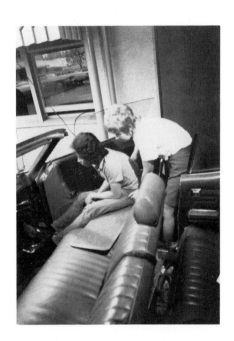
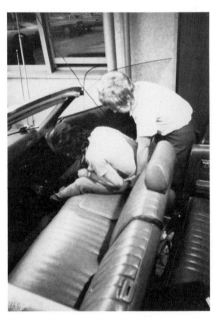
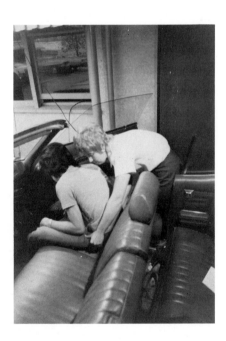

FIGURE 12-64

CAR TO WHEELCHAIR

Method 1. (Fig. 12-68) The helper places the sliding board well under the patient's buttocks. One hand holds the patient's shoulders and leans him away from the direction of travel. He is pulled over onto the chair by his belt.

Method 2. (Fig. 12-69) The patient is pulled into the chair over a bridge board by pulling on a strap threaded through a D-ring on a canvas and nylon belt. Balance is maintained with the helper's other hand holding the upper arm under the patient's axilla.

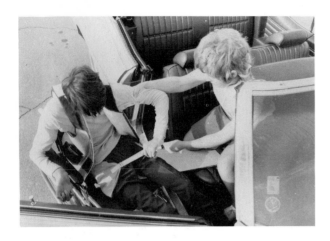
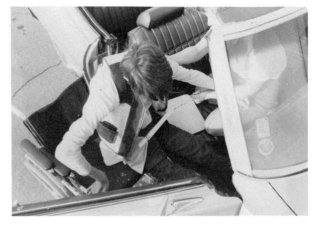

FIGURE 12-65

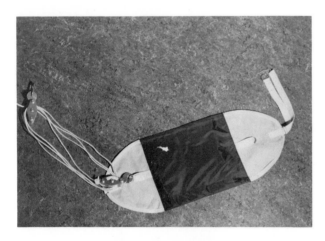

A

FIGURE 12-66

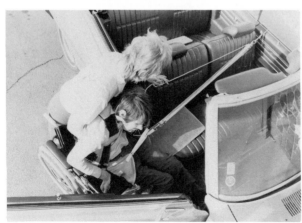
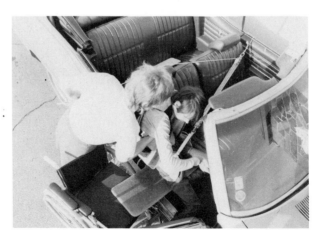

B

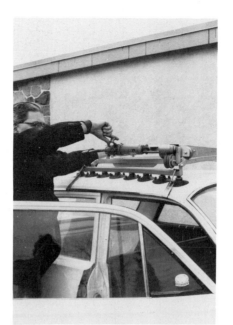
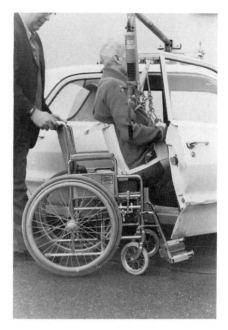

FIGURE 12-67

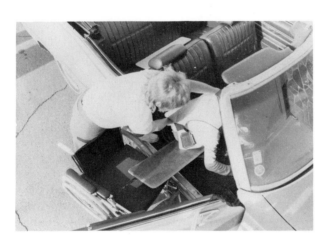
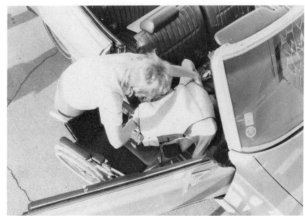

FIGURE 12-68

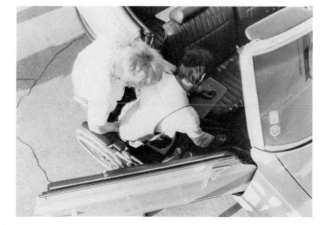

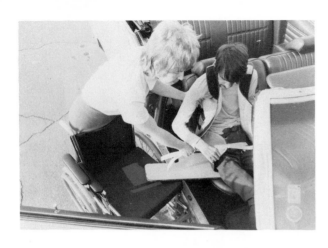

FIGURE 12-69

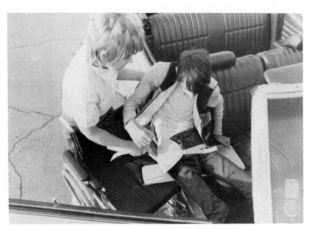

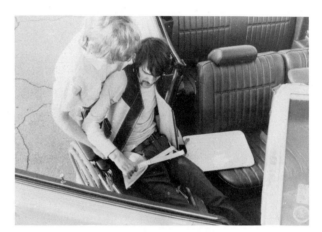

Method 3. (Fig. 12-70) The pulley system may be used to slide the patient out of the car. The pulley may be hooked to a ring on the car door or to the door handle. The other end is hooked to the D-ring on the canvas belt. It may be necessary to maintain the patient's balance with one hand.

LIFTING THE WHEELCHAIR INTO THE CAR

Method 1. (Fig. 12-71) The helper folds the chair, applies the brakes, and tips the chair so she can reach over and grasp the spokes below the axle and the front of the chair. Rocking back using a thigh as a fulcrum, the helper pulls the chair in tightly so the armrests are against her body and the chair is swung up and placed in the trunk. The trunk well may be filled in with plywood so that the chair is easier to lift out.

Method 2. (Fig. 12-72) A ramp may be made from plywood with padded angle brackets attached to hook over the edge of the trunk so that the chair may be slid up on the drive rim.

Method 3. A chair loader may be made from metal tubing. The bottom of the loader is bent to about 100° to form a lip to accommodate the folded wheelchair. The lip stays flat on the ground when the loader is leaned against the car

352

with a handle attached to the tubing at the bottom centre of the lip (Fig. 12-73A). The top ends are bent to provide both a holding fulcrum and legs. The lengths of the legs are determined by the depth of the trunk. The legs have small fixed wheels at the ends, which will roll along the floor of the trunk.

The folded chair is rolled onto the loader and the brakes are applied. One chair wheel and the handle are grasped together and raised until the loader wheels touch the trunk floor (Fig. 12-73B). The chair is now pushed into the trunk and left in position on the loader, ready for use when unloading.

Method 4. (Fig. 12-74) The chair may be loaded behind the front seats. The chair is folded, but the brakes are not applied. The chair is tipped back and the castors are placed over the doorsill. The chair is rolled into the car, but as the castors approach the transmission tunnel, the chair is tipped back with the castors high and the pushing handles resting on the car floor.

Method 5. The area in the car between the doorsill and the transmission tunnel may be filled in with plywood or hardboard, leaving a half inch ledge to prevent the chair from moving too much. The chair is rolled straight in and can remain with all four wheels on the floor (Fig 12-75).

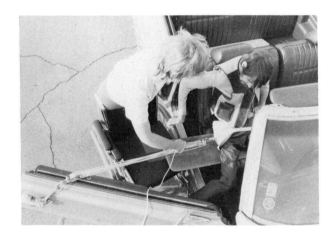

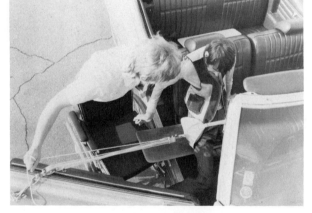

FIGURE 12-70

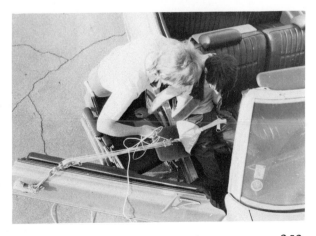

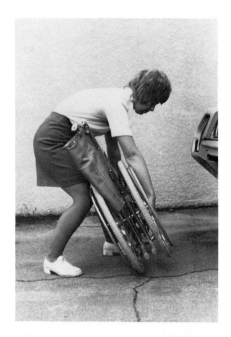
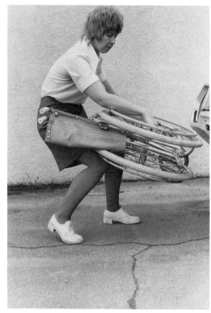
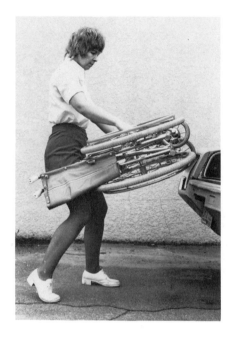

FIGURE 12-71

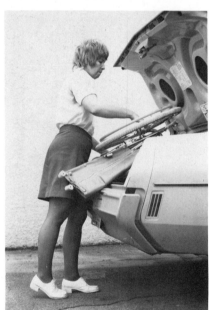

USING A VAN

The simplest possible method must be worked out for getting a patient in and out of a vehicle, even if this involves considerable expense for commercial hoists or lifts. Frequently a family will forego short expeditions or leave the patient at home if transfers are difficult. Freedom of movement is of the utmost psychological benefit to the patient and the family unit.

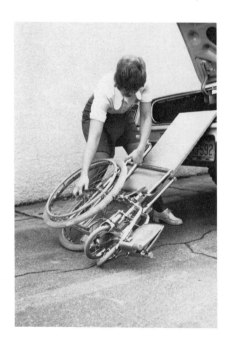
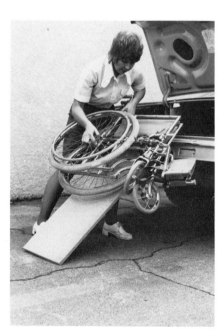

FIGURE 12-72

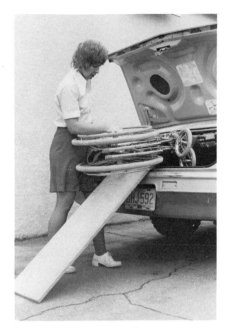

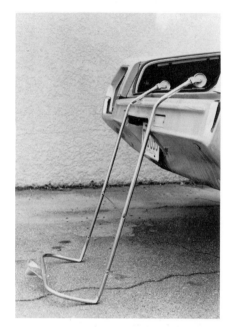

A

Use of a van is often the most practical method of transport because it eliminates the need to transfer the patient from the chair and the need to load the chair separately. The wheelchair should be fixed to the floor once loaded and the patient secured with a floor safety belt. A cross-over safety belt attached to the ceiling is also recommended.

Three of the simplest mechanical hoists are illustrated here. These hoists are equipped with limit switches so when the hoist is in position the motor cuts off. For safety, the mechanism locks if there is a power failure.

B

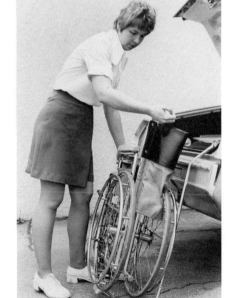
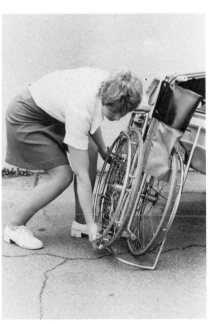
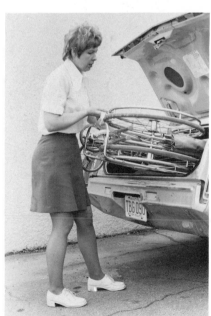

FIGURE 12-73

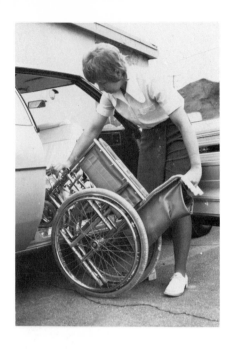
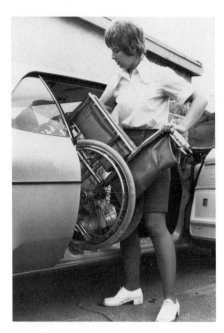
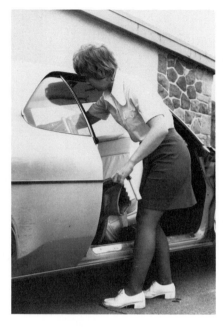

FIGURE 12-74

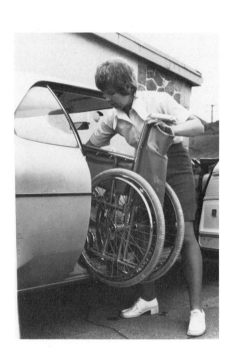
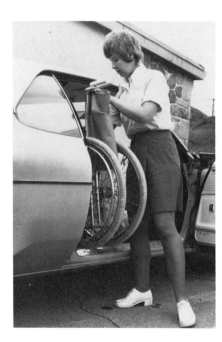

FIGURE 12-75

A powered ramp may be self-operated by some patients, using a joystick or button control (Fig. 12-76). The patient wheels over the leading edge onto the apron. When activated, the ramp will raise the patient and roll the chair into the van, allowing the chair to remain horizontal.

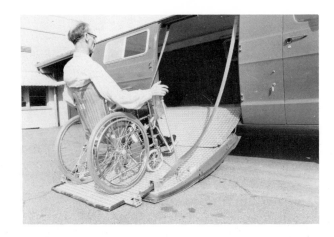
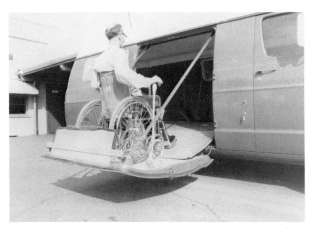

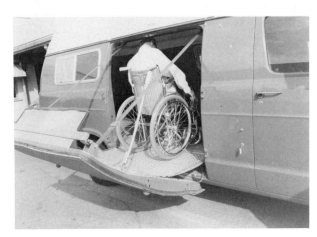
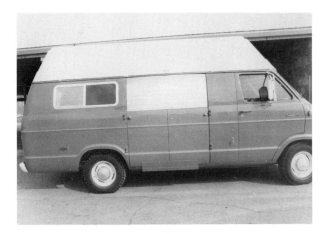

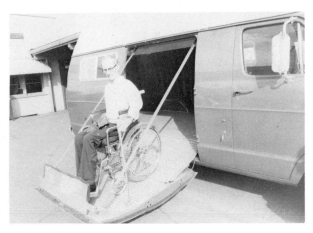

FIGURE 12-76

A powered elevator, which can be swivelled into place, requires very few moves from the helper. The chair is secured to the elevator floor; then the elevator is raised and swivelled into the van (Fig. 12-77).

Another type of powered elevator is usually installed at the rear of the van

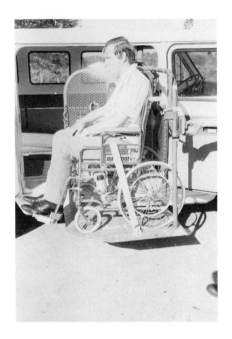
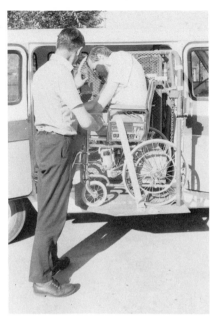
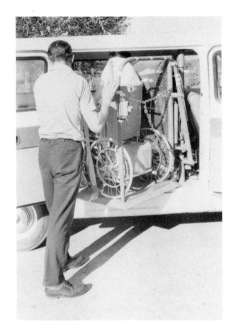

FIGURE 12-77

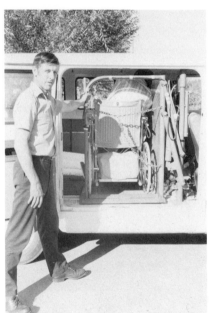

(Fig. 12-78). Once the elevator reaches the van floor height the patient must be pushed in, secured, the doors closed, and the elevator folded. These tasks are not difficult but they are time consuming.

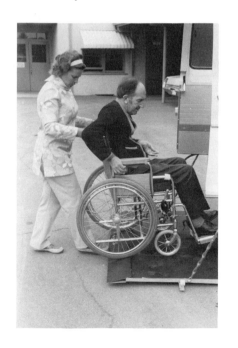
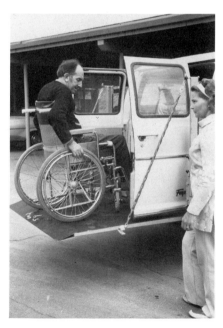

FIGURE 12-78

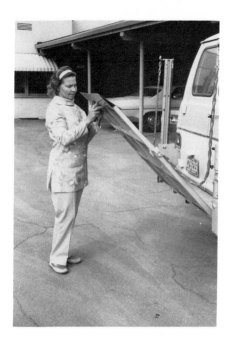 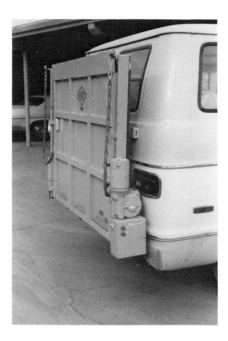

A metal ramp may be used if the helper is capable of pushing the chair up the grade safely. This model is attached to the floor of the van and can be folded to allow the door to be shut (Fig. 12-79). One ramp is on a slide so that the width can be adjusted (Fig. 12-80).

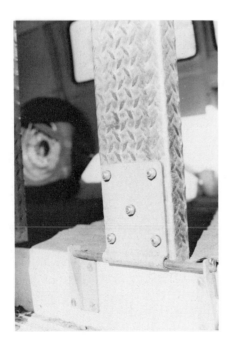 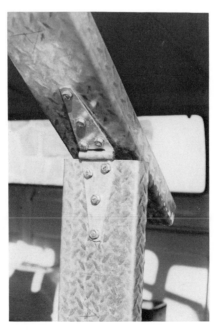 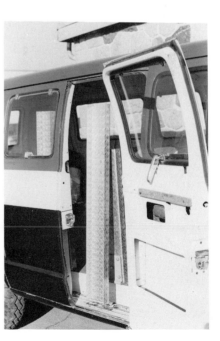

FIGURE 12-79

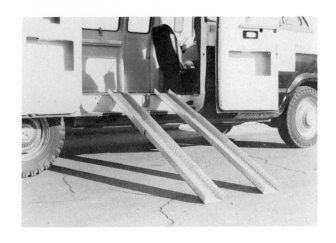

FIGURE 12-80

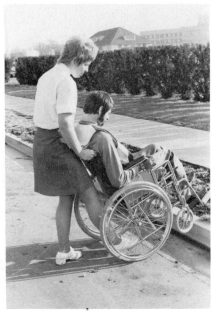

FIGURE 12-81

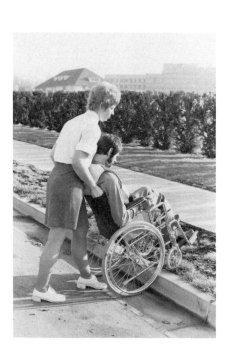

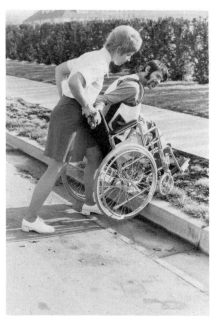

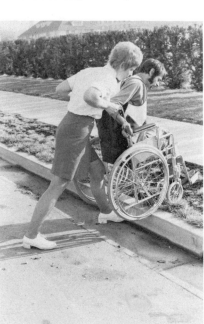

MOVING THE PATIENT BY WHEELCHAIR

Each patient must be prepared to instruct an inexperienced helper in easy and safe methods of controlling a chair. He will be wise to ask the helper to give him time to hook an elbow around the pushing handle first for extra safety.

MOUNTING CURBS

Curbs may be mounted from a direct forward approach or from the rear. In the forward approach (Fig. 12-81), the chair is tilted back by stepping on the tipping lever, and the front castors are placed on the sidewalk. The wheelchair is lifted and pushed to roll the rear wheels up over the curb. If the patient is able to lean forward once the castors are on the sidewalk, this will considerably reduce the weight on the back wheels.

When the chair is backed towards the curb and the rear wheels touch the curb, the chair is tipped back. The helper leans back to pull the chair up the curb (Fig. 12-82). She wheels the chair back so that the front castors will be on the sidewalk when she lowers the chair.

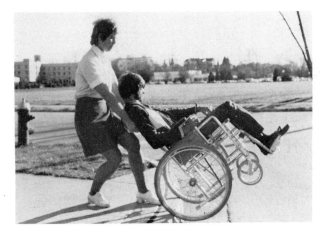 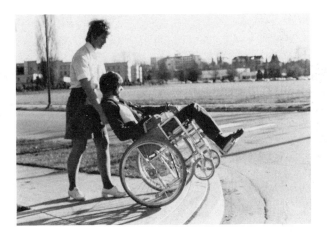

FIGURE 12-82

DESCENDING CURBS

Again, there are two methods for descending a curb. In one instance, the chair is turned on the sidewalk so that it faces away from the road (Fig. 12-83). The helper steps backwards off the curb and, pulling the chair towards her, lowers the back wheels onto the road. The chair is balanced on the back wheels and wheeled back far enough so that the footrests do not hit the curb. The chair is lowered onto the front castors; the helper uses a foot on the tipping lever to give control. It may be necessary to place a hand over the patient's shoulder while lowering the chair to prevent him from falling forward.

In the forward method, the chair faces the roadway and is tipped back with its tipping lever to balance on its back wheels. The chair is rolled over the curb

361

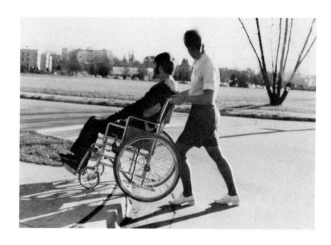

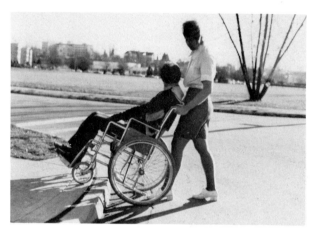

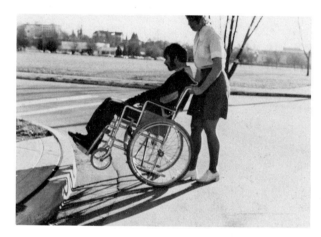

FIGURE 12-83

edge and pushed forward before lowering it onto its front castors (Fig. 12-84). It may be convenient to maintain the chair in a tipped position while crossing the road to avoid tipping the chair again at the next curb.

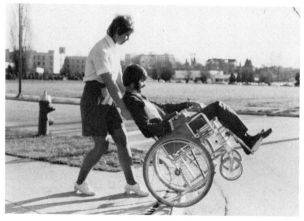

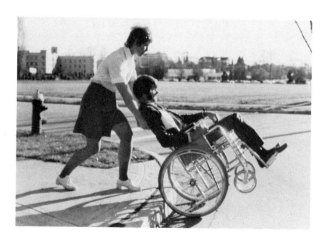

FIGURE 12-84

WHEELING OVER ROUGH GROUND

The chair should be tipped onto the rear wheels by stepping on the tipping lever. It may be pushed in this balanced position when the ground is rough or soft. If the terrain is very difficult it will be easier to pull the chair backwards in the tipped position.

WHEELING DOWN SLOPES

When a steep slope is descended, the chair should be reversed and brought down backwards with the castors on the ground (Fig. 12-85). This ensures that the patient does not fall forward and leaves the helper free to control the chair.

The chair may be pushed forwards if the slope is minor. It may be necessary to place one hand over the patient's shoulder to maintain the patient's balance (Fig. 12-86). If the slope levels abruptly, care must be taken not to snag the footrests when wheeling forwards.

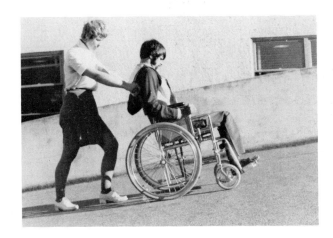

FIGURE 12-85

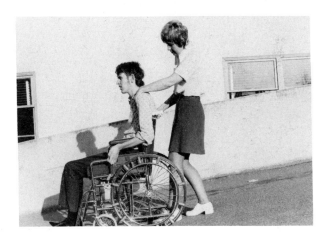

FIGURE 12-86

WHEELING UP SLOPES

When ascending a slope, the chair may be pushed forward in the normal manner (Fig. 12-87). The helper may reverse the chair and tip it back onto the rear wheels on steep slopes. By leaning back to pull and keeping the elbows straight while holding the pushing handles, the helper will gain a considerable amount of mechanical advantage (Fig. 12-88). On short steep slopes, the chair may be tipped well back (Fig. 12-89), and the chair pushed quickly up the slope to gain momentum, much like pushing a loaded wheelbarrow.

363

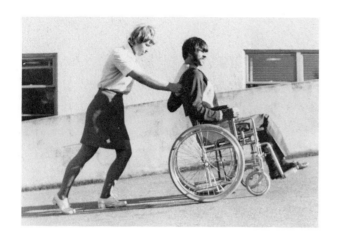

FIGURE 12-87

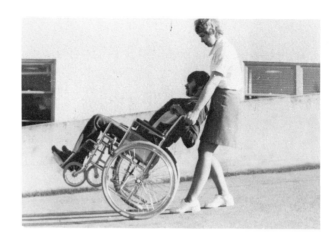

FIGURE 12-88

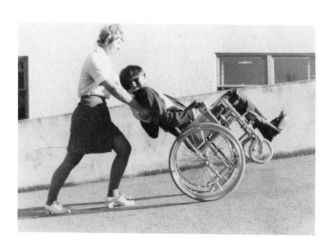

FIGURE 12-89

ASCENDING STAIRS

With practice, one person can ascend stairs with the patient in the wheelchair (Fig. 12-90). This is, of course, dependent on the weight of the patient and the strength of the assistant. The wheelchair is reversed and tipped back. The chair is then pulled to the stairs. The assistant mounts the stairs keeping one foot on the first step and one on the second. She pulls the chair up the first step keeping her elbows straight; then she moves her feet to the next step before proceeding. Any attempt to assist by lifting from the front will throw the helper at the rear off balance. If a second helper is available he may remain in front, prepared to hold the chair if necessary.

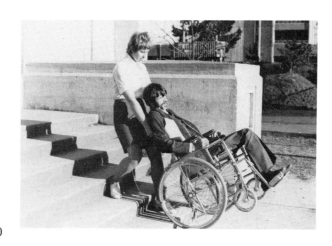

FIGURE 12-90

It may be necessary to carry the chair up the stairs if there are curves or corners in the stairway. The chair is faced away from the stairs and the rear assistant grasps the pushing handles and tips the chair back. The front assistant grasps the chair footrest supports and lifts the chair free of the stair. Both assistants proceed up the stairs in unison. When inexperienced persons are assisting they should be instructed to grasp parts of the chair that will not come loose. Removable arms, adjustable legrests and wheels are frequently grasped by the inexperienced. If the stairs width permits, four persons may carry a chair, one at each corner. This is less fatiguing if large numbers of chairs are to be moved.

DESCENDING STAIRS

The same positions used in ascending the stairs are used for descending the stairs.

Appendix

PUSHER MITTS

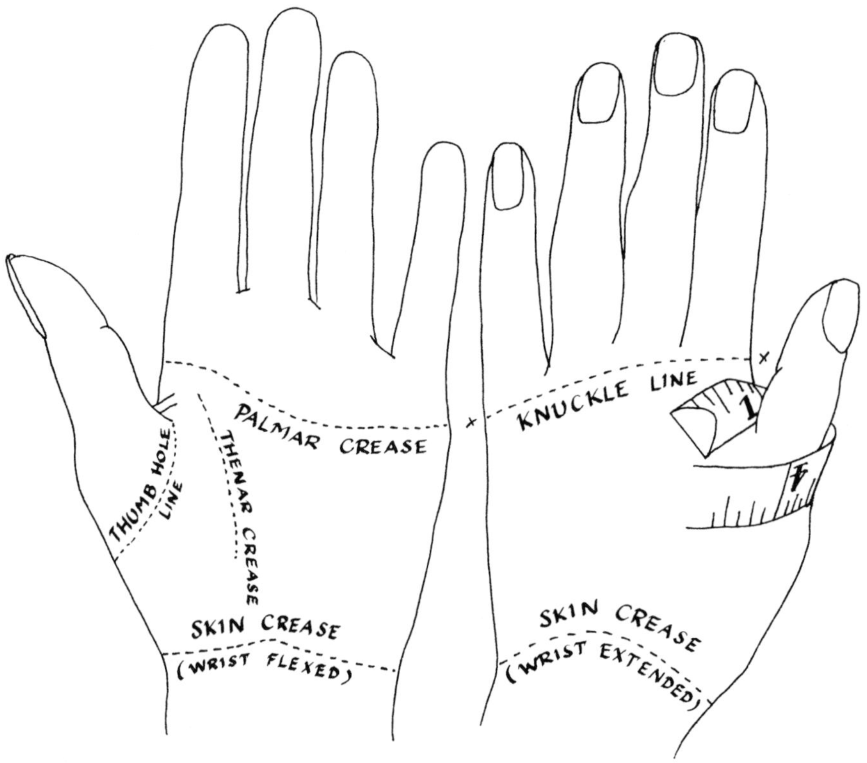
PALMAR CREASE
KNUCKLE LINE
THUMB HOLE LINE
THENAR CREASE
SKIN CREASE (WRIST FLEXED)
SKIN CREASE (WRIST EXTENDED)

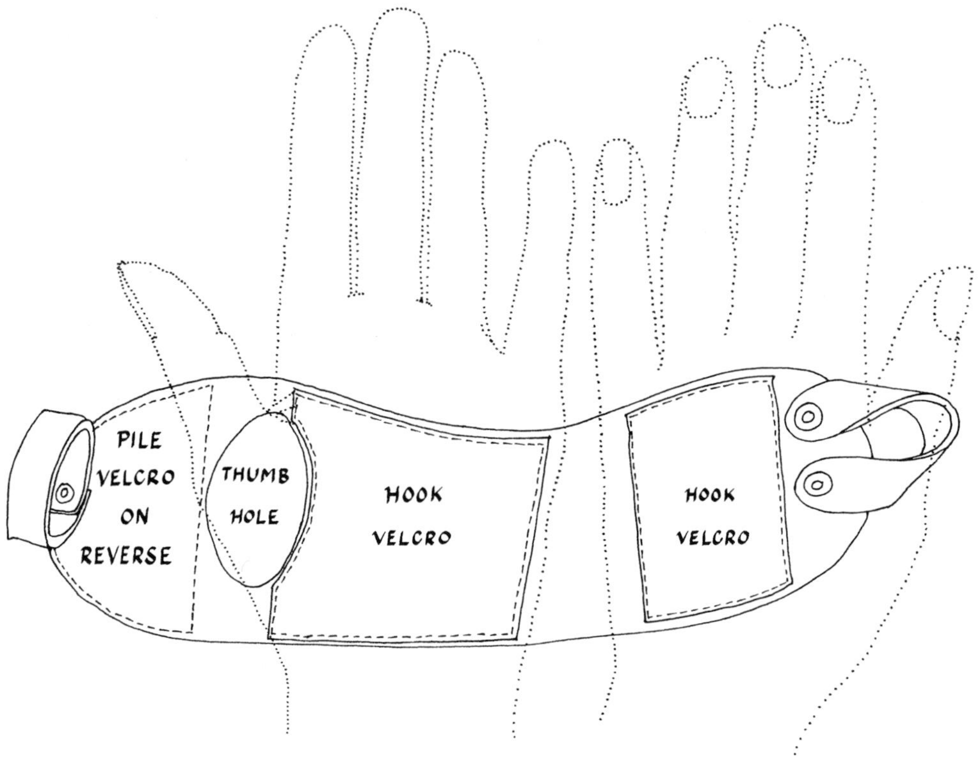
PILE VELCRO ON REVERSE
THUMB HOLE
HOOK VELCRO
HOOK VELCRO

CONSTRUCTION OF PUSHER MITTS

Pusher mitts are made of cowhide and velcro. The hand is placed palm down on a piece of paper to make a pattern. The outline of the hand is traced and the knuckle line and the wrist extension skin crease are sketched in. The hand is turned over, keeping the ulnar border on the paper. The outline of the hand is traced again and the palmar crease and the wrist flexion crease are drawn in. The pattern follows inside these lines with an overlap for fastening. Great care must be taken not to overlap the wrist flexion and extension creases; an abrasion can develop very quickly if the edge of the pushers mitt should rub against the skin.

The thumb hole should be as small as possible because the pushing area is often close to the thumb. It is simple to enlarge the hole if necessary. The thumb loop should be low around the metacarpal below the metacarpophalangeal joint, or it will tend to pull the thumb into hyperextension. The leather loop should be in contact with the skin all around the thumb. The fastening loop must provide room for the insertion of a finger or thumb.

Velcro is stitched to the cowhide. It may be replaced when it loses its friction value. The mitt may be made symetrical so that it can fit either hand, thus prolonging the life of the pushing surface.

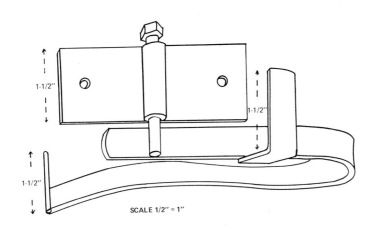

1-1/2"

1-1/2"

1-1/2"

SCALE 1/2" = 1"

SIDE-APPROACH SWING-AWAY BED HOOK
(viewed from under bed)

SIDE-APPROACH SWING-AWAY BED HOOK (top view)

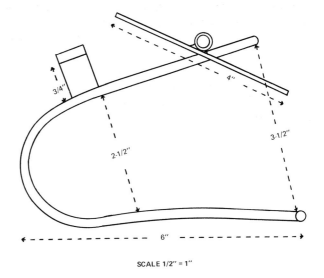

3/4"

4"

3-1/2"

2-1/2"

6"

SCALE 1/2" = 1"

SIDE-APPROACH SWING-AWAY BED HOOK

The hook part of the swing-away bed hook is made of 1/8 x 1/2-inch cold rolled steel. A 3/16 inch welding rod is brazed to the tip to prevent the hook from swinging under the bed out of reach.

About an inch from the other end a 5/16-inch bolt is brazed vertically to the outside of the hook. A 1/8 x 1-1/2 x 4-inch cold rolled steel plate has a 1-1/2 inch long 5/16-inch I.D. 1/2-inch O.D. tubing brazed vertically to the center to provide a bushing so that the bolt on the hook can be inserted. A lock nut keeps it in place. The stop is made of 1/8 x 1/2-inch cold rolled steel, bent and brazed to the underside of the hook.

The plate is bolted to the inside of the bed frame. The stop is also placed on the inside of the frame so that the hook will be stable when swung out ready for use. The location of the hook is established with the wheelchair in position and the patient ready for transfer.

FRONT-APPROACH BED HOOK

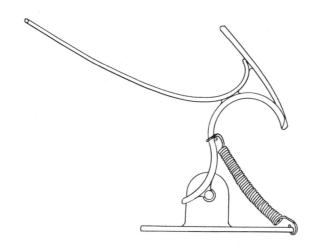

FRONT-APPROACH CHAIR BED HOOK

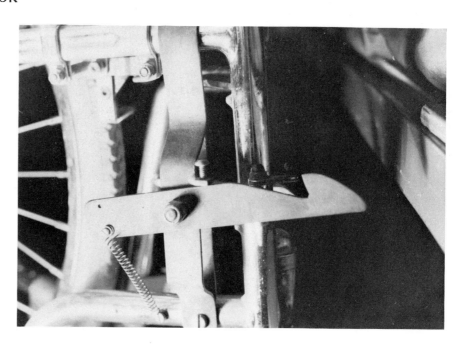

372

FRONT-APPROACH BED HOOK

This hook is used to lock the front upright of the wheelchair to the bed during a front-approach transfer. A right hook is shown from above. The drawing is reversed for the left hook, which must be used at the same time on the left upright of the chair.

The S-shaped hook is made of 1/8 x 1/2-inch cold rolled steel and 5/16 inch bolt is brazed to it vertically near one end. A 1-1/2-inch length of 1/8 x 1/2-inch cold rolled steel is brazed to the tip of the "S" and gently curved so that when the wheelchair front makes contact, it will cause the hook to swing back in position to spring in to lock around the chair front uprights. The bracket, which is bolted to the bed frame, is made of 1/8 x 1-1/2 x 2-1/2-inches of cold rolled steel. A U-shaped tongue is brazed to the bottom edge of the plate. A bushing is brazed to the underside of the tongue and a 5/16-inch hole drilled through the tongue using the bushing as a guide. Small holes are drilled for attaching a light spring. About 8 inches of 3/16-inch welding rod is brazed to the hook and bent so that it can be reached and used to release the hook.

FRONT-APPROACH CHAIR BED HOOK

These hooks are permanently attached to the wheelchair and are ready for use when the leg rests are swung away. Brackets are placed vertically and bolted to the top and bottom tubing of the chair frame so they do not interfere with folding. The hook is set in position so that, when the chair is wheeled against the bed, the hooks will engage under the bed frame. A stop is placed on the vertical bracket to prevent the hook from swinging past the horizontal. The springs at the rear of the hook rocker arms must be heavy enough to keep the chair locked to the bed during transfers. A light chain, cable, or nylon cord may be fastened to the back of the hook rocker arm and led to a position that allows the patient to reach and pull to release the hook.

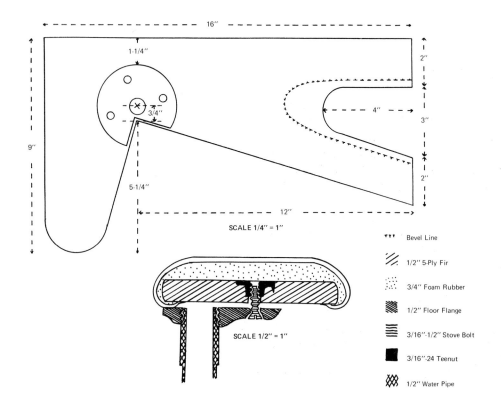

PADDED TRANSFER BOARD "A"

SCALE 1/4" = 1"

SCALE 1/2" = 1"

▼▼▼   Bevel Line

⟋⟋   1/2" 5-Ply Fir

⋰⋰   3/4" Foam Rubber

▨▨   1/2" Floor Flange

☰   3/16"-1/2" Stove Bolt

■   3/16"-24 Teenut

▩   1/2" Water Pipe

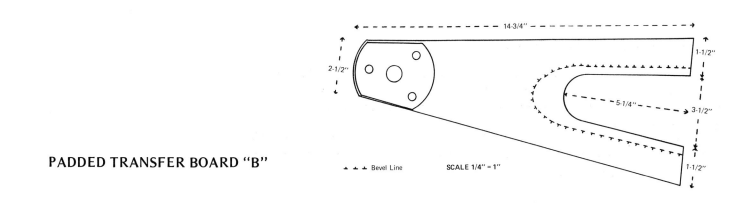

PADDED TRANSFER BOARD "B"

⊥ ⊥ ⊥ Bevel Line   SCALE 1/4" = 1"

CONSTRUCTION OF PADDED TRANSFER BOARD "A"

A plywood base is cut according to the pattern with the grain running along the length. The edges are slightly rounded and the underside of the wheel cutout is bevelled. The floor flange is cut, filed, and positioned. The T-nut holes are drilled and the T-nuts are inserted on the top of the board. A wide U-shaped leather gusset is cut and stapled at the bevel line under the board by the wheel cutout so that it bulges through to about 2 inches above the board, allowing the curve of the wheel to be accommodated.

Foam is glued over the board and around all edges before upholstering with slippery material such as nylon taffeta. A gusset will be required at the right angle by the floor flange. Care must be taken to maintain the height of the covering over the wheel cutout when the upholstery is pulled tight.

The floor flange is now bolted on. A 3-1/2-inch post is made of 1/2-inch water pipe which is threaded at one end, and turned down on a lathe for 2 inches at the other end to fit the front wheelchair arm socket. The measurement from collar to flange is usually 1 inch but may require adjustment so that the bridge board is the same height as the compressed wheelchair cushion. A tridon clamp may be used as an adjustable collar instead of the turned collar.

The pattern shows the underside of a board to fit on the left of the chair. It should be reversed for a right transfer.

CONSTRUCTION OF PADDED TRANSFER BOARD "B"

If a patient does not require the tongue, which extends the sliding surface between the front of the chair seat and the bed, a smaller version may be used. Advantages are that right or left transfers may be made using the same board and it may be useful for toilet transfers.

The construction of transfer board B is similar to A, except that an extra hole must be drilled at the front of the flange since two holes are eliminated when the sides of the flange are cut off.

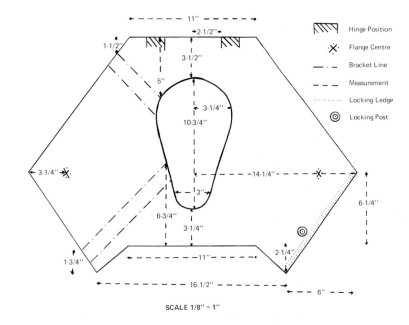

DELTA WING TOILET SEAT

Legend:
- Hinge Position
- Flange Centre
- Bracket Line
- Measurement
- Locking Ledge
- Locking Post

11"
2-1/2"
1-1/2"
3-1/2"
5"
3-1/4"
10-3/4"
3-1/4"
14-1/4"
3"
6-3/4"
3-1/4"
6-1/4"
1-3/4"
11"
2-1/4"
16-1/2"
6"

SCALE 1/8" = 1"

RAISED TOILET SEAT AND DELTA WING TOILET SEAT BRACKET

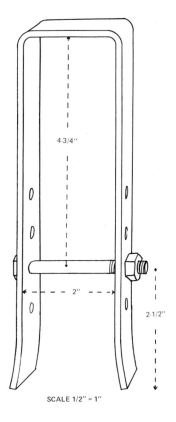

4-3/4"
2"
2-1/2"

SCALE 1/2" = 1"

376

CONSTRUCTION OF DELTA WING TOILET SEAT

In the pattern, the bracket lines and the locking ledge positions are shown on one side only for clarity. The seat is made of 3/4-inch plywood, and the edges and corners are rounded. The four brackets are placed on the toilet bowl and are adjusted until they are on the bracket lines as drawn on the pattern. The positions are marked so that the T-nuts can be fixed in the top of the seat. The T-nuts are also positioned for the floor flanges and the hinges.

The seat is padded with 1-inch foam carried down to cover all edges and upholstered with naugahyde. The naugahyde must be brought well under the seat at the hole. The underside is now covered. A back 18 x 12 inches of 3/4-inch plywood is cut and the T-nuts are placed for the hinges before it is upholstered. Cadmium plated 8-inch strap hinges are used, and both leaves are offset at right angles 1-1/4-inch from the hinge centre to allow the top to fold flat on the seat for easy transportation. Two 3/4-inch floor flanges to fit 3/4-inch water pipe are bolted to the underside, and two metal locking ledges 1/2-inch square and about 5 inches long are screwed to the underside of the seat under the edges of the wings.

A single leg is made of 3/4-inch water pipe and is threaded on one end, ready to be screwed into one of the flanges on the underside of the seat. The leg should be approximately 20-1/2 inches long but this should be checked before final cutting. Allowance must be made for the extra length of the crutch tip which is slipped over the pipe to protect the floor. A locking post is made of 1/2-inch water pipe turned on a lathe for 1 inch of its length to fit into the front arm socket of the wheelchair. The protruding pipe is measured so that with the addition of a crutch tip, the pipe will fit under the seat and catch behind the locking ledge. When in use, the leg is screwed into the flange on the side furthest from the patient. This seat is very useful for training purposes since it can be adjusted for transfer from either side.

CONSTRUCTION OF RAISED TOILET SEAT
AND DELTA WING TOILET SEAT BRACKET

The brackets are made of 1/8 x 1 inch cold rolled steel or aluminum alloy. The bolt is a 5/16-inch carriage bolt. A piece of I.V. tubing may be sleeved onto the bolt to protect the toilet bowl. The projecting ends may also be covered. Adjustment holes are 3/4 inch apart, centre to centre. Two holes should be drilled in the top for screwing to the underside of a toilet seat. One hole is drilled in the centre top if the seat is to be of a type that may be disassembled. In this case a metal plate is screwed to the underside of the toilet seat with a 5/16-inch bolt protruding through. The bolt fits through the hole at the bracket top and is fastened with a wing nut. This model allows the brackets to be swivelled slightly to adapt to different makes of toilet bowl.

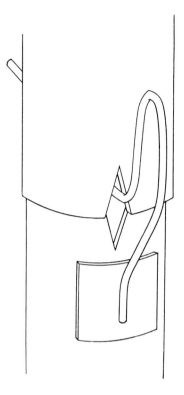

LOCKING MECHANISM OF THE SWING-AWAY GRAB BAR

HOIST SWING

14"

15-1/2"

23"

16-1/2"

8-1/2"

31"

SCALE 1/8" = 1"

378

CONSTRUCTION OF LOCKING MECHANISM
OF THE SWING-AWAY GRAB BAR

This drawing shows only the swing-away mechanism of the grab bar. The pin is brazed to a plate, which rests against the bar to keep the pin horizontal. The pin is bent, leaving room for holding so that it is easy to remove. The horizontal bar is welded to the sliding sleeve. The "V" slots are at opposite sides of both the upright bar and the sleeve. These cause the bar to be more stable as more pressure is applied to the bar and eliminate the movement found in a hold-and-through pin type.

CONSTRUCTION OF HOIST SLING

This sling is made of double canvas. The back is reinforced with corset bones sewn in vertically at 1-inch intervals, so that the back does not fold when dropped between the patient and the chair back. The straps are made of 3/4-inch nylon webbing. The buckles and dog leash clips are heavy duty, and the 3/4-inch D-rings are spot welded at the joint. Care must be taken to leave no bulky seams which could cause undue pressure.

Glossary

Abduction. Moving limb away from midline.

Adduction. Moving limb toward midline.

A-Frame. A track or bar running between the top of two A-supports.

Anaesthesia. Lack of sensation.

Anterior. In front.

Axilla (ae). Armpit/armpits.

Balkan beam. Bar over the bed running from head to foot.

Ball-bearing feeder. Commercially available mobile arm support that requires little effort to operate but needs a considerable amount of individual fitting.

Bridge board. Board to bridge a gap so that the patient can cross it. Also known as a transfer or sliding board.

Bumper. Rubber-tipped furniture guard at front of chair.

Cock-up splint. Splint to immobilize wrist in some extension.

Condom. Prophylactic rubber sheath worn on the penis, used in collection of urine.

Cord lesion level. Level where the cord is damaged; not necessarily where the vertebrae are broken or displaced.

Depression of shoulder. Pulling shoulder down.

D.I.P. joint. Distal interphalangeal joint, last finger joint.

Distal. Far, away from trunk. Opposite to proximal.

Dorsum. Back, i.e. dorsum of hand—back of hand.

Drive rims. Small rims outside wheelchair wheels, used for pushing.

Elevation of shoulder. Pulling shoulder up.

Extension. Straightening (usually). Opposite to flexion.

External rotation. Turn outward, i.e. external rotation of hip—leg and foot are turned out.

Extremities. Upper—Arms
            Lower—Legs

Fixed strap (sling). A strong loop of webbing or leather taped or bolted to a bar.

Flaccid. Lack of muscle tone, lack of spasticity, loose.

Flexion. Bending. Opposite to extension.

Flexor-Hinge splint. A lively splint that causes the fingers to meet the thumb when the wrist is extended.

Floating strap (sling). A strong loop of webbing or leather that moves freely on a bar.

Front bumper. Rubber-tipped furniture guard at front of chair.

Gatch frame. Bed frame that is divided into independent movable sections. May be used for raising a patient to a sitting position, etc.

Genitourinary apparatus. Tubing, bag, etc., for urine collection. Also known as genitourinary system and G.U. apparatus or system.

Grab bar. A bar, firmly fastened to a wall or floor, used as a hand hold.

Hamstrings. Muscles at back of thigh. They bend the knee and extend the hip.

Hanger. Fixture on wheel of wheelchair for fastening the drive rim.

Hyperextended. Extended beyond the normal position, i.e. extended beyond 180° at the elbow.

Ileostomy bag. An ileal bladder bag placed over the opening of a diversion from kidney to abdominal wall used to collect urine.

Iliac crest. Bony ridges at sides of abdomen. Outer portion of pelvis on either side.

Internal rotation. Turn inward, i.e. internal rotation of shoulder—back of hand placed on small of back.

Intrinsic muscles. Small muscles of the hand.

Ischial tuberosity. Bony protrusion under the buttock region.

I.V. tubing. Intravenous tubing.

Joint D.I.P. Distal interphalangeal joint, last finger joint.

Joint M.P. Metacarpophalangeal joint, joint at base of finger.

Joint P.I.P. Proximal interphalangeal joint, middle finger joint.

Lateral. Outside, away from midline. Opposite to medial.

Limit switch. Switch that cuts off automatically at predetermined point.

Long sitting. Sitting with legs straight on a flat surface.

Medial. Inside, near midline. Opposite to lateral.

M.P. joint. Metacarpophalangeal joint, joint at base of finger.

Natal cleft. Crease between the buttocks.

Palmar. Front, palm side of the hand.

Perineal crease. Crease formed where the buttocks meet the legs.

Phalanx (Phalanges). Bones of the finger/fingers.

P.I.P. joint. Proximal interphalangeal joint, middle finger joint.

Posterior. Behind, the back of.

Prone, pronated. Face down, palm down. Opposite to supine.

Protraction. Pulled forward, i.e. protraction of shoulder—the scapula moved forward on the chest wall.

Proximal. Near, close to trunk. Opposite to distal.

Pubis symphysis. Bony part at the base of the abdomen.

Quadriplegia. Some degree of impairment in all four limbs. Also known as tetraplegia.

Reflex. Movement that is not controlled voluntarily. Involuntary muscle response to nerve stimulation.

Retraction of shoulder. Draw shoulders back, i.e. retraction of shoulder—shoulder blades together.

Sacrum. Bony part at base of back.

Scapula. Shoulder blade.

Shoulder depressors. Muscles that pull the shoulder down.

Shoulder elevators. Muscles that pull the shoulder up.

Shoulder girdle. Collar bone, shoulder, shoulder blade, and the muscles that stabilize and move them.

Shoulder protractors. Muscles that pull the shoulders forward around the chest wall.

Shoulder retractors. Muscles that pull the shoulders back.

Sliding board. Bridge board, transfer board.

Sling. Usually a canvas support for use with hoists, etc.

Spacer. Metal tube separating the wheel and the drive rim of a wheel chair.

Spasms. A sudden, often violent, involuntary contraction of a muscle or a group of muscles.

Spasticity. A state of increase over the normal amount of tension in a muscle.

Spinous process. Piece of bone that protrudes, i.e. in the spine the bones that can be felt down the back.

Strap. Leather or webbing, sewn, rivetted, or buckled in a loop.

Supine, supinated. Face up, palm up. Opposite to prone.

Symphysis pubis. Bony part at the base of the abdomen.

Tenodesis. Normal flexion or extension of the relaxed fingers caused by movement of the tendons when extending or flexing the wrist.

Tetraplegic. Some degree of impairment in all four limbs. Also known as quadriplegia.

Thumb web. Web between thumb and first finger.

Tibial tuberosity. Part of bone just below and in front of the knee joint.

Tipping lever. Protruding bars at rear of the chair. Used by a helper's foot to tip the chair back.

Transfer board. Bridge board, sliding board.

Triceps. Muscle that extends the elbow.

Tridon gear clamp. Hose clamp, adjustable by a screw gear.

Trochanter. Bony prominence at top of thigh bone, hip.

Trolley. A cart, small table on castors, for use in mainly the kitchen.

Ulnar border (of hand). Side of the hand by the little finger.

References

The following listing of texts and articles dealing with the various aspects of rehabilitation is included for additional information.

Agerholm, M. (ed.): Equipment for the Disabled; An Index for Equipment. 4 Vols. ed. 2. Section 8; A 2 - D 9. National Fund for Research into Crippling Disease, London, 1966.

Barber, L. M., and Nickel, V. L.: Carbon-dioxide-powered arm and hand devices. Am. J. Occup. Ther. 23: 215, 1969.

Beard, J. E. and Long, C.: Follow-up study on usage of externally powered orthoses. Orthot. Prosthet. 24: 35, 1970.

Comarr, A. E.: Bowel regulation for patients with spinal cord injury. J.A.M.A. 167: 18, 1958.

Comarr, A. E.: Practical management of the patient with traumatic cord bladder. Arch. Phys. Med. Rehabil. 48: 122, 1967.

Frankel, H. L. F.: Bowel training. Paraplegia 4: 254, 1967.

Garrett, J. W., and Levine, E. S.: Psychological Practices with the Physically Disabled. Columbia University Press, New York, 1962.

Jackson, R. S.: Sexual rehabilitation after cord injury. Paraplegia 10: 50, 1972.

Jousse, A. T., McDonald, M., and Wynn-Jones, M.: Bladder control in the female paraplegic patient. Paraplegia 2: 146, 1964.

Kamenetz, H. L.: The Wheelchair Book. Charles C Thomas, Springfield, Illinois, 1969.

Klinger, J. L., Frieden, F. H., and Sullivan, R. A.: Mealtime Manual for the Aged and Handicapped. Institute of Rehabilitation Medicine, New York, 1970.

Licht, S.: Orthotics Etcetera. E. Licht, New Haven, Conn., 1966.

Pine, M.: Housing the Disabled. Design of the unit. Central Mortgage and Housing Corporation, Ottawa, 1970.

Safilios-Rothschild, C.: The Sociology and Social Psychology of Disability and Rehabilitation. Random House, New York, 1970.

Savino, M., Belchick, J., and Brean, E.: The quadriplegic in a university setting. Rehabilitation Record 12: 3, 1971.

Siegel, M. S.: The vocational potential of the quadriplegic. The Medical Clinics of North America 53: 713, 1969.

Symington, D., and Fordyce, W.: Changing concepts in the management of traumatic paraplegia. G.P. 32: 140, 1965.

Trombly, C.: Myoelectric control of orthotic devices: for the severely paralysed. Am. J. Occup. Ther. 22: 385, 1968.

Turner, J. (ed): Differential Diagnosis and Treatment in Social Work. The Free Press, New York, 1968.

Wheeler, H. W.: Planning Kitchens For Handicapped Homemakers. Rehabilitation Monograph XXVII, The Institute of Physical Medicine and Rehabilitation, New York University Medical Centre, New York, 1965.

Index

356 438